THE PRAEGER HANDBOOK OF OCCUPATIONAL AND ENVIRONMENTAL MEDICINE

THE PRAEGER HANDBOOK OF OCCUPATIONAL AND ENVIRONMENTAL MEDICINE

VOLUME

III   Practice Insights

Tee L. Guidotti, MD, MPH

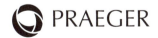

PRAEGER

AN IMPRINT OF ABC-CLIO, LLC
Santa Barbara, California • Denver, Colorado • Oxford, England

Copyright Acknowledgments

Material from two chapters adapted from Tee L. Guidotti. "Taking the Occupational History." *Ann Intern Med*. 1983; 199-4: 641–651.

Library of Congress Cataloging-in-Publication Data

Guidotti, Tee L.
  The Praeger handbook of occupational and environmental medicine / Tee L. Guidotti.
    p. ; cm.
  Includes bibliographical references and index.
  ISBN 978-0-313-35999-6 (set hard copy : alk. paper)—ISBN 978-0-313-36001-5 (vol 1 hard copy : alk. paper)—ISBN 978-0-313-36003-9 (vol 2 hard copy : alk. paper)—ISBN 978-0-313-38204-8 (vol 3 hard copy : alk. paper)—ISBN 978-0-313-36000-8 (set ebook)—ISBN 978-0-313-36002-2 (vol 1 ebook)—ISBN 978-0-313-36004-6 (vol 2 ebook)—ISBN 978-0-313-38205-5 (vol 3 ebook)
    1. Medicine, Industrial—Handbooks, manuals, etc. 2. Environmental health—Handbooks, manuals, etc. 3. Medicine, Industrial—Handbooks, manuals, etc. I. Title. II. Title: Praeger handbook of occupational and environmental medicine.
    [DNLM: 1. Occupational Medicine. 2. Environmental Health. 3. Environmental Medicine. 4. Occupational Health. WA 400 G948p 2009]
  RC963.32.G85 2010
    616.9'803—dc22   2009046237
ISBN: 978-0-313-35999-6
EISBN: 978-0-313-36000-8

14 13 12 11 10   1 2 3 4 5

This book is also available on the World Wide Web as an eBook.
Visit www.abc-clio.com for details.

Praeger
An Imprint of ABC-CLIO, LLC

ABC-CLIO, LLC
130 Cremona Drive, P.O. Box 1911
Santa Barbara, California 93116-1911

This book is printed on acid-free paper ∞
Manufactured in the United States of America

CONTENTS

Contents

VOLUME 3:

Practice Insights

17 DISEASES AND HEALTH PROTECTION

Diseases from occupational and environmental hazards represent failures of health protection. When a disease is discovered early, it may represent an opportunity for early treatment, but it always represents a warning that preventive measures are not working. The occupational and environmental medicine (OEM) physician, by virtue of medical knowledge, generally understands the disease process best and knows what to look for. The OEM physician is not necessarily an expert in treating these same diseases but does not have to be. That is what specialists are for.

Medicine is richly endowed with excellent clinicians, but there are few physicians who are effective in prevention and managing the social consequences of disease, which is the essence of the value that OEM brings to society. Oncologists concentrate on curing or managing cancer, not on assessing causation or preventing it, unless they have a personal interest and are motivated by commitment. OEM physicians concentrate on preventing and assessing the risk of causation of cancer and other diseases, not in treating them, unless they want to and are motivated by the rewards of patient care. Except for a few diseases that are uniquely occupational and require specialized skills to manage, such as lead toxicity in the adult sufficient to require chelation, the value the OEM physician brings is in understanding the cause, promoting primary prevention, recognizing the disorder early, limiting disability, and mitigating the consequences, not providing unique or specialized treatment or procedures.

Occupational and environmental diseases range over the spectrum of clinical medicine, involving every organ system. A limited number are relatively common, are important because of their associations, and present critical issues for the OEM physician beyond patient care. These are emphasized in this chapter. This chapter also emphasizes occupational diseases over environmental because the workplace is the site of greatest risk.

Occupational diseases usually present more of a diagnostic dilemma than occupational injuries. In practice, the distribution of occupational diseases in North America can be approximated by the "rule of halves" (Figure 17.1), a general approximation that is useful in planning occupational health services. This rule of thumb states that the distribution of occupational diseases in a large working population in a diversified economy tends to be divided roughly as

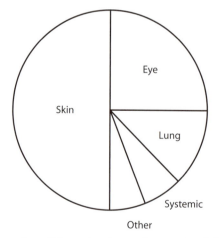

Figure 17.1. The proportion of the major classes of occupational disease can be approximated by the "rule of halves," which is useful for planning purposes.

follows: skin disorders account for roughly half of all occupational diseases, eye disorders roughly half of the remainder (or one-quarter), lung disorders half of that (or one-eighth), and half of the residual is systemic toxicity problems. The remainder tends to be a mix of many types of problems. This general approximation holds true as a rule of thumb for industrialized communities but may be distorted somewhat in smaller communities in which a single dominant industry presents an unusual hazard, such as coal mining.

Environmental diseases are generally more familiar to the physician outside OEM. At the level of regulatory control in most developed countries, overt disease caused by environmental exposure is rare. More common is aggravation of existing disorders, especially asthma, by environmental triggers, such as ozone or mold allergens. Environmental hazards are likely to play their most important role as risk factors in multifactoral diseases, such as the contribution of lead to behavioral disorders in children or of air pollution to low lung function. Environmental hazards are more likely in general to have an effect on children than adults.

In the discussion to follow, special emphasis is placed on occupational dermatoses, lung diseases, and toxic conditions because of their frequency, noise-induced hearing loss because of its frequency and the ease of prevention, and cancer because of its high frequency in certain occupational groups and its high visibility as an occupational health problem. Eye disorders are usually treated by specialists or physicians already trained for the practice and are not discussed in detail here.

Toxic disorders are an important class of occupational disease, but with a few specific exceptions, systemic toxicity is dealt with elsewhere in this book, usually where the agent is first introduced and discussed, generally Chapter 2 or 10.

This chapter does not provide detailed guidance on treatment. The reader is referred to the American College of Occupational and Environmental Medicine's *Occupational Medicine Practice Guidelines* (referred to as the *ACOEM Practice Guidelines*, or *APG*) or other authoritative references on management for treatment guidance.

CLINICAL APPROACH

The practice of clinical occupational medicine seldom changes because of advances in medicine. Occupational medical practice changes little because of the introduction of new drugs and treatment. Rather, practice is changing with the changing economy, the introduction of new industrial processes, and changes in the workforce. The North American economy continues to move in the direction of domination by service occupations. The manufacturing sector frequently introduces new and different products and processes that create different workplace conditions.

Patterns of occupational disease change with the introduction of new and sometimes exotic chemicals and, even more importantly, the adaptation of chemicals that were frequently encountered in the past in new applications in which their hazards were not recognized. It is not uncommon in occupational medicine to see old hazards reappear in new workplaces. Arsenic, for example, was so closely associated with mining and smelting that it never occurred to technology wizards in microelectronics, with a very different mindset, that it would be a problem, as it became in the early days of the semiconductor industry. Indeed it is a truism of occupational medicine that exposures never truly disappear from the workplace—they reappear in new technologies, where they are often overlooked until they begin to cause problems.

Likewise, old hazards tends to reappear in the evaluation of new, or at least newly appreciated, risks as more is learned about mechanisms of disease. Previously, arsenic was known to cause groundwater contamination from natural sources and at those levels was associated with a risk of bladder, skin, and lung cancer. Now, arsenic is known to be associated with cardiovascular disease and neurocognitive impairment, as are mercury and lead.

Occupational medicine is more than the identification and treatment of diseases and injuries. It is fundamentally involved in the prevention of these disorders. Prevention, however, is usually easier and more readily undertaken if one has an understanding of what is being prevented. This chapter will concentrate on the identification and understanding of important occupational diseases.

Five questions will be answered:

1. What are occupational disorders?
2. How does one recognize them?
3. How does one evaluate them?
4. What does one do when one finds them?
5. Who is available to help the physician in evaluating occupational disorders?

Occupational diseases are disorders that arise directly out of the workplace, working conditions, and exposures, including physical hazards that occur at work. By extension, they may include disorders that arise from work that is not part of an employment relationship, such as avocational work (hobbies or volunteer work), or from military or civil service, that share the same conditions and causes. The definition is important because there are other diseases that may be triggered, aggravated, or exacerbated but not caused at work; these diseases are usually called "work-related diseases." Many other diseases may be important with respect to the capacity to work but are not caused by workplace conditions. These distinctions are very important with respect to diagnosis, recognition, compensation, and prevention. For example, asthma that arises *de novo* from sensitization to a chemical used on the job is an occupational disease, and failure to recognize this will put the patient at risk if exposure continues; it is compensable under workers' compensation and can best be prevented by removing the antigen or reassigning the worker. Asthma that arises in a worker unrelated to their work may be made worse by exposure to irritants on the job, including exposures that would not bother most people; it is treated differently under many workers' compensation systems, and in the individual case controlling the level of exposure may be all that is needed. Asthma that has no correlation with working conditions may be a health problem for the worker and a serious cause of lost productivity in the workplace; it is not compensable under workers' compensation and at most would require an accommodation (in the United States, under the Americans with Disabilities Act).

Occupational diseases come to the attention of the physician through correlating the occupational history, which is discussed in considerable detail in Chapter 15, with clinical findings. The occupational history permits one to develop an exposure profile for the individual and in the format provided allows one to obtain information on the workplace, on hobbies, and on avocational exposure and exposure in the home.

Chapter 15 presents a guide for incorporating the occupational history and exposure profile into the clinical assessment and using resources available to physicians for interpreting the findings. This stage is comparable to the traditional medical process of deriving a differential diagnosis and then ruling in or out each possibility.

One evaluates occupational disorders by methodically considering each of five points:

1. Structural changes
2. Functional changes
3. Diagnosis and pathophysiology
4. Exposure circumstances
5. Behavioral causes (i.e., why exposure was allowed to occur)

Structural changes are often the first clue to the possibility of an occupational association with a disorder. For example, the evaluation of occupational lung disease often begins with changes in tissue structure as reflected in the chest film. Structural changes may be the only evidence of a lesion, and one may not be able to document functional impairment in the individual. This is usually the case, for example, with early stages of a pneumoconiosis.

Functional changes must be evaluated in order to assess the degree of impairment that may be present and to determine if the structural change has progressed to the point of interfering with the worker-patient's ability to function, either on the job or in daily life. Examples of functional assessment are spirometry and exercise testing. At times structural changes are not at all evident or at least are invisible to our clinical methods of detection and in such circumstances functional changes may be the only way to document the presence of an occupational disorder. This is particularly true in the case of occupational asthma.

The medical diagnosis of an occupational disorder is often less important in occupational medicine than it might be in nonoccupational practice. Diagnosis is important to give an indication of prognosis and helps to define treatment. Other than systemic toxicity, however, most occupational diseases are treated generically, not with targeted therapy. Structural or functional changes may be more significant in identifying the proper category of occupational disorders, regardless of the specific diagnosis. On the other hand, in the occupational setting a diagnosis, however firm, is not sufficient in the evaluation of the patient. As a practical matter, causation analysis and functional assessment, which are usually subsidiary in general medicine, are at least as important as the clinical diagnosis. Causation is absolutely required because without a conclusion regarding etiology and the agent or exposure responsible, the link with work cannot be made, compensation cannot be considered, and prevention cannot be undertaken. The functional assessment is as or more important than a definite diagnosis because it establishes the basis for compensation and fitness to work. The diagnosis, however, does not necessarily have to be exact to guide treatment or to initiate a claim.

Identification of the specific agent or hazard that caused the disorder is only half of the description of etiology. Causation in occupational cases also requires a definition of the circumstances of exposure, with an indication of what the individual may have been exposed to and why that particular individual came into contact with the hazard. A comprehensive description of the exposure circumstances requires an understanding of the job requirements, the conditions of work, and at times, behavioral factors related to how the individual or co-workers perform on the job and the policies of management. The level of detail that may be required parallels that of the fitness-to-work evaluation (See Chapter 18.) These issues are seldom described in as much detail in the evaluation of personal health problems.

Many resources are available to help physicians in interpreting the occupational history, evaluating occupational disorders, and establishing the diagnosis and functional assessment in treating these occupational disorders. In addition there are many other occupational health professionals, occupational health nurses, occupational hygienists, safety engineers, ergonomists, radiation health professionals, audiologists, toxicologists, epidemiologists, risk and liability control personnel, and vocational rehabilitation councilors who are usually only too glad to assist the physician in evaluating a case either on a consultation basis or more often in an informal basis by telephone. These occupational health professionals constitute a valuable resource for the physician. A little advance preparation in getting to know them and where they are in the community often becomes exceedingly useful in an emergency or when in sorting out a difficult case. Occupational medicine is one field of medicine in which the team approach works well and in which the physician cannot expect to do everything alone.

Environmental medicine has fewer resources to draw on than occupational medicine, because the field has not been as well defined. The member clinics of the Association of Occupational and Environmental Clinics (www.aoec.org) represent a resource for consultation in both occupational medicine and environmental medicine that is reliable and firmly in the mainstream of medicine. For children, the national network of Pediatric Environmental Health Specialty Units (described in Chapter 12) are essential sources of information and only a telephone call or email away.

DERMATOSES

Occupational skin disorders are the most common type of occupational disease, comprising a third to half of all occupational diseases seen by physicians. Occupational skin disorders are much more common than available statistics would indicate because they are unlikely to be brought to medical attention unless they become severe or uncomfortable. They are often seen in service industries, such as hairdressing, healthcare, and restaurants (among bartenders, dishwashers, and food handlers) as well as in manufacturing. While rarely life-threatening, occupational dermatoses may be quite distressing to the patient and are usually easily preventable. When severe they can be disfiguring, depressing, and a limitation on earnings.

The management of occupational dermatoses is similar to that of the same skin disorders in nonoccupational settings, with the additional feature that effective prevention and control depends on identifying the occupational cause of the disorder and protecting the worker from contact with the responsible agent. (See Chapter 14 for personal protection of the skin.)

The skin is a complex organ with a massive surface area and is uniquely accessible to examination. Although the skin provides an effective barrier to most physical and chemical exposures, it is not completely impermeable and represents a major pathway of absorption. (See Chapter 2.) The skin presents a number of host defenses that resist local injury, including buffering of pH within a narrow range, immune mechanisms, cooling by vasodilation, mechanical protection against abrasion (by the stratum corneum), protection against ultraviolet radiation (by the pigmented melanocytes of the basal cell layer), and antimicrobial activity (fatty acids that inhibit bacterial and fungal growth on the skin surface).

The diagnosis of occupational dermatoses begins with the history and inspection. The changes are generally easily visible and often appear sharply delineated in areas of the body uncovered by work clothes: neckline, wrist, or face. The history of the reaction is important, as local contact dermatitis may generalize in the "id" reaction, involving distant sites not obviously related to the circumstances of exposure. Occasionally, usually in oil acne, the eruption may be on parts of the body covered by saturated clothes or occluded by heavy clothing in an environment of heat and humidity. The inside of work gloves may become contaminated during careless use, producing a dermatitis on the hands despite a history of using personal protection. The history of the initial response of the rash may be useful if it is clearly associated with job duties or time in the workplace; often, however, recurrent dermatoses become relatively persistent and may not go away with time off work. It may take weeks for a severe contact dermatitis to heal after exposure ceases. The medications used to treat the dermatitis occasionally may aggravate it or change its presentation.

Factors that aggravate occupational dermatoses, or make it more likely that an exposure will result in a dermatitis, include heat, moisture, physical abrasion, pressure, and occlusion. All these factors may be present in the case of tight gloves or ill-fitting work clothes. Excessive dryness may also cause skin problems. Some measures ostensibly taken to protect the skin may make the dermatitis worse. Frequent hand washing, for example, may cause chapping, cracking, loss of oils, and exacerbated dermatitis.

Prevention of occupational dermatitis rests on good hygiene and the use of personal protection, including impermeable but cool and comfortable gloves, kept clean on the inside, and work clothing, including aprons. Barrier creams are oil-based substances applied to exposed parts of the body to prevent irritation of the skin. They are marginally useful but quickly lose their protective action with time and activity. Barrier creams can be used within gloves for added protection, especially if the glove itself is thought to be part of the problem. (Personal protection is described in Chapter 14.)

Treatment of occupational dermatoses is specific to the type of dermatitis and similar to that of other dermatitides. Control of exposure to irritants and allergens and any aggravating factors is the key to management, however. Treatment is seldom very effective if exposure and irritation persist.

Acute Skin Injury

Acute irritant skin injury resembles a burn and can be exceptionally severe (see Chapter 16). These "chemical burns" occur as a consequence of contact with strong acids (for example, plating solutions), strong bases (for example, cement or ammonia), or highly reactive chemicals (for example, ethylene oxide or potassium permanganate). Prolonged immersion in solvents, which extract lipids from the skin, may cause a similar clinical picture, often accompanied by cracking and fissuring. The chemical burn usually begins with erythema, pain, and pruritus and may develop blisters or ulcers. Injury in these cases penetrates to the dermis and may cause severe scarring. Recovery may be accompanied by disfiguring hyperpigmentation in persons with pale skin or either hyper- or hypopigmentation in persons of color. Repeated exposure to more dilute strong irritants or to solvents may result in chronic skin changes, either resulting in a hypertrophic dermatitis or skin atrophy and nummular dermatosis, which is characterized by skin hypertrophy.

One strong irritant deserves special mention because of its extreme hazard. Hydrofluoric acid (HF) is heavily used in the semiconductor industry for etching silicone chips and removing surface oxides, in the oil industry as a fraccing agent and for maintenance of reaction vessels, in metallurgy to remove impurities and oxides from steel (a process known as "pickling"), and as a fluorine source in making fluoropolymers. HF is a weak acid in chemical terms, but when the acid dissociates it forms fluoride ion (F^-), which has a strong affinity for calcium and penetrates cell membranes very efficiently. An HF burn causes deep and spreading tissue injury that is very difficult to contain and manage. HF burns begin with erythema and swelling and, while they may not initially look very bad, may progress over hours to blanching (extreme pallor), blistering, and excruciating pain, out of all proportion to the visible sign of injury. HF burns may easily lead to necrosis and extensive tissue loss, and because of fluoride's affinity for calcium in bone they may demineralize bone underneath the skin destruction, which can result in loss of fingers and toes. Amputation is sometimes required. Treatment, to be initiated as early as possible, is calcium gluconate as a surface gel (which has to be prepared at the time using KY Jelly ® or a similar product because it is no longer commercially available), as a dilute solution for eye irrigation, by tissue infiltration within and beyond the obviously affected skin area, and if necessary by intra-arterial injection, which may save body parts. Any OEM physician who could possibly be called upon to manage an HF burn is advised to receive special training in their treatment (provided at no cost by manufacturers of HF) and to maintain an appropriately large supply of calcium gluconate at the ready.

CONTACT DERMATITIS

"Contact dermatitis" comprises 75 percent of occupational skin disorders. Of this, approximately 80 percent is due to local irritation and 20 percent is due to an allergic response to specific antigens. Atopic individuals are much more likely (by 13–14 times) to experience contact dermatitis of either type, not just allergic contact dermatitis, than nonatopic individuals. Both allergic and irritant contact dermatides are aggravated by heat, humidity, and physical abrasion.

An "irritant contact dermatitis" may take many forms, but usually presents as eczema or changes in pigmentation. The irritation may come from relatively prolonged contact with a weak irritant, which may be almost any compound in the workplace. The most common irritants are acids, bases, solvents, soaps, and detergents. The latter four tend to extract oils and lipid from the skin, creating a dry, chapped rash. Once the surface of the skin is broken, a rash tends to perpetuate itself, especially with frequent hand washing. Agents used to cleanse the skin may perpetuate the irritation. Abrasive (usually pumice-containing) soaps, waterless hand cleansers, and solvents are particularly troublesome in this regard and should be avoided once the dermatitis appears. An irritant contact dermatitis frequently results from the cumulative effect of several irritating exposures. Although sometimes refractory, irritant contact dermatitis can usually be managed by reducing the sum total of irritant exposures and often allows continuation of work activities with personal protection or reduced exposure.

"Allergic contact dermatitis," or eczema, is a Type III immunologic reaction to a specific antigen. Common sensitizers include nickel, disulfiram (a rubber constituent), epoxy and other resins, and organic dyes. Once an individual is sensitized to an antigen, minimal contact thereafter produces a reaction. This makes management much more difficult, in general, than for irritant contact dermatitis and almost always requires avoiding the antigen entirely. Fortunately, antigens encountered in workplaces tend to be relatively weak and often require considerable time to provoke sensitization. A dermatitis occurring within the first month on a new job is unlikely to be allergic in nature. This is important because effective control of allergic contact dermatitis is often more difficult than that of an irritant effect if the worker cannot avoid contact with the sensitizing agent in the workplace. A rash occurring several weeks to months after beginning a new job or after the introduction of a new chemical into the workplace may be either an allergic or irritant mechanism. Sensitization to perfumes and cosmetic constituents sometimes produce an allergic dermatitis that may appear at home or at work, confusing evaluation. Persons with a history of eczema may be at risk for the id reaction, in which the dermatitis generalizes to involve previously normal skin, often in areas distant from the initial eruption. This can create a very confusing clinical picture.

"Patch testing" to evaluate allergic contact dermatitis is a useful tool in occupational medicine with appropriate standardization of practice and in experienced hands. Patch testing is an important but limited diagnostic tool in the evaluation of occupational dermatoses. The kits, or "trays," with which patch testing is conducted do not contain all possible occupational antigens for every workplace situation and are more likely to miss an antigen than to register a false positive. Thus, patch testing should normally be considered confirmatory if positive rather than definitive evidence against an occupational association if negative. It is useful in identifying specific allergens to which the worker has become sensitive. In theory, exposure to that substance can be avoided subsequently. The antigen is supplied in a diluted solution that is applied to the skin in the form of a saturated piece of gauze or cellular discs, under an occlusive dressing, usually on the worker's back in groups of 23. Localized eczematous reactions occur in the presence of allergy within 48–72 hours in most cases or up to 96 hours in a minority of reactions.

Patch testing is conducted following a set of strict international guidelines using standard solutions standardized by the American Academy of Dermatology. It is possible to formulate solutions of allergens not included in the standard kits, especially when the material is water-soluble or can be obtained in the form of metal salts. There are serious limitations to patch testing as a diagnostic procedure, however. False positive tests can occur on highly reactive skin and with the application of substances that are also irritants. Workers can become newly sensitized to allergens during the course of patch testing to chemicals they tolerated previously. False negatives can occur, especially if the worker is under treatment or the solution is not standard. Patch testing only indicates the presence of a specific allergic reaction; it cannot rule out an irritant contact dermatitis or, indeed, an allergic contact dermatitis resulting from exposure to an allergen that does not happen to be included in the panel used. Patch testing should be performed in a suitably equipped facility by a dermatologist or allergist familiar with internationally standardized protocols and with the limitations of the technique. Because it is time-consuming and often inconclusive, patch testing is not performed by many dermatologists and may be hard to arrange.

Figure 17.2 presents a characteristic example of allergic contact dermatitis in a thirty-two-year-old man at a pressed wood plant. He developed this eczematous rash from exposure to resin dust compounded with glue containing glutaraldehyde; subsequently he also developed occupational asthma with wheezing following exposure. Patch testing showed a 3+ reaction to glutaraldehyde.

"Contact urticaria," resulting from sensitization to allergies involved by skin absorption, is a relatively uncommon reaction expressed as local hives. Generalized urticaria can occur after inhalation of an allergen, usually in the context of a respiratory reaction. However, urticaria often occurs with no cause identified.

Strong irritants, such as acids, alkalis, and highly reactive chemicals such as ethylene oxide, are not as likely to cause contact dermatitis as they are to cause an obvious chemical burn, blistering, or ulceration.

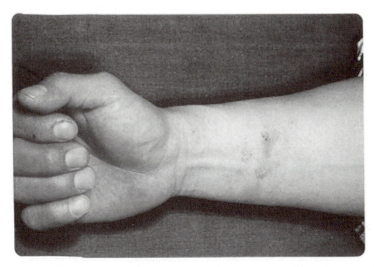

Figure 17.2. Allergic contact dermatitis in a thirty-two-year-old worker sensitive to glutaraldehyde in the glue used in a pressed wood plant. He also had occupational asthma, with bronchospasm following exposure. Note the distribution of the rash in the exposed area between glove and sleeve.

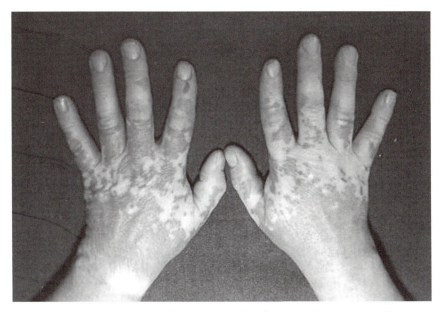

Figure 17.3. Depigmentation and hypertrophic skin changes in the hands of a fifty-three-year-old spray painter who had frequent skin contact with solvents.

Chronic or persistently recurrent dermatitis may lead to secondary effects, such as hypo- or hyperpigmentation and hypertrophy. Figure 17.3 shows the effect of chronic, recurrent solvent exposure on the hands of a spray painter.

Other Dermatoses

Other dermatoses are noteworthy as clues to an occupational exposure. Photosensitization may appear as an acute sunburn or eczema on exposed areas of skin, often accompanied by conjunctivitis. This occurs most commonly in occupations involving heavy exposure to coal tar products, such as roofing, but has also been seen in workers exposed to light-cured acrylic and vaporized epoxy resins and among bartenders, pickers, and grocery store workers who handle produce, principally celery and limes, that are bruised and infected with a common fungus which secretes a type of psoralen that is photosensitizing.

"Oil acne" or "oil folliculitis" is often associated with exposure to greases and lubricating oils in settings in which washing is inconvenient or work clothes become saturated. It usually appears on the hands and forearms because of exposure in these areas. Hair follicles are often inflamed and occluded as a first sign.

"Chloracne" is a persistent and often severe form of nonpostular acne, usually affecting the face, especially in the preauricular area. Chloracne reflects systemic exposure to chlorinated cyclic hydrocarbons (e.g., pentachlorophenol, PCBs, furans, and dioxins). Exposure to these agents usually occurs in one of a few specific situations: an industrial accident involving chemical reactions, poor manufacturing processes, application of wood preservatives, burning of preserved wood, and exposure to chemical wastes. Unlike oil acne, chloracne is a sign of significant systemic toxic exposure and may be associated with other effects of exposure, such as hepatic disorders and neuropathies. It tends to be refractory to treatment. Suspicion of chloracne merits referral to a dermatologist, evaluation by a toxicologist or OEM physician, and close follow-up.

A common ulcerating occupational dermatitis is a reaction to chromium. Typically, "chrome ulcers" present as punctate, persistent open sores on the hands that are very slow to heal. They may appear in workers handling cement, which contains small amounts of chromium (see Figure 17.4).

Skin cancer is a serious occupational health problem, mostly related to work out of doors. The nature and distribution of skin cancers among workers at risk parallels that of the general population and reflects primarily exposure to ultraviolet light. The risk of skin cancer, including melanoma, can be reduced significantly by protecting clothing and the provision of shelter for workers outdoors. Photosensitizers, such as coal tar products (which are concentrated polycyclic aromatic hydrocarbons), play an important role in some industries, enhancing the initiating effect of UV radiation.

Systemic exposure to arsenic is associated with basal cell carcinoma and squamous cell carcinoma, both invasive and in situ (known as Bowen's disease). These may be associated with the characteristic nonmalignant skin rash of arsenic, hyperkeratotic skin changes that are usually most obvious on the palms and plantar surface.

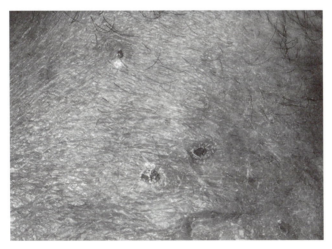

Figure 17.4. Chrome ulcers on the hands of a man who handled dirt contaminated with potassium chromate; they are usually associated with handling cement.

Numerous specific skin disorders are associated with particular occupations; others are cutaneous signs of systemic disease that may have an occupational cause. Agricultural, food, and forestry workers are particularly susceptible groups for dermatoses. Causes of dermatitis in these occupations may include sensitization to certain pesticides, photosensitization (as noted above), irritation by contact with poison oak or ivy, insect bites, or exposure to common solvents and chemicals. Infectious occupational dermatoses may also be seen in forestry, agriculture, food, and forestry workers, including Lyme disease, sporotrichosis (classically seen in horticulture after the skin is pricked by rose thorns), and erysipeloid. The clinical presentation of dermatoses in agricultural and forestry workers is often modified by sun exposure, heat and humidity, and the improper use of protective equipment, which may actually retain sensitizing or irritating agents next to the skin if the inside of gloves, masks, or clothing becomes contaminated.

Occupational dermatoses may also be caused by mechanical factors, such as friction (calluses, abrasions, exacerbation of psoriasis), pressure (blistering, ulcers), and minor trauma. Exposure to vibration, heat, and cold may result in specific cutaneous manifestations, as described in Chapter 9. Penetration by foreign bodies, including fibrous glass, asbestos fibers, or metal fragments, often leads to granuloma formation and palpable nodules. Recovery from inflammatory conditions often leads to pigmentation changes and may be cosmetically troublesome.

RESPIRATORY DISEASES

Table 17.1 summarizes the common benign and malignant occupational and environmental diseases of the respiratory tract and thorax most likely to be encountered in OEM practice. As a practical matter, occupational lung disorders are most critical to understand, and the rest of this section will be devoted primarily to lung disorders and primarily to occupational hazards because the greatest hazard is in the workplace. However, it should be recognized that upper airway disorders occur commonly, especially associated with atopy and irritation, and may be associated with the usual symptoms of cough, rhinitis, and sometimes voice changes.

Diseases of the pleura, because of its inaccessibility except by lymphatic transport, occur primarily in response to asbestos.

Within the lung, the disorders of greatest concern in OEM are the "pneumoconioses" (dust-related diseases of the lung), airway disorders (asthma or bronchitis and their variants), "hypersensitivity pneumonitides" (a class of immune-mediated responses to inhaled antigens), "toxic inhalation" (an acute syndrome associated with

Table 17.1. Disorders of the Respiratory Tract in Occupational and Environmental Medicine

	Benign	Malignant
Upper airway (except larynx)	Rhinitis, sinusitis, septal perforation	Nasal and sinus cancer, pharyngeal cancer
Larynx	Laryngitis, dysphonia, stridor, obstruction, polyps	Laryngeal carcinoma
Lower airways (bronchi, bronchioles)	Bronchoconstriction, asthma, bronchitis, chronic obstructive airway disease, bronchiolitis	Bronchogenic carcinoma
Parenchyma, (alveoli)	Pneumoconioses, emphysema, hypersensitivity pneumonitis, pneumonia	(Usually metastatic)
Thorax (pleura)	Pleural fibrosis (plaques and diffuse thickening), acute pleural effusion of asbestos, "rounded atelectasis" syndrome	Mesothelioma, metastatic disease

diffuse alveolar injury), and cancer of the lung and pleura. "Inhalational fevers" (acute, self-limited febrile illnesses associated with inhalation of zinc or copper) are characterized by a transient infiltrate but are really more transient systemic toxicities than lung disorders. (Inhalation fevers are discussed briefly in Chapter 10.)

Expressions of Lung Injury

The lung has a limited repertoire of change. The patterns of expression of lung injury are limited by the structure and functional possibilities of the organ. Occupational and environmental lung diseases mimic many if not most nonoccupational disorders. Depending on the mechanism of the response to the inhaled toxic agent, the disease may result in a restrictive or an obstructive defect and a malignant or a benign process and will primarily affect the airway or the parenchyma. Some occupational lung disorders have extrapulmonary manifestations even in the absence of malignancy. Indeed, the range of structural and functional abnormalities produced by occupational exposures embraces most of the clinical spectrum of pulmonary medicine.

The lungs are highly vulnerable to injury from the dusts and gases in the atmosphere. To protect the delicate structures of the lower respiratory tract, the human lung is protected by elaborate defense mechanisms. These defense mechanisms may be compromised or overwhelmed by occupational exposures, leading to various types of occupational lung diseases.

Toxic agents that may be inhaled can be categorized as either particulate (solid) or nonparticulate (gas). Toxic exposures in the workplace are often a mixture of gaseous and particulate compounds, as in exposure to welding fumes or combustion exhausts. In many cases gaseous compounds are carried adsorbed onto the surface of particles. In such dual exposures the toxic substances on the particle are carried much more deeply into the lower respiratory tract than they would otherwise penetrate. The clinical expression of the toxic reaction is determined by the dose received, the pathophysiology of the response, characteristics of the host, and the presence of modifying factors such as other exposures and infectious agents. Chapter 2 discusses inhalation toxicology in more detail.

Inhaled dust is rapidly cleared by the highly effective centripetal mucociliary stream, which removes a prodigious burden. A relatively small quantity of residual dust is left behind for phagocytosis by alveolar macrophages. The macrophages, having engulfed the individual particles, may migrate on the alveolar surface or interstitially to the edge of the mucociliary escalator (this process is not well understood), or they may migrate interstitially. Although interstitial migration probably drains into lymphatic system for the most part, a significant amount of dust is trapped in local concentrations at the coal dust macules, where presumably drainage is impaired or overwhelmed or reaches an anatomic "dead end." These transport mechanisms may be impaired by inflammatory respiratory disease, by simultaneous exposure to irritant exogenous agents, which may be ciliostatic, or by exposure to other particulates, which may saturate the phagocytic capacity of the macrophages.

Macrophages release proteases and inflammatory products that cause local damage and initiate a dysfunctional repair mechanism by fibroblasts. Phagocytosis of even inert particles, such as latex beads, by alveolar macrophages is enough to release small quantities of lysosomal enzymes into the surrounding milieu. Dusts that are refractory to digestion and that initiate cytotoxicity, such as silica, cause more release. These include collagenase, elastase, plasminogen activator, and lysosomal hydroxylases. Thus, alveolar macrophages may not be activated by ingesting inert particles such as carbon, but they are stimulated to release, inadvertently as it were, potentially locally destructive enzymes. This is reasonable in a system evolved to dispatch microorganisms, but it is counterproductive in dealing with inert particles. Furthermore, partially denatured protein is chemotactic, so that the cellular reaction perpetuates itself. The schema in Figure 17.5 illustrates the

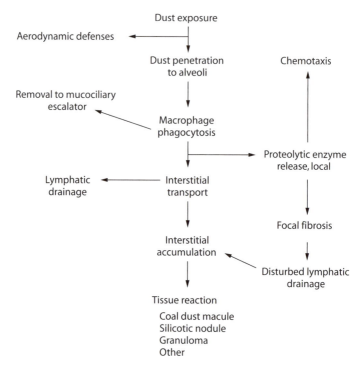

Figure 17.5. Fate of inhaled particle penetrating to lower respiratory tract.

common mechanism for reacting to dust deposition in the lung, in this case the formation and extension of the coal macule in coal workers' pneumoconiosis.

Focal fibrosis and focal emphysema may result, which contributes to an obstructive component of dust-related disease. There are opportunities for individual variation implied by this schema. Miners with α_1-antitrypsin deficiency, for example, will have more extensive local destruction than otherwise, but this combination is obviously rare. The avidity and efficiency of macrophages in clearing mycobacteria have a genetic component.

Nonparticulate, gaseous toxic agents penetrate into the respiratory tract depending on how soluble they are in water. The mucosa of the respiratory tract absorbs and removes most readily toxic gases that are water soluble. Host defense mechanisms against infection and particulates, especially the mucociliary escalator and alveolar macrophage, are very vulnerable to the effects of toxic gases, and their efficiency is often considerably reduced after exposure. Cigarette smoking exposes the lungs to the toxic agents in cigarette smoke, interferes with the mechanisms of host defense, and often interacts with other toxic exposures to produce more severe toxicity than could otherwise occur.

Clinical Assessment

The evaluation of occupational lung disease must address five essential questions:

1. What is the nature of the process?
2. What exposure in the patient's employment may have been responsible?
3. What is the prognosis of this condition and what ultimate level of disability accompanies the natural history of the disorder?
4. What can be done to control or limit the disease process?
5. Are other persons in the same workplace likely to be affected, now or in the future?

The first question, on the nature of the lesion, requires a description of the structure, function, and malignant potential of the process. Structure is usually evaluated by chest film (increasingly supported by high-resolution CT scanning), function by pulmonary function tests, and malignant potential by biopsy or cytopathology. The radiological findings provide evidence of the nature of the process, such as fibrosis, when it affects the lung's gross structure. Few occupational lung diseases have characteristic findings on chest film, although asbestosis and silicosis do have pathognomonic signs, as will be described. Functional impairment, such as airway obstruction, can be assessed by history or best by spirometry. Determination of malignancy requires tissue or cytologic confirmation, although radiological evidence may be very convincing.

The second question, concerning exposure, is often apparent from the occupational history. A history of exposure to a known carcinogen, a fibrogenic dust, or a potent sensitizing agent should be considered for significance in light of the presenting symptoms and the known effects of the agent. Identification of the agents helps to suggest a prognosis and is essential for establishing eligibility for compensation. Defining the cause may contribute to future preventive measures. The clinical management of individual patients may or may not be affected by identification of the agent.

The third question, on prognosis and disability, depends on the agent responsible and on the functional status of the patient. Silicosis and asbestosis, the two most common pneumoconioses of the over 200 known, both produce serious restrictive disease that will often advance regardless of future exposure. Most other pneumoconioses produce structural abnormalities on chest film greatly out of proportion to the modest changes they cause in pulmonary function and usually stabilize or may even regress after exposure ceases, presumably because of mobilization of dust and remodeling of fibrosis.

The fifth question, on the risks to other workers, is critical. Other employees who worked in the same plant may be at risk for the same outcome. The physician should always inquire about the health of co-workers, the number of employees in the workplace, and whether the hazard is still present.

Pneumoconioses

The pneumoconioses are diseases characterized by the deposition of dust in the lung and the pulmonary response to its presence. As is the case with tuberculosis, the lung's intrinsic reaction is a key part of the development of the disease. Usually, this consists of an inflammatory reaction, usually low-grade, that may or may not lead to extensive fibrosis. The degree of fibrosis that results varies with the properties of the dust. Silica and the fibrous silicates, such as asbestos or zeolite, cause intense fibrotic reactions. Carbon black or iron oxide provoke only small and localized reactions. Coal dust, the other common pneumoconiosis, falls in between depending on the composition of the coal. Some pneumoconioses are also associated with immune responses that modify their presentation and add new mechanisms of action: silica (which has a strong association with autoimmune disorders), beryllium (which produce a sarcoidosis-like response), and hard-metal disease (which, as a result of the cobalt content of the alloy, is associated with occupational asthma). Others may be associated with direct toxicity if the dust is soluble.

Pneumoconioses caused by metals of high atomic number (which are dense to x-rays) present an exaggerated appearance on chest film. They usually appear first as dense, multiple-nodular opacities. Correlation between radiological patterns and functional impairment is often poor. Function is usually preserved, as measured by routine spirometry, until the disease becomes advanced. The usual pattern of functional impairment in an advanced pneumoconiosis is restrictive, but mild obstruction may occur, especially when there is also a bronchitis. The identification of a pneumoconiosis and its differentiation from idiopathic interstitial fibrosis, sarcoidosis, the interstitial pneumonias, or cancer is sometimes possible only by open biopsy. It is important in such cases to notify the pathologist receiving the tissue when a pneumoconiosis is expected. Special techniques are often required to identify the type of dust in a pneumoconiosis and the diagnosis can be overlooked even by experienced pathologists.

The evaluation of a suspected pneumoconiosis begins with the chest film. The simple PA chest film is a clinical tool of remarkable usefulness, particularly in the evaluation of occupational lung disorders. Most pneumoconioses appear first as multiple, rounded nodules in the lower lung fields. Silicosis, although it presents first as rounded nodules, occurs first in the upper lung fields. Asbestosis presents irregular nodules. Otherwise, the pneumoconioses have a relatively uniform appearance that resembles sarcoidosis.

Over the years, experience with the radiographic diagnosis of occupational lung disease has led to the appreciation of perceptual problems on the part of film readers and their resolution by adopting certain conventions. The standard system for communicating the morphology, nodularity, and severity of radiographic changes in cases of suspected pneumoconiosis is the so-called "ILO Classification of the Radiographic Appearance of the Pneumoconioses." (ILO stands for International Labour Office.) This system is based on a psychological process of dealing with uncertainty in the mind of the physician reading the chest film. This necessarily involved system uses four basic categories expanded into a twelve-point scale reflecting and actually using to advantage the uncertainty of classification in the mind of the reader. For example, for a film that is probably category 2 but for which the reader considered assigning category 1, the reader would indicate 2/1. The biggest difficulty with the ILO system comes in distinguishing between 1/0 and 0/1, since this represents the dividing point between presumed normal and presumed diseased. The system also provides an interpretation by the type of density observed, assigning a series of small letter designations depending on the shape, regularity of margins, and size of the densities. The system was designed and is used for classifying films for epidemiological purposes but has been adopted in the United States for certain purposes in determining eligibility for compensation. It is not appropriate for use in clinical diagnosis, since its use requires that the diagnosis already be made, but it is useful for staging. The ILO Classification, and most definitely the "B-reader program," which is the testing program managed by the National Institute of Occupational Safety and Health (NIOSH) for proficiency in applying it, is now based on obsolete technology. The conventional PA chest film on which it is based is rapidly becoming obsolete and even unavailable in many centers, replaced by digitized films. Guidelines for application of the ILO Classification to digital films are now available and a complementary classification system for HRCT (high-resolution computed tomography) has been proposed but is not universally accepted.

Pulmonary function in the pneumoconioses, generally, is mildly irritating for most dusts and may contribute to obstructive lung disease. For the fibrogenic dusts that are the major cause of serious disease, function varies with the stage of the disease. In the earliest stages of most pneumoconioses, there may be mild obstructive changes due to airway irritation, even for benign dusts such as graphite. As the disorder progresses, some component of airway obstruction progresses due to focal emphysema, but it is almost always masked and overwhelmed by a progressive restrictive change due to the advancing fibrosis.

Reactions to Fibrogenic Dusts

The most important pneumoconioses in terms of frequency, medical management, and poor prognosis are the fibrogenic dusts, which induce scarring in the lung: the pneumoconioses arising from exposure to asbestos ("asbestosis"), crystalline silica ("silicosis"), and coal dust ("coal workers' pneumoconiosis") are historically and still today by far the most common fibrogenic dusts to which workers are exposed. The dusts responsible are minerals sharing silica as a common chemical element but with very different composition, chemical and physical properties, and potency in causing fibrosis in lung tissue. Silica is silicone dioxide in various forms, usually nearly pure α-quartz in crystalline form. Noncrystalline silica is not so potently fibrogenic. (Hereafter in this section, "silica" will refer to crystalline silica.) Asbestos, which exists in many forms, is a silicate, with additional constituents. Coal dust is a complex mixture of predominantly carbon with some mineral composition and is more potently fibrogenic the greater the proportion of silica, although its pathology is distinctly different.

In each case, the dust, once inhaled, is picked up by defensive cells of the body, specifically the alveolar macrophage. The alveolar macrophage has as its mission to search out and destroy foreign and potentially threatening bits of matter, such as bacteria. It does so by a variety of physical and chemical reactions more appropriate to killing bacteria than digesting particles of mineral origin. The incidental release of protease and intracellular oxidizing agents damages the surrounding lung tissue.

The effects of the inhaled dust on the macrophage are also a critical aspect of its toxicity. In the case of these two dusts, the reactions of the macrophage to the dust create more damage than the dusts themselves might otherwise. The macrophage is itself killed or severely damaged by its encounter with the silica dust particle, by mechanisms that are still under investigation. The damaged cell, directly or indirectly, stimulates fibroblasts, the cells that lay down collagen, the rope-like substance that is the basic element of connective tissue, in an exuberant and abnormal way, resulting in scarring and stiff abnormal tissue in the interstitium, the structural tissue of the lung, between the walls of the alveoli. However, the pathologic features of the three dust diseases are very different.

In silicosis, the dust and its accompanying macrophage find their way directly and by lymphatic channels into the interstitial space, which tends to run alongside blood vessels in the lung. The scarring that takes place occurs in the interstitium in the form of a mass of rope-like fibers that thicken and stiffen the formerly delicate interstitial tissue. In addition, collections of dust-laden macrophages and certain lymphatic drainage areas become centers of particularly active

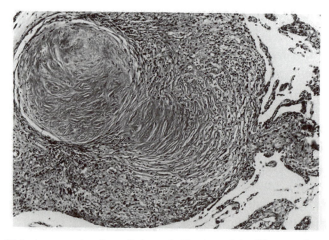

Figure 17.6. An exceptionally well-formed silicotic nodule. (Photograph courtesy of Dr. Jerrold L. Abraham.)

fibrosis. This is the origin of the "silicotic nodule," a characteristic feature of silicosis not found in asbestosis or any other pneumoconiosis (Figure 17.6). These central areas thicken, coalesce with adjacent nodules, and become the centers of an extensive web of fibrosis that radiates out from the nodules. As the nodules grow larger, the tissue at the centre dies from ischemia, or lack of blood-born nourishment. This results in a thickened, almost glassy appearing center in the middle of the nodule, which otherwise resembles a fingerprint due to the whorled tangle of rope-like collagen fibers.

There is a characteristic lesion of coal workers' pneumoconiosis, the coal dust macule, but the fibrosis is not as exuberant and the fibrosis is not organized in a concentric pattern as in silicosis.

By comparison, asbestosis is a ragged and irregular disease, resulting in extensive patches of fibrosis in the interstitium. The macrophage bearing an asbestos particle is greatly impeded in its ability to pass through the interstitial space and lymphatic channels compared to the macrophage bearing silica particles. That this would be so can be understood by simple geometry. Asbestos particles are long and thin and may get stuck while passing through narrow channels. Silica and coal dust particles, although irregular, are more nearly spherical. The contrast is like a person getting onto a crowded escalator carrying a beach ball (a particle of silica or coal dust) or carrying a ladder (asbestos). Many more asbestos particles get stuck in the interstitium. When they do travel considerable distances in the lymphatic channels, they cause considerable fibrosis wherever they tend to collect. The pleural surface, the tissue lining the thoracic cavity and its viscera, tends to trap asbestos fibers and so is particularly subject to this injury, leading to fibrosis in the form of pleural plaques and the risk of cancer.

Silicosis and Silica-Related Disease

Silicosis is an ancient disease that continues to occur today in numerous occupations, although it is entirely preventable. Worldwide, silicosis is the most prevalent serious occupational lung disease, mostly in less economically developed countries where the resulting illness is a cause of significant disability and an economic drag on development. Although the incidence of obvious silicosis has declined in developed countries and it has been effectively eliminated in Western Europe and Canada, there are still over one hundred deaths every year from the disease in the United States and much unrecognized morbidity because of underreporting and lack of recognition of silica-related diseases beyond classical silicosis.

Silica dust is intensely fibrotic, producing a characteristic microscopic lesion called the "silicotic nodule," a nidus of focal fibrosis surrounding a lymphatic deposition of silica dust, each of which may grow into a large, whorled fibrotic mass and coalesce with one another. The chest film appearance begins as isolated opacities against a normal lung parenchyma that progresses over years to a reticulonodular infiltrate and further progresses over months and years to severe fibrosis, formation of bullae, fibrotic masses, and calcification of the lymph nodes and parenchymal masses (see Figure 17.7). Two pathognomic radiological features of severe silicosis are calcification of enlarged hilar nodes in a thin oval or elliptical pattern ("eggshell" calcification) and retraction and fibrosis of the parenchyma at the apices into dense crescents concave toward the hilum ("angel wings," a mordant reference not only to the sign's appearance but to its significance as a harbinger of death). Silicosis can be characterized by radiological stages and by variants characterized mostly by the rate of progression.

"Simple silicosis" is characterized by isolated rounded opacities, usually first visible in the upper lung fields. As it progresses, simple silicosis is characterized by proliferation of rounded small opacities resembling miliary tuberculosis or sarcoidosis (with which it is frequently confused), gradually increasing in density and dispersion among the lung fields (Figure 17.7). The effect is something like white sand scattered on the chest film. The parenchymal lesions may be associated with hypertrophy of the hilar lymph nodes, which later calcify around the periphery. At times, the lymph node hypertrophy can be extreme, and rare cases may not show parenchymal opacities on the chest film at all early on. (Figure 17.8 demonstrates such a

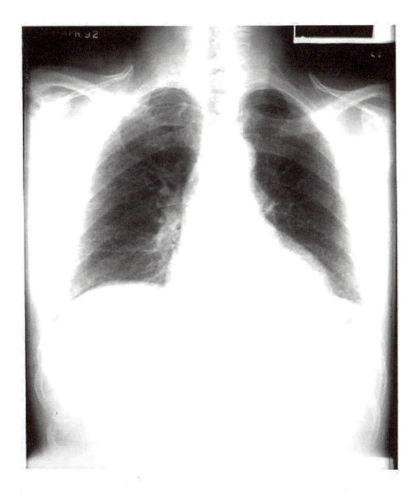

Figure 17.7. Early simple silicosis. (Reproduced with permission of the American Academy of Family Practice.)

case, which resembles sarcoidosis; the diagnosis must be made by biopsy.) There is often a thin dense ring of calcification around the lymph nodes—so-called egg shell calcification characteristic of silicosis that is only rarely seen in other conditions such as sarcoidosis. Progression of the disease is associated with increases in

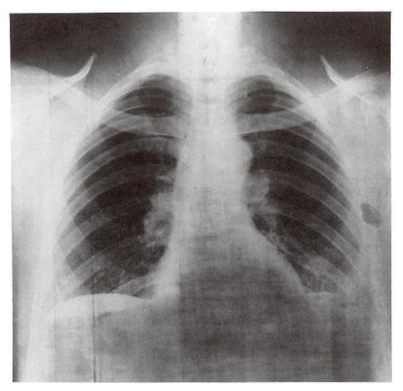

Figure 17.8. Silicosis, biopsy proven, presenting as hilar lymphadenopathy.

the size and number of opacities (see Figure 17.9). Simple silicosis is usually not associated with significant respiratory impairment.

In "complicated silicosis," which is often and historically more correctly called "conglomerative" or "chronic nodular silicosis," the silicotic nodules coalesce into a fibrotic mass and a confluence of opacities on the chest film ("progressive massive fibrosis" is a term more historically correct for coal workers' pneumoconiosis). This leads to contraction of the upper lobes, traction emphysema, and bullae, which contrast against the densely fibrotic parenchyma and create the "angel wing" pattern (see Figure 17.10). Clinically, this massive fibrotic reaction in the lungs leads to dyspnea and progressive restrictive disease. There may also be a concealed obstructive

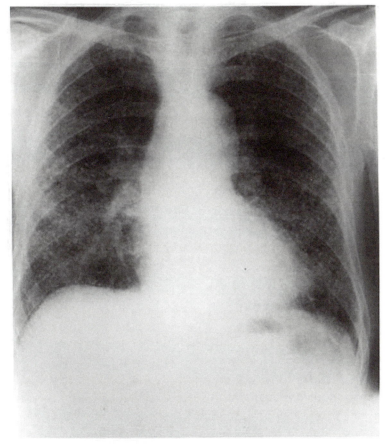

Figure 17.9. Advanced simple silicosis. Note micronodular opacities, hyperplastic lymph nodes, and calcification of hilar nodes.

component reflecting some underlying emphysema or COPD (chronic obstructive pulmonary disease). Unlike asbestosis, there are few physical signs that accompany even advanced silicosis; rales and clubbing are generally absent. Ultimately, respiratory failure and right heart failure (cor pulmonale) may result. Eventually, the outcome of advanced conglomerative silicosis is respiratory failure and cardiopulmonary arrest if the disease continues to progress. There is no way to modify progression of the disease.

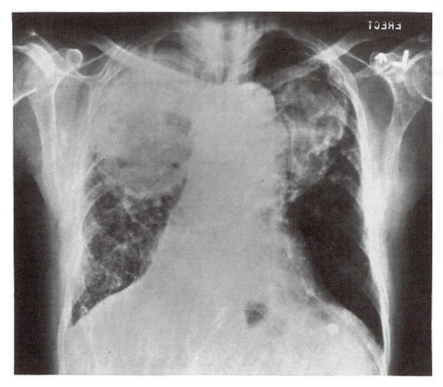

Figure 17.10. Conglomerative silicosis in a high-performance ceramics worker; the patient compounded the material, which included silica, for the tiles on the heat shield of the Space Shuttle. (Reproduced with permission of the American Academy of Family Practice.)

"Accelerated silicosis" is a form of silicosis that is rapidly progressive and passes through the simple and complicated stages within a few years or even months. It is associated with heavy dust exposure and carries a very poor prognosis. Accelerated silicosis usually occurs in outbreaks associated with abusive working conditions. This form of silicosis is thought to have been responsible for most of the deaths of the workers in the "Hawk's Nest" water tunnel disaster of 1930–1931 at Gauley Bridge, West Virginia, the worst industrial disaster in American history. The last reported outbreak in North America came in 1988 in a cluster of cases among oil field sandblasting workers in Texas.

Patients with silicosis who are already infected with the tubercle bacillis, other mycobacteria, or similarly behaving organisms (such as actinomycetes) are very susceptible to opportunistic infection, most commonly reactivation of tuberculosis. The resulting, distinct condition of "silicotuberculosis" can become a devastating, swiftly progressive fibrotic process that, untreated, resembles a malignancy. The diagnosis of silicotuberculosis is suggested when there is a change in the rate of progression of silicotic nodules on the chest film so that the disease appears to be accelerating or when there is onset of systemic symptoms such as fever, weight loss, or new cough (especially hemoptysis). The infection tends to favor upper lobes and may develop early when fibrosis is not far advanced. The recovery of acid-fast bacilli from sputum may be difficult because the mycobacterial burden is much less than in other forms of tuberculosis; repeated sputum induction and even gastric washings may be required. *Mycobacterium tuberculosis* is the most common organism, atypical mycobacteria are becoming increasingly common (*Mycobacterium kansasii, Mycobacterium avium-intracellulare*), and a similar condition occurs with opportunistic infection by *Acinetobacter spp.* (See Figure 17.11, which is an advanced case of silicotuberculosis with infection by *M. kansasii*.) Deep fungal infections (aspergillosis, cryptococcosis, sporotrichosis) and nocardiosis have also been described. Silicotuberculosis tends to be refractory to treatment due to poor penetration into the fibrotic mass by antibiotics. Often, patients require life-long suppression using triple therapy.

"Acute silicosis" is a distinct disease, characterized by an alveolitis that occurs early in the disease due to overwhelming silica dust exposure, which produces a clinical picture resembling diffuse alveolar injury. Patients rarely survive to progress to more chronic forms and so the pathology does not feature the typical lesions of silicosis. Acute silicosis, or silica-induced alveolar proteinosis, is associated with massive outpouring of proteinaceous debris and fluid into alveolar spaces, presumably as a consequence of acute inflammation and diffuse alveolar injury. The chest film appears

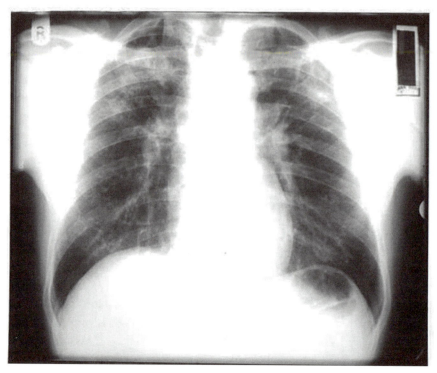

Figure 17.11. Silicotuberculosis with an atypical mycobacterium, infection due to *Mycobacterium kansasii.*

much like a slowly evolving pulmonary edema or adult respiratory distress syndrome (ARDS) but without any obvious precipitating cause. Acute silicosis may respond in part to lavage and administration of high-dose steroids, but is still generally fatal since respiratory failure supervenes due to continued accumulation of debris and lipoproteinaceous material in the airspaces. Occasionally acute silicosis is complicated by opportunistic infection. In view of the extremely poor prognosis and tendency for this form of silicosis to be seen in young workers because of the circumstances of exposure, the physician must consider transplantation and other heroic measures. Like accelerated silicosis, it has been associated with multiple fatalities among workers who have been heavily exposed at the same site.

Silicosis may be associated with other silica-related disorders, such as systemic sclerosis (including scleroderma, the skin manifestations), the combination of which is called Erasmus' syndrome, and its characteristic nephritis, a more benign nephritis with proteinuria, and airway obstruction, although the pattern of advanced silicosis is always predominantly restrictive. (See Figure 17.12, the chest film of a man with biopsy-proven silicosis, showing mostly hilar changes including calcification of nodes,

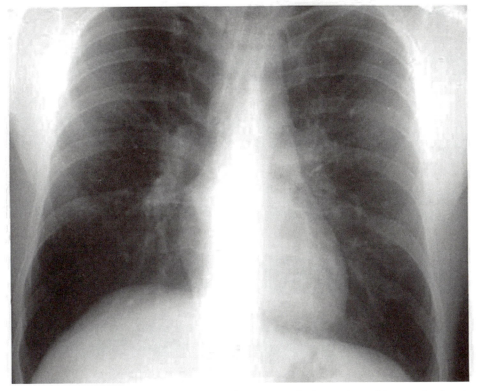

Figure 17.12. Silicosis, with early eggshell calcification on right, in a patient with systemic sclerosis (Erasmus syndrome) and nephropathy.

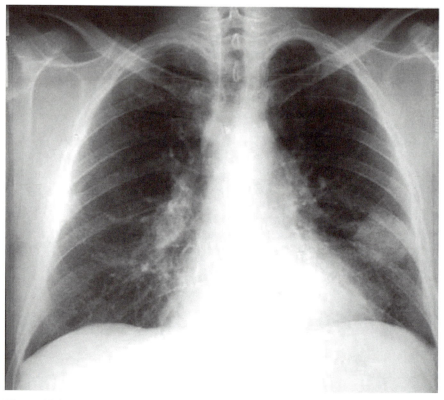

Figure 17.13. Lung cancer in a worker with advanced simple silicosis and hilar changes.

who had systemic sclerosis and classic scleroderma, with proteinuria and early CRST nephropathy.)

Silica exposure, and therefore these disorders, is also associated with an elevated risk of lung cancer. (See Figure 17.13. A single case does not establish an association, of course, but this case illustrates the presentation of lung cancer against a background of parenchymal and hilar silicosis.) This elevation is associated with significant exposure to crystalline silica but does not seem to require radiological silicosis and is interactive with cigarette smoking, although not to the same degree as asbestos.

Asbestosis and Nonmalignant Asbestos-Related Disorders

This section discusses only nonmalignant respiratory diseases related to asbestos, which are growing less common because there are fewer people living today who had asbestos exposure in the 1970s and before when exposure levels were high. Even so, there are many prevalent cases among older workers and occasional new cases. The Centers for Disease Control and Prevention (CDC) has determined that the total burden of asbestosis in North America is probably at its peak at the current time, because of the latency of the disease, which requires a decade or more to develop, depending on the intensity of exposure.

Exposure to asbestos in a young person today is most likely to occur in poorly managed asbestos abatement activities. Asbestos as a hazard is discussed in Chapter 10; asbestos-related malignancy is discussed in the section on occupational cancer. Although there is an on-going debate about the relative potency of chrysotile compared to the amphiboles in causing these cases, there is no serious controversy over whether chrysotile can cause these disorders. A unified approach to the diagnosis of nonmalignant asbestos-related disease, with standardized criteria, has been developed by the American Thoracic Society and is now in its second revision (see Table 17.2).

"Asbestosis," sometimes called "white lung" colloquially, is a functionally serious pneumoconiosis, lethal in its advanced forms, resulting from the inhalation of large quantities of asbestos fibers. Asbestosis should never be used as a general term for a history of exposure to asbestos or for other asbestos-related conditions. The term is specific to the interstitial fibrotic lung disease. Even so, asbestosis usually occurs in association with other nonmalignant asbestos-related disorders and is a strong risk factor for malignancy, which may not be easily detectable because of the chest film changes of the underlying pneumoconiosis

Asbestosis is a widespread interstitial fibrosis that develops first in the lower lung fields as a pattern of "irregular opacities,"

Table 17.2. The Approach to Nonmalignant Asbestos–Related Respiratory Disorders

2004 Criterion and Guidelines	How to Satisfy the Criterion
Evidence of structural change, as demonstrated by one or more of the following:	Demonstrate the existence of a structural lesion consistent with the effects of asbestos. This criterion is almost always satisfied by chest film in the first instance.
• Imaging methods • Histology	Chest film, HRCT, and possibly future methods based on imaging. Criteria for identifying asbestosis on microscopic examination of tissue have been developed by the College of American Pathologists. Biopsy is seldom required to make diagnosis of nonmalignant asbestos–related disease and may be contraindicated in advanced diseases due to risk of pneumothorax.
Evidence of plausible causation, as demonstrated by one or more of the following:	Latency for asbestosis is typically ten to twenty years or more. Exposure was higher in the workplace in the 1970s and earlier.
• Occupational and environmental history of exposure (with plausible latency)	See Chapters 8 and 15. Bystander and passive exposure may occur. The most likely contemporary exposure for young people is in asbestos abatement activities that are not in compliance with the OSHA Asbestos Standard or other applicable standards.
• Markers of exposure	Sufficient to establish asbestos exposure if no other cause of pleural disease demonstrated. The chief marker of exposure is the presence of pleural plaques.
• Recovery of asbestos bodies	Asbestos bodies are asbestos fibers that are coated with protein and hemosiderin as a result of macrophage ingestion. They may be demonstrated through sputum examination, bronchoalveolar lavage, biopsy (rarely required), or autopsy. Individual asbestos fibers are rarely visible by light microscopy during examination of tissue, even when numerous.

Exclusion of alternative diagnoses	Nonmalignant diseases resembling asbestos-related disease should be ruled out clinically: sarcoidosis, idiopathic interstitial fibrosis, IV drug-injection fibrosis, systemic sclerosis and other rheumatological lung diseases.
Evidence of functional impairment, as demonstrated by one or more of the following:	Functional assessment is not required for diagnosis but is part of a complete evaluation, in order to monitor progression and to quantify impairment.
• Signs and symptoms (including crackles)	Signs and symptoms are not specific for the diagnosis of asbestosis but are associated with significant impairment. The progression or new onset of respiratory symptoms is evidence of diminished reserve and decompensation. Cor pulmonale and right heart failure is a late change and a poor prognostic sign.
• Change in ventilatory function (spirometry)	Typical pattern is early irritation and trend to low-grade obstructive change and small airway effects, usually still within range of normal function, which are soon overwhelmed in advanced disease by progressive restrictive change.
• Impaired gas exchange (reduced diffusing capacity)	Low diffusing capacity for carbon monoxide is relatively sensitive and often reduced early in the progression of asbestosis, but it is not specific to asbestosis.
• Inflammation	Bronchoalveolar lavage is not necessary for diagnosis and is rarely performed but would show inflammation while asbestosis is active. Histology not required but may be indicative.
• Exercise testing	Useful for work capacity evaluation and for early detection of impairment.

Source: Adapted from the American Thoracic Society.

which sometimes resemble little threads or lint on the chest film. The characteristic opacities are short, squiggly, or irregular lines that often link together rather than the smooth, discrete,

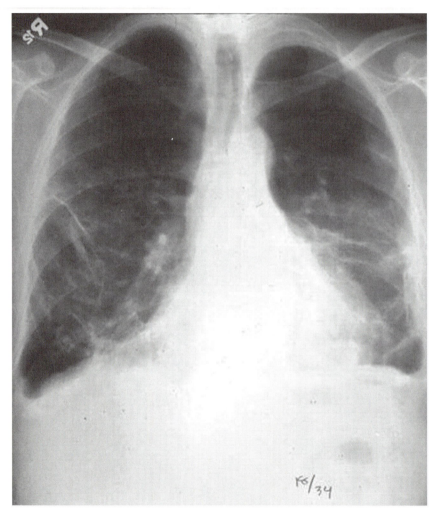

Figure 17.14. Asbestosis at an advanced stage. Note fibrotic changes, irregular pleural border and diaphragm, shaggy heart border, and blunted costophrenic angles, all of which are typical. Source: Ad Hoc Committee [on Update of 1986 Criteria for the Diagnosis of Nonmalignant Asbestos-Related Disease: Guidotti TL, Miller A, Christiani D, Wagner G, Balmes J, Harber P, Brodkin CA, Rom W, Hillerdal G, Harbut M, Green FHY]. Diagnosis and initial management of nonmalignant diseases related to asbestos. *Am J Respir Crit Care Med*, 2004;170:691-715. Reproduced with Permission from The American Journal of Respiratory and Critical Care Medicine, American Thoracic Society.

rounded opacities of other pneumoconioses. Over time, these coalesce into fibrotic streaks and bands (see Figure 17.14). The lung becomes progressively scarred and stiff. The natural history of the disease is progression of the restrictive impairment, sometimes to total disability, and a high risk of bronchogenic cancer, whether asbestosis is visible on the chest film or not. Asbestosis usually has many accompanying features on chest film that reflect pleural and pericardial changes, including diaphragmatic calcification (which results from pleural plaques on the diaphragm), blunted costophrenic angle (due to pleural fibrosis), and a "shaggy" (ill-defined) left cardiac border (which results from composite shadows of fibrosis and the pericardium). Examination of individuals with asbestosis may reveal clubbing, crackles, and tachypnea.

The management of asbestosis is supportive and preventive; patients with asbestosis may experience serious and sudden decompensation in the event of intercurrent pneumonia. The disease is not associated with smoking, but smoking clearly makes the symptoms worse and management more difficult. For this reason, and because there is an interaction between smoking and asbestos exposure for cancer risk, quitting smoking is even more critical for such patients than for other smokers.

All but the earliest irregular parenchymal changes are usually accompanied by characteristic pleural signs on the chest film (shown well in Figure 17.14). These result from a transient, painless pleuritis that occurs early in the natural history of asbestos-related disease but is almost never observed radiologically unless captured by accident. Pleural changes alone do not define asbestosis, nor do they indicate a risk of mesothelioma beyond confirming the fact of asbestos exposure. "Pleural plaques" are discrete fibrotic regions of the parietal pleura visible on the chest film as an irregular pleural border from the side and as polygonal lesions overlying the lung fields face on. Pleural plaques tend to calcify over time. On the diaphragm they appear as rectangular-stepped discontinuities or streaks of calcification. They can be very large and dramatic (as in

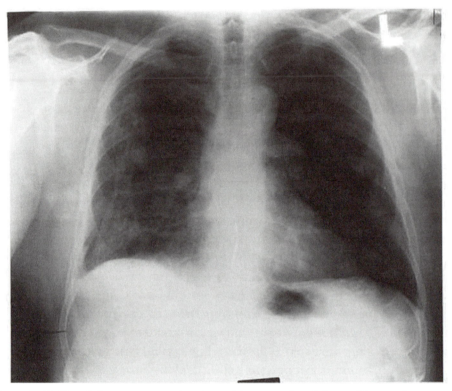

Figure 17.15. Pleural plaques, most prominently on right postero-lateral chest wall, in a worker exposed to asbestos. Source: Ad Hoc Committee [on Update of 1986 Criteria for the Diagnosis of Nonmalignant Asbestos-Related Disease: Guidotti TL, Miller A, Christiani D, Wagner G, Balmes J, Harber P, Brodkin CA, Rom W, Hillerdal G, Harbut M, Green FHY]. Diagnosis and initial management of nonmalignant diseases related to asbestos. *Am J Respir Crit Care Med*, 2004;170:691-715. Reproduced with Permission from The American Journal of Respiratory and Critical Care Medicine, American Thoracic Society.

Figure 17.15) or tiny and ill-defined, bilateral or unilateral, over-lying a single rib (the usual location), or extending across several intercostal spaces. Pleural plaques often occur in isolation and serve as reliable markers (in the absence a history of chest trauma or tuberculosis) of past exposure to asbestos. "Pleural thickening" is a more diffuse fibrotic change in the pleura, without a discrete border. Pleural changes due to asbestos almost never cause symptoms or functional impairment.

Less common effects of asbestos exposure on the pleura include benign pleural effusion (the transient pleuritis described above) and rounded lung syndrome. Benign pleural effusion does not appear to be a premalignant lesion and behaves much like the effusions associated with primary tuberculosis. "Rounded atelectasis" or "folded lung" presents as a round, comet-shaped pleural-based mass with the "tail" pointed toward the hilum. (Figure 17.16 shows this, in the left mid-lung field.) This mass forms when a peripheral segment of lung becomes atelectatic and due to the traction of fibrosis rolls up on itself, caught between thickened visceral pleura and interlobar fissure. Rounded atelectasis is often mistaken for lung cancer but has a characteristic appearance on HRCT, with curved blood vessels, air trapping, and attachment to the pleura, as in Figure 17.17.

Asbestos bodies (asbestos fibers encrusted with protein and iron from cellular activity) are usually abundantly visible when they are

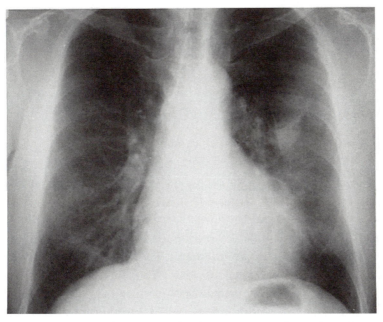

Figure 17.16. Rounded atelectasis, a peripheral mass consisting of parenchyma distorted by pleural fibrosis; this is not a lung cancer. Source: Ad Hoc Committee [on Update of 1986 Criteria for the Diagnosis of Nonmalignant Asbestos-Related Disease: Guidotti TL, Miller A, Christiani D, Wagner G, Balmes J, Harber P, Brodkin CA, Rom W, Hillerdal G, Harbut M, Green FHY]. Diagnosis and initial management of nonmalignant diseases related to asbestos. *Am J Respir Crit Care Med*, 2004;170:691-715. Reproduced with Permission from The American Journal of Respiratory and Critical Care Medicine, American Thoracic Society.

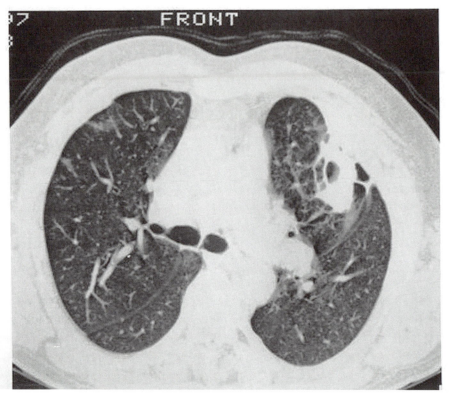

Figure 17.17. CT scan of same patient as in Figure 17.16, showing details of the mass: air trapping, contorted blood vessels, attachment to pleura. Source: Ad Hoc Committee [on Update of 1986 Criteria for the Diagnosis of Nonmalignant Asbestos-Related Disease: Guidotti TL, Miller A, Christiani D, Wagner G, Balmes J, Harber P, Brodkin CA, Rom W, Hillerdal G, Harbut M, Green FHY]. Diagnosis and initial management of nonmalignant diseases related to asbestos. *Am J Respir Crit Care Med*, 2004;170:691-715. Reproduced with Permission from The American Journal of Respiratory and Critical Care Medicine, American Thoracic Society.

searched for under the microscope (Figure 17.18). They are also markers of exposure to asbestos.

Airways are also affected by asbestos exposure, as a result of interstitial fibrosis in the adjacent alveoli. Chronic obstructive airway disease caused by asbestos may be clinically significant in some cases and adds an obstructive element to the primarily restrictive impairment of asbestosis. Early on, there may be a relatively pure detectable obstructive component on spirometry, but as the disease progresses the restrictive pattern soon becomes overwhelmingly predominant.

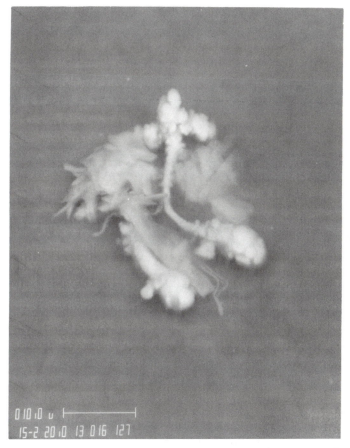

0 10 ı0 u
15-2 20 ı0 13 0 l6 l2l

Figure 17.18. Asbestos body visible in lung tissue on a scanning election microphotograph. (Photograph courtesy of Dr. Jerrold L. Abraham.)

Coal Workers' Pneumoconiosis and Less Fibrogenic Dusts

"Coal workers' pneumoconiosis" (CWP), or "black lung," is probably the best-known dust disease of the lung because of historical associations with mining communities. The characterization of CWP as a distinct pneumoconiosis came slowly because the historically recognized lung disease of coal miners ("miner's phthisis") was often confounded in epidemiological studies and complicated in individual cases by silicosis, cigarette smoking, and a high prevalence of tuberculosis and histoplasmosis in coal mining regions in North America, especially Appalachia. It has been recognized for decades, however, that CWP is a distinct disease with a tendency to develop into a more aggressive fibrotic form; the functional impairment in nonsmoking miners is obstructive and is initially somewhat less than for other fibrogenic dusts but can progress into severe restrictive disease.

CWP and other lung diseases associated with underground coal mining are declining in frequency as a result of dust suppression in mines but have not been eliminated in the United States. CWP also remains an important and common occupational lung disease in developing countries.

The medical diagnosis of CWP almost always depends on the chest film. Only rarely is biopsy justified but the diagnosis may be made by direct examination of tissue at autopsy to qualify the surviving family for benefits. As noted, CWP has its characteristic histological lesion, the coal dust macule, a fibrotic nodule, less dense than the silicotic nodule, surrounding an arteriole and packed with black "anthracotic" particles left behind by macrophages that migrated to that location.

The chest film in CWP begins, as do most pneumoconioses, with scattered rounded opacities, predominantly in the lower lung fields initially. Figure 17.19 demonstrates the typical chest film appearance of CWP. The interpretation of the chest film in CWP relies on the occupational history, since there is no pathognomonic sign for early CWP. However, the natural history of CWP is distinct from that of other pneumoconioses. CWP progresses through stages, first as "simple CWP," in which the opacities remain discrete and lung function is preserved, and then, when any one mass reaches one centimeter in diameter, to "complicated" CWP, in which they coalesce into complex, structured disc-like lesion that appears in the upper lung fields, and restrictive changes become apparent. As these lesions grow by accretion of smaller opacities, they may form very large, much denser masses. This is called "progressive massive fibrosis" and is associated with restrictive

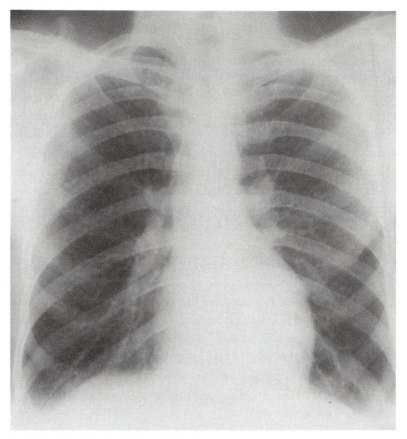

impairment, pulmonary hypertension, a high risk of right heart failure, and a poor prognosis. Complicated CWP has disappeared in North America but was once all too common where coal was mined underground.

It is not clear why CWP should project a radiological shadow in the first place, since coal is mostly elemental carbon. A density of 0.4 g/cm³ is required for coal dust to be barely visible on the chest film, and the total lung burden of dust in the lung is far lower than what

Figure 17.19. Simple coal workers' pneumoconiosis in a 55-year old retired Japanese anthracite miner. Reprinted with permission from "Occupational Lung Diseases," February, 1984, *American Family Physician*. Copyright © 1984 American Academy of Family Physicians. All Rights Reserved.

would be required to produce shadows by density of dust alone. This strongly implies that the origin of the "interstitial" pattern of small nodular opacities characteristic of CWP is local tissue reaction.

There is no practical method of detecting or quantifying coal dust in the lung of the living patient other than by x-ray film. Sputum production of coal pigment is compatible with a recent acute exposure but says nothing about the cumulative lung burden.

The potency of coal dust in inducing changes in the lungs is reflected in the "rank" of the coal, which is its silica content and which is a complex function of the geologic characteristics of the coal seam. Higher-rank coal, such as anthracite, is more fibrogenic than bituminous coal, which in turn is more fibrogenic than lignite (brown coal). The rank and density of coal reflects the compaction and mineralization of fossil wood and plant matter over millennia.

The pathology of CWP involves the bronchiole, the arteriole, and the alveolar wall. The characteristic pathologic finding in CWP is the coal dust macule, a discrete (occasionally confluent) nonindurated focus of black pigment macroscopically under the visceral pleura and on the cut surface of lung parenchyma. The macules tend to constrict and efface arterioles that run through them. Microscopically, the coal dust macules are typically in various stages of development. The carbonaceous pigment is mostly intracellular in macrophages and may remain present ten years after cessation of exposure. The macrophages are concentrated in the peribronchial and periarterial interstitium, trapped by local fibrosis. The distribution of macules follows the known patterns of peribronchial and periarterial lymphatic drainage, and draining nodes typically show heavy accumulations of pigment. Limited dilatation of the respiratory bronchioles is common, in a pattern compatible with centrilobular emphysema, but without bronchiolitis.

With so many structures involved, one might expect that simple CWP would have a profound effect on ventilation, perfusion, and gas exchange. Surprisingly, it usually does not. In general, coal miners have slightly lower forced vital capacities (FVC) and one-second forced expiratory volumes (FEV_1) than do nonminers; these changes usually do not become statistically significant until the miners have worked underground thirty years or more. The FVC and FEV_1 are lowest, on the average, for anthracite miners and less reduced for bituminous miners but are not markedly reduced in any large population sample of working miners. Cigarette smoking obliterates any differences in the degree of small airway disease associated with simple CWP. Diffusing capacity is within normal limits for nonsmoking miners with simple CWP. When the disease converts to progressive massive fibrosis, however, the advancing restrictive process comes to overwhelm the earlier, more modest changes.

"Caplan's syndrome" is the association of CWP with rheumatoid arthritis; it can occur with other pneumoconioses. Caplan's syndrome probably represents one particularly well-defined end of the spectrum of autoimmune disorders caused by altered self-antigens in the damaged lung. Anti-lung antibodies and other manifestations of autoimmunity are common in the pneumoconioses generally, particularly CWP.

Toxic Inhalation

Toxic inhalation is a general term for a pattern of deep-lung injury produced by a variety of gases that penetrate to the deep lung, including ozone (O_3), phosgene ($COCl_2$), chlorine (Cl_2), nitrogen oxide (NO_2, not to be confused with nitrous oxide, N_2O, or nitric oxide, NO), hydrogen fluoride (HF) (see Table 17.3). Exposure to these gases at the levels required to produce this condition is usually the result of accidental release, uncontrolled chemical reactions, or fires. Some of these gases, particularly phosgene, chlorine, and nitrogen dioxide, are generated when plastic furnishings and interior design fixtures burn, as in a hotel fire. In such combustion situations, cyanide (CN) and carbon monoxide (CO) are also released and may contribute to toxicity. Several gases uncommonly encountered in industry and agriculture may cause toxic inhalation, with other systemic toxicity: silane (SiH_4), phosphine (PH_3), hexafluoroacetone

Table 17.3. Some Toxic Gases Associated with Diffuse Alveolar Injury

Oxidant gases (nitrogen dioxide, ozone, phosgene, hyperbaric oxygen)
Sulfur dioxide (rare because of low penetration to deep lung)
Chlorine
Ammonia
Hydrogen sulfide
Hydrogen fluoride
Heated mercury, cadmium (not to be confused with metal fume fever)

(F_3CCOCF_3, found in the semiconductor industry), and methyl bromide (CH_3Br, bromomethane) and sulfuryl fluoride (SO_2F_2), used as fumigants. Nickel carbonyl is discussed at the end of the subsection because of its unusual characteristics.

Historically, the most common toxic inhalation was silo filler's disease, which resulted from exposure to nitrogen dioxide released during the incomplete fermenting process during storage in a large, deep silo (see Figure 17.20). When agricultural workers entered the silo a few weeks after filling it with harvested grain (especially maize, because it is rich in tryptophan, a nitrogen source), they would encounter the brownish gas and experience the characteristic symptoms described. Greater awareness and changes in agricultural practices have mostly eliminated the disorder. (Silo filler's disease is not to be confused with farmer's lung, a hypersensitivity pneumonitis.)

The mechanism of toxic inhalation involves inhalation of a gas that is either not readily dissolved in water, and so penetrates to the deep lung at a high concentration, or inhalation of a soluble gas at such a high exposure that it reaches a high concentration at the alveolar level regardless. In addition to incidental irritation of the upper airway (and usually eyes), the gas irritates the bronchial mucosa causing severe cough and may induce acute bronchospasm and damages to the bronchiolar mucosa on the way down. Once the gas has penetrated to the alveolar level, it injures the delicate alveolar wall, damages the barrier between the vascular space and first the interstitium and then

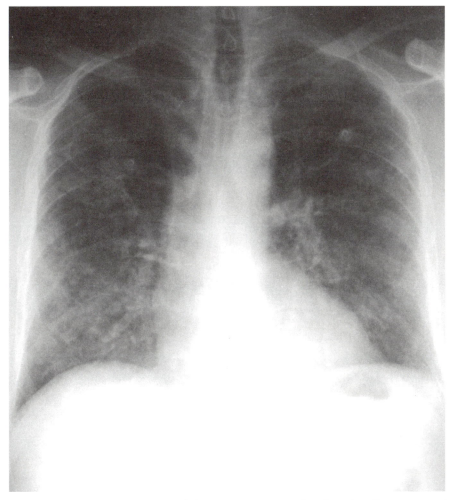

Figure 17.20. Silo filler's disease, toxic inhalation due to nitrogen dioxide, with infiltrates representing pulmonary edema. Reprinted with permission from "Occupational Lung Diseases," February, 1984, *American Family Physician*. Copyright © 1984 American Academy of Family Physicians. All Rights Reserved.

the alveolar space, and may cause pulmonary edema. This "diffuse alveolar damage" results in a relatively slow process by which fluid passes under vascular pressure from the alveolar capillary bed into the alveolar wall as interstitial edema and then later breaks through under pressure into the alveolar space as pulmonary edema. If the patient recovers, the diffuse alveolar injury may be repaired in a dysfunctional manner, with scarring and interstitial fibrosis. Injury to small airways may also result in overly exuberant fibrosis that overgrows the wall of the airway, leading to bronchiolitis obliterans (not to be confused with bronchiolitis obliterans organizing pneumonia, which is different), in which small airways disappear because they are absorbed into the inflammation around them, which leads to fixed airway obstruction and chronic impairment.

As a consequence of this sequence of events, these agents produce a relatively stereotyped clinical picture, with a predictable but not always complete sequence of events:

1. Acute bronchospasm and dyspnea develop at the time of exposure. Usually the subject is removed from the exposure by co-workers, who may also be affected if they do not stop to use self-contained breathing apparatus.

2. Unless overwhelmed, the victim will often appear to recover from the initial symptoms.

3. About four to twelve hours later, severe dyspnea may develop as a result of pulmonary edema caused by diffuse alveolar injury that may not have been appreciated at the time of initial exposure. The pattern of pulmonary edema on chest film is similar to that of the adult respiratory distress syndrome, or "capillary leak," rather than pulmonary edema due to congestive heart failure. The time lag reflects the migration of fluid from the vascular to the alveolar space and represents the onset of alveolar pulmonary edema.

4. After the patient recovers from the acute process and the delayed development of pulmonary edema, their recovery may be interrupted by the onset of refractory shortness of breath weeks later. This would be due to bronchiolitis obliterans. A chest film may show a hyperlucent lung and air trapping.

5. Much later, interstitial fibrosis may occur, with the characteristic pattern of "honeycombing" (interstitial fibrosis) on the chest film.

The management of patients with toxic inhalation is primarily supportive. This form of pulmonary edema is similar to adult respiratory distress syndrome (ARDS) and is familiar in the intensive care unit. One-third of such patients die.

The single greatest clinical mistake in such cases is not to recognize the potential for pulmonary edema. Patients have been sent home from the emergency room only to die in their bed hours later. Pulmonary edema due to toxic inhalation is life threatening and leads to mortality in about one-quarter of cases historically. Among those who survive the pulmonary edema, an unknown fraction will then develop the obliterative bronchiolitis. A few develop bronchiolitis without experiencing pulmonary edema. There is no effective treatment for obliterative bronchiolitis after it is fixed. However, as it develops the process may be arrested with steroids, which are sometimes required for prolonged periods. The small airways or bronchioles have in the aggregate a much greater cross-sectional area than the larger airways associated with asthma. There are, of course, many more of them. As a result, their obstruction does not interfere significantly with airflow until very many are involved. This means that the disorder is largely silent until the condition is far advanced. Symptoms of cough and shortness of breath may not be associated with the degree of the patient's impairment in pulmonary function. These symptoms relate more closely to the fibrotic changes occurring in the tissue than the obstruction of the airways.

Two precautions should be followed in every suspected case of toxic inhalation. First, the patient must be observed through the period of risk for pulmonary edema, normally in a hospital. At the very least, a responsible adult must stay with the patient in order to return the patient to medical attention immediately if dyspnea develops. Second, exposure to other toxic agents must also be considered, particularly in cases of fire or explosion. The most important gases in such multiple exposures are carbon monoxide and hydrogen cyanide, but pesticides, hydrogen sulfide, volatile organic compounds that depress the central nervous system, or other chemicals may be present, depending on the circumstances of the exposure.

An organic metal compound, nickel carbonyl $(Ni(CO)_4)$, causes an unusually treatable form of toxic inhalation, with elements of systemic toxicity. Nickel carbonyl produces a similar pattern of pulmonary edema and is often associated with fever, leukoytosis, and headache; it is most often encountered in nickel plating and case-hardening operations in treating steel and in nickel refining. Urinary nickel levels confirm the diagnosis. Specific treatment with disulfiram, parenterally if necessary, may be life-saving by reducing biologically available nickel following exposure. This condition is quite rare.

Occupational Asthma

Asthma is, of course, very familiar to any clinician. However, occupational and environmental asthma require new ways of thinking about this disorder and an expanded definition of asthma. Usually asthma of whatever type presents as wheezing, cough, and shortness of breath, occurring repeatedly in isolated episodes, often immediately following exposure to a recognizable allergen. However, there are many variations. Airflow obstruction may become chronic (although still variable), and a restrictive defect may develop as a result of air trapping. Asthma may also present as a bronchitis, without discrete episodes of bronchospasm.

Asthma can be considered to be a disease with many variations, which has been the predominant view in clinical medicine, or a collection of individual disorders all characterized by reversible obstruction of air flow, latent or active airway reactivity, and some degree of inflammation of the airways. Occupational and environmental asthma is most usefully thought of as an umbrella term for a group of related disorders involving the response of airways to triggers and conditioning factors in the work environment. Intensive study of occupational asthma, in particular, in recent years has expanded medical knowledge of asthma in general and its mechanisms.

"Environmental" asthma hardly needs to be qualified as such because environmental factors are so well known to play a major role in triggering asthma from any cause: environmental allergens (most often molds, dust mite, cockroach, and animal antigens), air pollution (particularly ozone, as a trigger for asthmatic episodes), dampness (a known independent risk factor for respiratory symptoms in homes), chemical irritants (passive cigarette smoke, strong fragrances especially those rich in aldehydes, volatile solvents, and gasoline), dust (acting as a nonspecific irritant), and cold, dry air (which provokes cold-induced and exercise-induced asthma). This does not mean that asthma is caused exclusively by environmental exposures in the first instance, however. Asthma is clearly a complex process that begins with a genetic predisposition, is conditioned by environmental factors (which may include air pollution), is shaped in its expression by either sensitization (to allergens in the surrounding environment, acting by a very specific hypersensitivity response) or irritants (acting by a nonspecific mechanism), and triggered or perpetuated by environmental exposures acting on a persistent underlying condition of inflammation and airway reactivity. Whether the case in question is "extrinsic" asthma (the classic immediate hypersensitivity variety typically seen in childhood) or "intrinsic" (the more variable variety occurring in adulthood), asthma is so closely linked with environmental influences that it practically defines an environmental disorder.

"Occupational asthma" as a term of art refers to reversible airway disorders arising from or triggered by factors in the workplace and embraces a broad range of symptoms, including the classic immediate hypersensitivity reaction of allergic asthma, immediate bronchospasm due to airway provocation, an isolated late response that sometimes presents as sleep disorder, and combinations and variations of these presentations. A wider variety of airway responses than are typically seen in conventional asthma is common to occupational asthma. As well, the spectrum of incomplete or partial responses is more complete because symptoms that characterize asthma (especially cough and shortness of breath) are commonly seen in workers with underlying reactive airways but who have not been given the formal diagnosis of asthma, because the disorder is predominantly upper airway and may not present with wheezing. These patients may have allergic rhinitis or allergic sinusitis and are usually atopic. Sometimes they had asthma in childhood and think that they have "outgrown" it. (As children grow into adulthood, the increase in diameter of their airways reduces obstruction to airflow but airway reactivity remains.)

Occupational asthma is easiest to understand in terms of its relationship to exposures in the workplace. One of the most important practical distinctions to be made is between conditions induced by a sensitizer (antigens) and those induced by irritants. The former is more difficult to manage because a sensitized individual experiences an immune response after exposure at very low levels, well below occupational health standards, and personal protective equipment is often insufficient to control symptoms, usually leading to medical removal that may involve disruptive reassignments, lost jobs and opportunities, and lost income. The latter usually involves moderate to heavy exposure to only moderately irritating gases, solvents, or aerosols (highly irritating inhalants cause toxic inhalation), can often be managed by ventilation of personal protective equipment, and only requires medical removal as a last resort.

Occupational asthma includes the following airway disorders as they relate to workplace exposures:

- New-onset asthma
  - Sensitizer-induced (immediate or delayed response)
  - Irritant-induced
- Provocation and aggravation of preexisting asthma and airway reactivity
- Reactive airway dysfunction syndrome (RADS)
- Cold- or exercise-induced asthma
- Airway reactivity secondary to hypersensitivity pneumonitis

Cold air- and exercise-induced asthma are the same phenomenon, provoking the airway response due to dry air passing over the moist bronchial mucosa, either because of low moisture content or hyperventilation and exertion. This causes drying and cooling of the airway and stimulates vagal receptors, which release mediators from mast cells for an otherwise conventional asthmatic response of bron-chospasm. Cold air and exercise provoke an immediate response, but once exposure or exertion stop, air flow rapidly corrects.

Airway reactivity associated with hypersensitivity pneumonitis is discussed above in the subsection on pneumonitides.

Principles of evaluation in occupational asthma involve a detailed work history that documents the onset of respiratory symptoms and any association with work activity. Symptom diaries are very useful for this purpose. Spirometry establishes levels of function, but because asthma by definition is variable, any one tracing cannot accurately determine baseline impairment. Methacholine challenge is rarely necessary to confirm that airway reactivity exists but is occasionally necessary to ensure that it will be recognized for insur-ance or compensation purposes. Pre- and post-shift pulmonary function studies may demonstrate a big incremental loss in airflow and may also confirm the diagnosis but do not identify the respon-sible exposure.

Treatment for all forms of occupational asthma is conventional, as for other forms of reactive airway disease. Avoiding known sensitiz-ers completely and reducing or eliminating any and all irritant exposure is the mainstay of prevention and maintenance. Personal protective equipment may be effective and may allow the worker to continue around irritant exposures but is usually insufficient to prevent responses from sensitizer-induced occupational asthma.

The management of compensation for occupational asthma can be difficult. It is often difficult to support a claim without identification and documentation of a particular trigger (either sensitizer or irritant), although it may not be possible to be that specific in the workplace. Because asthma is by definition highly variable and pulmonary function may be normal between events, impairment ratings tend to be low. The assumption is usually made that because the disorder is episodic and depends on triggers, it does not have to be disabling. This is not necessarily true, if the inciting exposure is technically necessary for a particular job or career that represents the worker's usual occupation or that requires substantial training or education. There may be substantial dislocations in the injured worker's functional capacity that are not reflected in the ultimate impairment rating and in his or her life and career path that are not reflected in the resulting disability ratings.

Sensitizer-Induced Occupational Asthma

Sensitizer-induced occupational asthma involves an allergic response to a specific antigen, either a low-molecular-weight hapten (such as an isocyanate or trimellitic anhydride) that binds to a carrier molecule (such as albumin) to form a complete antigen or a high-molecular-weight molecule, often a protein (as in the case of baker's asthma). Sensitization can occur at any level of exposure but is more likely with high exposure levels. Thereafter, however, low levels are sufficient to trigger a hypersensitivity response. Sensitizer-induced asthma may present as an immediate hypersensitivity reaction, when the response is mediated by reaginic antibody, mostly IgE. It may also present as a delayed, leukotriene-mediated response that occurs hours after exposure. Individuals with atopy are more likely to become sensitized on or off the workplace, but a personal or family history of atopy or allergies is not sufficiently predictive of future risk to exclude an otherwise fit worker from a job involving exposure to known sensitizers.

Patterns of airway reactivity may be complicated and mixed in occupational asthma. As noted, at least two types of reactions may occur, singly or in combination. The immediate hypersensitivity reaction is a typical acute asthmatic episode. The delayed hypersensitivity reaction may occur several hours after exposure, consists of dyspnea, cough, and sometimes wheezing, and often interferes with sleep. The delayed reaction may be overlooked entirely in the patient's evaluation or may be falsely attributed to an antigen present in the home. The delayed reaction is thought to be mediated by leukotrienes, a class of mediators of bronchial smooth muscle contraction different from those responsible for the immediate reaction.

Management depends critically on identifying the sensitizing agent in the workplace. Table 17.4 lists common sensitizers. This is by no means a complete list and only hints at the diversity of sensitizing agents. The easiest agents to identify are those that trigger the familiar immediate hypersensitivity reaction soon after exposure. Such conventional allergic sensitizers include animal secretions, ethylene diamine, grain dusts, detergent enzymes (now encapsulated and no longer likely to be a problem), epoxy resin curing agents, and virtually any organic or low-molecular-weight compounds, including metals such as platinum salts.

A few sensitizers produce reactions by mechanisms that are not typical of the common immediate hypersensitivity reaction, such as grain dust, wood dust, formaldehyde, pharmaceutical agents, and the isocyanates (most potently toluene diisocyanate, which has been

Table 17.4. Examples of Common Sensitizing Agents in Occupational Asthma

Low molecular weight
  Isocyanates (entire class; most potent is toluene diisocyanate, abbreviated TDI)
  Trimellitic anhydride
  Metal salts
  Epoxy resins
  Fluxes (used in cleaning joints for welding, brazing; historically colophony, a resin, was most potent)
  Persulfate
  Aldehydes
High molecular weight
  Pharmaceuticals
  Animal proteins (laboratory historically animal dander most potent)
  Latex (cross-reacts with avocado, banana proteins)
  Cereals
  Seafood (crab antigen most potent)
  Proteolytic enzymes (historically, when used as additives in detergents)
  Wood dust constituents (hardwoods generally more potent)

withdrawn for most purposes), a particularly potently sensitizing family of chemicals used in the production of polyurethane plastics and many paints and coatings. In such cases, the responses may be mixed, with immune, irritant, and toxicological (direct-acting) mechanisms each playing some role. These variant reactions are induced by minute quantities of the antigen, in contrast to those induced by irritant gases or the reactions that result in the hypersensitivity pneumonitides. Dual and variable responses are usually associated with slower recovery times and are relatively refractory to conventional treatment of asthma.

Certain agents tend to produce unusual airway reactions. Exposure to cotton dusts in textile milling and weaving may result in byssinosis ("brown lung"), a slowly developing and sustained reaction lasting several hours and variably associated with chronic changes. Western red cedar dust, a particular problem in the sawmills of the Pacific Northwest and British Columbia, may cause episodic bronchospasm in a cyclic pattern recurring over several days. Grain dust asthma is a complicated response that includes a persistent inflammatory condition and possibly variable responses to different antigens within the dust and its contaminants. Laboratory animal asthma is a particularly severe and rather common form of occupational asthma that carries an unacceptably high risk of systemic anaphylaxis; it occurs among animal handlers in research laboratories and is incompatible with continued employment once it develops. Latex allergy is often expressed as occupational asthma and has become a critical management issue in the healthcare sector, affecting the lives and careers of many nurses.

The history alone may be diagnostic in immediate hypersensitivity reactions induced by a single agent used only intermittently in the workplace. Sensitizer-induced occupational asthma can be difficult to evaluate in delayed, dual, or mixed responses. Allergy tests, including skin tests, RAST (radioallergosorbent), and patch tests, are usually helpful in such cases but are often limited in their application in occupational asthma because standard preparations of the suspect chemicals may not be available. Allergic precipitins, the demonstration in the serum of the patient of precipitating antibody to a particular antigen, are only helpful in suspected cases of hypersensitivity pneumonitis, not occupational asthma, and are developed by many workers who never develop symptoms.

Confirmation of the diagnosis can in theory be obtained by bronchial challenge in cases of immediate and late hypersensitivity reactions but test chambers and laboratories conducting antigen-specific bronchoprovocation are scarce. This is not a commercially viable test because it requires a specialist working in a dedicated, controlled clinical setting using titrated, quantified doses of the suspected antigen aerosolized for inhalation by the patient, following a very meticulous protocol that often requires several hours on successive days. Unless the test is undertaken for research purposes, there are not enough patients to justify the cost of setting it up. There is also a question of liability if the subject has an adverse reaction or is inadvertently sensitized by the test.

A useful substitute test to confirm the diagnosis and identify the agent, one that can be performed in the office, is spirometry before and after the patient reproduces his or her workplace exposure by performing the same job using the same materials. (This is presumed acceptably safe if the worker has already done it as a daily routine.) Detection of the late reaction is especially difficult and may require observing the patient in the office for many hours. Spirometry before and after the work shift may also suggest occupational asthma by reductions in air flow, but small changes in pulmonary function should not be overinterpreted. There is a normal diurnal variation in the peak flow of about 10 percent, more in persons with asthma (in addition to the usual variability in air flow from other triggers), such that lower readings in the afternoon are to be expected. Another useful technique is to provide the patient with a portable peak flow meter and to have the patient record his work duties, symptoms, and peak flow measurements every two hours for two weeks. The resulting patterns can be very revealing. Figure 17.21 shows the pattern in a thirty-seven-year-old tile setter whose asthma was triggered by exposure to the tile cement and grouting.

Once the offending agent is identified, it may be possible to avoid exposure through sound industrial hygiene measures or by changing work practices. More often, the worker must be reassigned to other duties that do not involve exposure to the offending agent, particularly when the mechanism is immunologic.

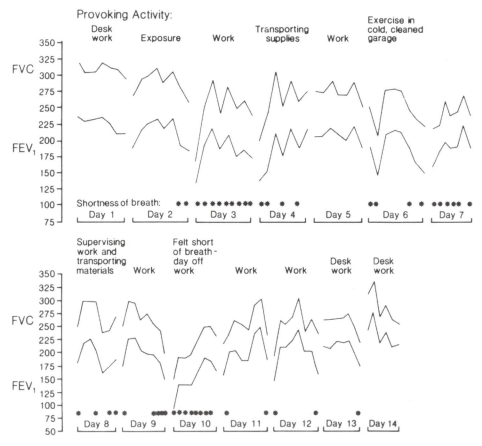

Figure 17.21. Occupational asthma in a thirty-seven-year-old tile and terrazzo setter, whose airway response followed exposure to tile cement or grouting. This graph shows pulmonary function at two-hour intervals during the waking hours over a two-week period in winter. Reaction is not seen on all days, but marked drop in lung function clearly seen following work on several occasions and in response to cold air.

Irritant-Induced Occupational Asthma

Irritant-induced occupational asthma is more common than sensitizer-induced occupational asthma and may be caused by any irritating exposure. This type of occupational asthma can best be visualized as a continuum from "irritant-induced aggravation of preexisting asthma" (resulting in bronchospasm acutely or perpetuating inflammation chronically) to "irritant-induced new-onset asthma" (in which the irritation induces the airway reactivity in the first instance), and "reactive airway dysfunction syndrome" (RADS), a more severe condition in which airway reactivity arises de novo from airway injury. These distinctions are very important in terms of management, prognosis, and compensation eligibility and management, but there is some degree of overlap.

A well-known example of irritant-induced new onset asthma was called "hot wire asthma" or "meat wrapper's asthma." It occurred when meat was wrapped in plastic wrap locally in supermarkets. The early apparatus used a hot wire to cut through the wrap, but the temperature was set too high. The plastic was degraded by the high temperature, releasing irritating fumes. Readjusting the temperature to melt through the wrap, rather than disintegrate it, solved the problem with no inconvenience or loss of productivity.

Irritant-induced aggravation of preexisting asthma ("aggravational asthma" for short) is very common and entirely nonspecific. This is a condition experienced by almost any worker with asthma, hay fever and allergic rhinitis, bronchitis, or for that matter, other airway disorders such as emphysema, who encounters a moderately irritating exposure in the workplace. The irritant exposure makes the existing symptoms of asthma worse in two ways, initially by provoking airway response and over the longer term by adding to the inflammation. Aggravational asthma is usually self-limited, and the worker returns to baseline after avoiding further irritant exposure, which may take a few days. Any irritant exposure will aggravate reactive airways in these circumstances, and all irritating exposures should be removed or reduced, including and especially at home. In a very few cases in which the worker's underlying asthma is especially brittle and difficult to manage, aggravation may result in an exacerbation or functional decompensation. Recovery may be prolonged or may only reach a new, lower baseline. The great majority of cases are self-limited.

Irritant-induced occupational asthma of all types is more likely to be associated with a longer term or repetitive exposure to a moderately irritating gas, dust, vapor, or solvent than a brief exposure to a strong irritant, which is more likely to be associated with toxic inhalation. The irritants that induce occupational asthma are much less reactive and are tolerated in the short term. They act by lowering the threshold for bronchial reactivity because of irritation and subsequent inflammation in the airway, sometimes resulting in a sustained nonspecific bronchitis and at other times airway reactivity when provoked by an irritant trigger. Individual susceptibility varies greatly, but the reactions induced by the irritant effects of these agents are generally milder than in sensitizer-induced asthma (with the exception of RADS) and require heavier exposure than those mediated by immunologic processes. Confusingly, some chemicals are both sensitizers (at low concentrations) and irritants (at high concentrations), acting by either mechanism in different patients and causing confusion in the individual case: examples include formaldehyde, isocyanates, and trimellitic anhydride.

Once irritant-induced new onset occurs or aggravation of preexisting asthma becomes severe, the clinical picture is no longer specific. Any low-grade irritant then makes symptoms worse, by provoking cough and chest discomfort. Such patients cannot tolerate side-stream cigarette smoke, fragrances, candles, or other sources of irritating exposures, but this is entirely nonspecific. It is a reflection of the underlying airway reactivity, not a specific or generalized chemical "sensitivity."

Further on the continuum or irritant-induced occupational asthma is reactive airway dysfunction syndrome (RADS). The diagnosis of RADS was originally based on a set of criteria developed by Stuart Brooks, who discovered it. The essential elements are:

- No previous history of respiratory disorder or atopy
- Onset after a single, specific event of exposure

- Exposure to a gas, smoke, dust, or fumes that has irritant potential at a high concentration
- Onset of symptoms within twenty-four hours and persistence for more than three months
- Symptoms consistent with asthma (cough, dyspnea, wheezing) requiring medical attention
- Airflow obstruction on spirometry

(Additional criteria reflected the use of this formulation for selecting patients with the disorder for clinical research.) These criteria are probably overly specific for the disease and therefore not sensitive enough (see Chapter 5 for an explanation of these terms). In other words, they probably exclude some injured workers who probably merit the diagnosis in clinical terms, but those they include are very likely to be true cases of RADS. For example, there is no obvious reason why a history of respiratory disorder or atopy would preclude the diagnosis of RADS in an individual, because there is no reason that someone with preexisting asthma or allergies would not get RADS; such conditions would not protect against RADS. Brooks's criteria make the exclusion only in order to isolate the disorder and to assemble a relatively homogeneous group of subjects for research purposes. This is an example of a case definition developed for research purposes being misapplied as clinical diagnostic criteria. RADS is really a result of airway injury independent of prior history. In a reaction to the restrictiveness of these criteria, some clinicians have swung to the opposite pole and diagnose RADS liberally after any irritant exposure. This is unfortunate because the natural history of RADS is different from other forms of irritant-induced asthma and so the distinction should be maintained.

RADS is properly diagnosed as the sequela, by history, of a single, discrete event sufficient to induce a persistent inflammatory process that manifests itself as the new onset of airway reactivity. The circumstances of exposure are not obscure, subtle, or easily forgotten;

cases often follow confined-space incidents in which exposure is moderately intense.

Although the management of RADS follows conventional treatment for asthma, the prognosis is highly variable. Several years of airway hyperactivity, with asthma symptoms and variable air flow, can be expected, and some patients never recover normal airway function. RADS is often associated with upper airway problems (sometimes called "reactive upper [airway] dysfunction syndrome," or RUDS), presenting as obstructive sleep apnea.

Hypersensitivity Pneumonitis

"Hypersensitivity pneumonitis," known in the United Kingdom as "extrinsic allergic alveolitis," occurs when a sensitized individual inhales large quantities of an antigen in the form of a respirable dust that is retained in the lung for some period after being inhaled, although it can be induced by small-molecular-weight chemicals that act as haptens (including the familiar isocyanates and trimelletic acid anhydrides). The lung mounts a T-cell mediated immune reaction that persists because the antigen is not rapidly cleared. The characteristic symptoms of hypersensitivity pneumonitis are dyspnea, fever, chills, and cough, developing over several hours or days. Repeated exposure to the same antigen leads to an inflammatory alveolitis, interstitial fibrosis, and ultimately to a restrictive defect. An immediate hypersensitivity reaction may occur together with the delayed reaction in some cases, resulting in wheezing and air flow obstruction in addition to the more chronic or subacute symptoms. Clubbing is common.

There are over 300 known forms of hypersensitivity pneumonitis, many of them quite rare, and undoubtedly more to be discovered in the future. They are usually given highly descriptive names, such as "cheese worker's lung" (caused by the mold *Penicillium casei*), "chemical worker's lung" (caused by any one of several chemical agents), and "humidifier/air conditioner lung" (caused by exposure to thermophilic actinomycetes in forced-air ventilation systems) but are sometimes given more esoteric names, such as "bagassosis" (caused by exposure to molds on crushed sugar cane, which is called bagasse) and "suberosis" (caused by exposure to molds growing beneath the bark of cork trees, inhaled by workers harvesting cork). Common antigens that produce this condition include molds and actinomycetes of many varieties, detergent enzymes, pharmaceutical agents, minute arthropods such as mites, and dust from vegetable matter, such as grain, or animal material, such as aerosolized droppings and proteins in droppings from birds. Confusingly, certain low-molecular-weight, incomplete antigens that also cause occupational asthma may cause hypersensitivity pneumonitis, including toluene and methylene diisocyanate (Figure 17.22) and trimellitic anhydride. Exposures resulting in a hypersensitivity pneumonitis may occur in many settings, but characteristic histories are exposure to dust from the renovation of old buildings, bird breeding, handling any number of powdered products, and performing maintenance work where powdered waste collects.

Farmer's lung (Figure 17.23) is the best-studied hypersensitivity pneumonitis and was a historical disorder of practical importance in rural areas with damp climates. The exposure involves farmers handling moldy hay. Farmer's lung is caused by a specific antigen of *Saccharopolyspora rectivirgula* (previously *Micropolyspora faeni*), a thermophilic actinomycete (not a true mold). Tests for serum antibody for farmer's lung and a few similar hypersensitivity pneumonitides are available from many laboratories as a panel, but there is not a general test for hypersensitivity pneumonitis. A positive test means that the patient is mounting an antibody response to one of the five or so antigens but does not conclusively demonstrate that that particular antigen is causing the pneumonitis, and a negative result only means that the patient is not mounting an antibody response to one of the antigens in the panel. The second most common hypersensitivity pneumonitis is "bird fancier's lung," which involves sensitization to bird proteins and is seen most often among pigeon hobbyists.

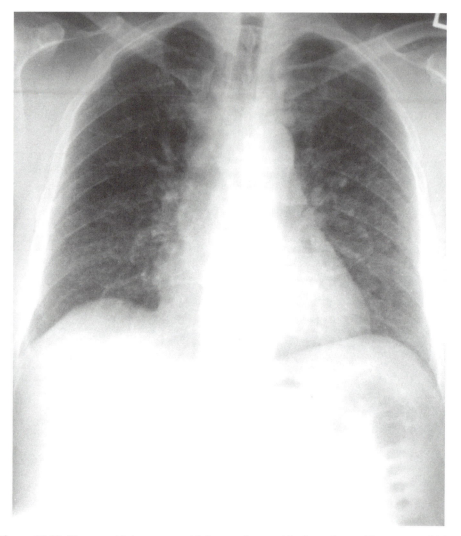

Figure 17.22. Hypersensitivity pneumonitis in a worker sensitized to toluene diisocyanate, which is also a cause of occupational asthma. Reprinted with permission from "Occupational Lung Diseases," February, 1984, *American Family Physician*. Copyright © 1984 American Academy of Family Physicians. All Rights Reserved.

Patients with hypersensitivity pneumonitis characteristically experience acute symptoms of fever, chills, and shortness of breath, then develop a patchy pulmonary infiltrate, reduced diffusing capacity, oxygen desaturation at rest or exercise, and a leukocytosis.

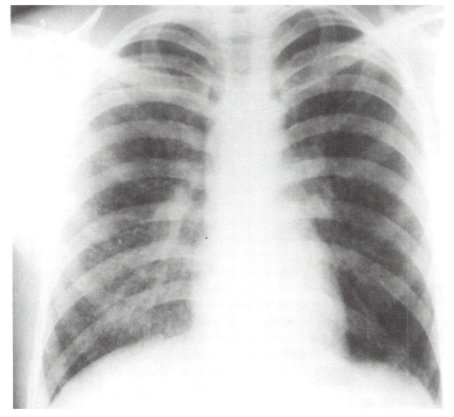

Figure 17.23. Farmer's lung, a hypersensitivity pneumonitis. Note reticular pattern and patchy infiltrate. Reprinted with permission from "Occupational Lung Diseases," February, 1984, *American Family Physician*. Copyright © 1984 American Academy of Family Physicians. All Rights Reserved.

These patients usually recover quickly in the hospital or if removed from the environment and deteriorate on returning to the setting as the disease returns, with crackles and persistent shortness of breath. If exposure persists, the pneumonitis becomes chronic and interstitial fibrosis results, leading to honeycombing and a restrictive defect.

This is one of the most rewarding serious pulmonary diseases to identify but often requires detective work. Identification and control of exposure to the offending antigen usually results in complete resolution of a potentially grave disease.

Industrial Bronchitis

Workers in dusty occupations, particularly steel workers and grain handlers, may develop a nonspecific chronic bronchitis, which in the older literature is called "industrial bronchitis." Cigarette smoking may aggravate the bronchitis, and smoking-induced bronchitis and cough is obviously the leading alternative diagnosis. This used to be thought of as more or less benign, but recent studies have demonstrated reduced lung function and an increased risk of obstructive lung disease among workers exposed to dusts of many kinds, including those previously thought to be of little health significance and known as "nuisance dusts." This disorder has not been as systematically studied as other occupational lung diseases but would be expected to fit the same pattern of higher risk among workers with atopy and a history of allergy as is observed with most airway disorders.

Fume Fevers

Fume fevers are systemic disorders resulting from transient effects of mediator release after inhalation. There are two common types of fume fever, both involving mixed pulmonary and systemic reactions to inhaled toxic agents. The pulmonary manifestations are transient and consist of fleeting infiltrates. The disease is a self-limited but highly unpleasant reaction, subjectively similar to influenza, developing an hour after exposure to the offending agent and lasting less than forty-eight hours.

Metal fume fever results from exposure to hot metal fumes, known to include zinc, copper, and cadmium and possibly other metal fumes. An acute, influenza-like illness results consisting of nausea, fever and chills, malaise, myalgias, and leukocytosis. Metal fume fever is most often seen when inexperienced welders try to weld or cut metal that is galvanized or of mixed composition. Within the welding trade, many workers drink milk as a folk treatment or prophylaxis against metal fume fever, but there is no evidence for its efficacy.

Polymer fume fever is a similar influenza-like reaction resulting from the pyrolysis products of chlorofluorcarbon polymers, usually when particles settle on cigarettes, burn, and the fumes are inhaled. Polymer fume fever can be prevented by banning cigarette smoking in the workplaces where products containing these polymers are fabricated.

Metal fume fever must not be confused with the much more serious condition of toxic inhalation, which may result from exposure to high concentrations of cadmium or nickel fumes or from high concentrations of volatilized mercury or lead. Polymer fume fever should also not be confused with "meat-wrappers' asthma," a problem of bronchospasm and irritant bronchitis resulting from the inhalation of fumes generated when polyvinyl chloride film wrapping was cut using a hot wire and discussed under irritant occupational asthma.

HEARING CONSERVATION

Loss of hearing has a profound effect. The auditory system is the primary channel of communication by which a person learns speech and monitors the accuracy of their own speech production, develops language skills, and adjusts to the immediate social environment. Inability to hear the sounds of speech progressively isolates an individual from social interaction. This often leads to feelings of paranoia, frustration, anger, intolerance, loneliness, depression, and inadequacy. It may also lead to frustration and impatience on the part of those dealing with the impaired person.

A major cause of hearing impairment in adults is exposure to excessive noise in the workplace. The OEM physician may become involved when testing programs are introduced into the community or when workers are identified as having impairment of hearing. The most constructive role of the OEM physician is to educate the patient on the importance of hearing conservation, to reinforce compliance with personal hearing protection measures, and to support appropriate rehabilitative intervention for the worker already suffering from hearing loss that is impairing communication abilities.

The hearing mechanism is a series of energy transducers, converting energy from acoustical to mechanical, to hydromechanical, and ultimately to electrochemical forms of nerve impulses that can be handled by the brain (Table 17.5). The weakest link in the chain is the conversion of hydromechanical energy to neuronal stimulation. The site where noise exposure is most likely to cause damage is the organ of Corti, in the cochlea. Each delicate hair cell and the neuron or neurons it stimulates is "tuned" to respond best to one fixed frequency. Exposure to repetitive and overly intense continuous noise injures and eventually destroys the delicate hair cells of the auditory sensory receptor.

Hearing impairment is classified clinically as conductive, sensory, neural, mixed, or central. (This is an oversimplification because some conditions such as presbycusis may have components of one or more types of loss.) Special audiologic studies are needed to distinguish among sensory, neural, and central auditory problems. Noise-induced hearing loss is sensory, with some component of neural.

Occupational noise-induced hearing loss is a relatively pure sensory impairment and follows a predictable sequence of events. First, there is a "temporary threshold shift" (TTS) in sound detection. Immediately after exposure and for minutes to hours afterward, the exposed subject cannot hear at the usual level of sensitivity. The TTS phenomenon usually affects frequencies between 3000 and 6000 Hz, which tend to be those about half an octave above the primary frequencies found in most environmental noise. A broader spectrum may be affected with exposure to more intense noise. When the subject's hearing acuity no longer recovers, it becomes a "permanent threshold shift" (PTS). In industrial situations, PTS centers around 4000 Hz. The loss of hearing acuity becomes greater with continued exposure and affects a broader range of frequencies, particularly on the low end of the spectrum. The impairment may become so severe that the individual cannot hear adequately in the critical range of

Table 17.5. Conversion of Energy in the Hearing Mechanism

Anatomic Location	Form of Energy	Medium of Energy Conduction	Type of Impairment If Interrupted
Outer ear			
External auditory canal	Acoustic pressure waves	Air	Conductive
Tympanic membrane	Mechanical vibration	Diaphragmatic motion	Conductive
Middle ear			
Ossicular chain★	Mechanical linkage	Mechanical	Conductive
Oval window	Mechanical displacement	Mechanical to fluid	Conductive
Inner ear			
Cochlea	Hydraulic wave	Cochlear fluid	Sensory
Organ of Corti	Nerve receptor stimulation	Neuronal transmission	Sensory
Acoustic nerve (cranial nerve VIII)	Nerve conduction	Neuronal transmission	Neural
Central nervous system			
Brainstem, temporal lobe			
Auditory cortex and association cortex	Nerve conduction	Neural and synaptic	Neural

★ The malleus, incus, and stapes.

frequencies needed to interpret human speech, 500–2000 Hz. At this point, the individual is severely disabled and may no longer be employable. The rate at which noise-induced hearing loss worsens is determined by the level of noise exposure, the duration of exposure, and individual susceptibility, which cannot be predicted.

Noise that may be damagingly loud can be recognized by several characteristics: (1) normal conversation levels of speech cannot be maintained at a distance of three feet between speakers, (2) tinnitus may occur upon termination of the noise, and (3) a sensation of "dampened" or less acute hearing follows termination of the noise (the TTS).

Hearing is evaluated by determination of hearing threshold levels at octave intervals from 250 to 8000 Hz, resulting in a graph called the "pure tone audiogram." A pure tone air/bone conduction audiogram can distinguish between conductive and sensorineural loss but cannot positively identify the cause of the impairment. Pure tone audiometric patterns of noise-induced hearing loss are generally characteristic, however, because they are centered on one frequency, 4000 Hz, where the organ of Corti is most susceptible to injury. The profile of noise thresholds is also usually symmetrical for both ears. Unilateral hearing loss is unlikely to be occupational in origin, unless firearms are used on the job or the worker habitually works with a noise source on one side only.

Noise-induced hearing loss usually starts with a distinct sensorineural "notch" in the audiogram centered at 4000 Hz. Over time, this hearing defect deepens and widens with continued exposure. Noise-induced hearing loss is not flat across all frequencies. Figure 17.24 shows examples of pure tone audiograms resulting from noise-induced sensory hearing loss. Audiograms should be performed only after the subject has been off work and isolated from exposure to loud noise (80 dBA or above) at least overnight, to avoid confusion introduced by a TTS.

Audiograms are highly sensitive tests that should be performed only by professional audiologists or certified technicians in acoustic booths or quiet rooms. The certifying agency for hearing conservation specialists is the Council for Accreditation in Occupational Hearing Conservation. Like all specialized laboratory tests, abnormal audiograms should be interpreted by qualified professionals.

In any individual case, hearing loss may be the result of other causes, most commonly presbycusis, otosclerosis, cerumen impaction,

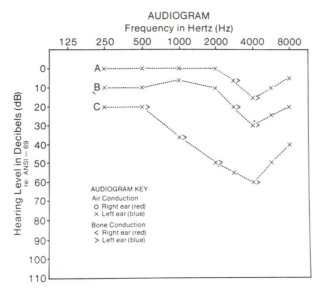

Figure 17.24. Typical audiometric configurations for noise-induced hearing loss as a function of years of exposure to high workplace noise levels: A (1-2 years), B (5-9 years), C (40 years). Results are given for one (left) ear only to show progression of the disorder. Reprinted with permission from "Hearing Conservation and Occupation Exposure to Noise," October, 1983, *American Family Physician.* Copyright © 1983 American Academy of Family Physicians. All Rights Reserved.

ototoxic drugs, middle ear effusions, and Meniere's disease. A characteristic audiogram with or without tinnitus in the absence of other symptoms, particularly dizziness, in a worker exposed to noise on the job for several years is rarely anything other than noise-induced hearing loss.

Impact noise produces barotrauma and acoustical injury based on the pressure wave. This may be associated with hearing loss across a much wider range of frequencies.

CANCER

The common feature of all occupational cancers is that they can be prevented. Because cancer is the second leading cause of years of life lost in developed countries (because on average it affects people at a younger age than heart disease) and because the risk increases with aging, prevention of cancer has become a priority in modern society.

Environmental Causes of Cancer

Cancers associated with personal choices of lifestyle, such as cigarette smoking, contribute the greatest fraction of preventable malignancies in North America. Cancers associated with occupational exposures, such as chemicals known to be carcinogenic, are a much smaller fraction of preventable cancers but are of particular concern to society since they are all theoretically preventable. Occupational causes of cancer typically require a latency period of over twenty years (there are many exceptions) until clinical appearance of the malignancy. Occupational causes of cancer are preventable and affect certain identifiable groups disproportionately. Some carcinogens associated primarily with occupational exposures, particularly asbestos and radon, may contribute importantly to national or regional cancer rates because of the widespread distribution of the hazard, the large number of workers exposed, the potential for wider exposure among the general population, and a synergistic effect with cigarette smoking. Environmental causes of cancer, such as radon (lung cancer), arsenic (skin, lung, and bladder), polycyclic aromatic hydrocarbons (PAHs, see Chapter 10) from combustion and in particulate air pollution, and background ionizing radiation place many more people at much lower levels of risk.

Passive cigarette smoke leads as the environmental carcinogen contributing most to the cancer burden. Radon and its daughters together are the most important environmental carcinogen of natural origin causing lung cancer. They are considered to be the two most important environmental causes of lung cancer in nonsmokers. (See Chapter 10 for a complete discussion.) Particulate air pollution is also associated with a risk of lung cancer in urban areas, but it is low in magnitude compared to occupational risks and far below active cigarette smoking. Arsenic, which is normally encountered as a natural contaminant in groundwater, is associated with cancers at multiple sites, as previously noted.

Occupational Cancer

The burden of disease represented by occupational cancer was initially estimated, based on data from the 1970s, at 4 percent. Contemporary estimates are higher, because of the greater number of asbestos-related malignancies, methodological limitations in the original studies by Doll and Peto (in 1981), the original estimates being based on a narrow selection of cancers (of six types), conservative assumptions about the contribution of occupational causes to common cancers, and the attribution of interactive (synergistic) effects to smoking as the primary cause in the Doll and Peto studies rather than occupational exposure. Contemporary estimates face their own uncertainties, however, and there is no consensus. The true picture is complicated because occupational exposures such as asbestos often interact with cigarette smoking to increase further the risk of lung cancer. Factors such as heredity, diet, and possibly medication may greatly modify an individual's risk of cancer following exposure.

Certain occupational groups, however, may have an unequivocal and greatly increased risk of specific cancers, as has been shown historically for pipefitters (asbestos), dye workers (aniline dyes), and chemists. Some occupational cancers are rare in the general population and seldom seen without a history of exposure to a particular carcinogen, such as hepatic angiosarcoma (vinyl chloride) and mesothelioma (asbestos). Most occupational cancers are common cancers in which occupational exposure to carcinogens contributes additional risk against a background rate, such as lung and bladder cancer. Others demonstrate an elevated risk against a low background rate and can be particularly difficult to evaluate, such as individual non-Hodgkin lymphomas and soft-tissue sarcomas, which probably have different occupational associations.

Workers' compensation claims for cancer are underrepresented (based on expected cancers for known causes such as asbestos), usually disputed (except for mesothelioma), and often insurmountably difficult to prove. As a consequence, the true burden of occupational cancer is greatly underestimated. There are many obstacles to identifying occupational cancers in population studies, as noted in Chapters 2 and 3. Cancer risk is highly age specific and rises exponentially after fifty years of age. Latency may be twenty years or more for a solid tumor (less for leukemias and bladder cancer), and the elapsed time overlaps the increase in risk due to age and is further confounded because the effect of a carcinogen also depends on age at first exposure. Misclassification bias, with respect to the cause of death, the diagnosis of cancer, occupational history, and death certificate data are often compounded by inaccuracies due to the age of the worker at the time of diagnosis, since many cases occur after retirement. Exposure assessment on a scale of decades is very difficult, and interactive effects are extremely difficult to quantify, impossible in small populations. Confounding due to smoking, lifestyle, and other occupational exposures is usual. These obstacles to evaluation in populations spill over to the assessment of causation in the individual. A compatible latency period, documentation of exposure, absence of other plausible causes outside of occupation, and consideration of confounding apply to the assessment of individual cases as well. The mere presence of a known carcinogen in the workplace proves little. No one is harmed if a carcinogen is tightly contained or kept from direct contact with the worker.

Table 17.6 lists occupational exposures known or strongly suspected to cause cancer in humans. Many chemicals, such as 4-aminodiphenyl and β-naphthylamine, were known early to be carcinogenic and have been withdrawn from commercial use. Some chemicals, such as dioxin, are known carcinogens in animal studies but do not show the same level of carcinogenic activity in humans, presumably because of differences in affinity for the molecular receptor. Arsenic is known to be a human carcinogen, but animal studies have not reproduced the carcinogenic effect

Table 17.6. Known or Highly Suspect Carcinogens in the Workplace

Substance	Where Encountered
Asbestos	See Chapter 10
Silica	See Chapter 10
Coke oven emissions	Steel mills, coke ovens (includes benzene and BCME)
3,3'-Dichlorobenzidine	Pigment manufacturing, polyurethane production
Radium, radon, radon daughters	Subsurface mining, accumulation in houses
4,4'-Methylene-bis	Plastics manufacturing: elastomer, epoxy resins, polyurethane foam
(2-chloroaniline) Uranium and radon	Underground mining
β-Naphthylamine	Chemical, dyestuffs, rubber industries
Ultraviolet light	Ubiquitous; working outdoors.
Auramine and magenta	Dye manufacturing (withdrawn from commerce)
Carbon tetrachloride	Very widespread
Benzidine	Clinical pathology laboratories; chemical dyestuffs, plastics, rubber, wood products
β-Propriolactone	Plastics, chemical, pharmaceutical industries
Vinyl chloride	Petrochemical, plastics, rubber industries
Chloromethyl methyl ether (CMME)	Chemical industry
Bis(chloromethyl) ether (BCME)	Chemical industry, nuclear reactor fuel processing
Ethyleneimine	Chemical, paper, textile industries
N-Nitrosodimethylamine	Chemical, rubber, solvent, pesticide industries
Chloroprene	Synthetic rubber industry
Trichlorethylene	Solvent and degreasing agent (withdrawn)

(*Continued*)

Table 17.6. (*Continued*)

Substance	Where Encountered
Benzene	Solvent and chemical constituent
Polychlorinated biphenyls	See Chapter 10
Chloroform	Chemical, pharmaceutical, textile, solvent industries
Acrylonitrile	Plastic, textile industries
Leather dust	Leather goods industry
Wood dust	Hard wood furniture industries
Chromate (hexavalent)	Electroplating, metal products, photography
Nickel subsulfide	Mining and smelting
Ionizing radiation	Medical and industrial x-ray
Arsenic	Mining, smelting; groundwater (natural contaminant)
Cutting oils	Machining, metal-working trades
Hydrazine	Mechanical applications, pharmaceutical industry
Ethylene dibromide	Foodstuffs (fumigation), gasoline additive

because of differences in metabolic pathways. At any given time, two or three dozen chemicals are under active review for carcinogenicity, but many more are being evaluated by commercial, industry, or research laboratories.

The PAHs are a particularly important class of chemical carcinogens (see Chapter 10). They are products of low-temperature combustion and found in coal tar and other complex mixed hydrocarbons. They are found in a very wide range of occupational settings, including foundry work, firefighting, steelmaking (historically in coke ovens, which have largely been replaced in steelmaking), and aluminum reduction (as a constituent of the electrodes in "pot rooms"). The risk that they confer for initiation is compounded by their effects as a promoter and by their effect of photosensitizing the skin and enhancing the effect of exposure to ultraviolet radiation, particularly in roofing and road building. PAHs are also important constituents of tobacco smoke and air pollution, both of which are important in the risk of cancer. They are associated with a very wide range of cancers, including lung, bladder, skin, and kidney. The PAHs demonstrate the drawbacks of taking the Bradford Hill criteria (see Chapter 3) too literally.

The International Agency for Research on Cancer (IARC) is the scientific body that reviews the evidence for carcinogenicity of a compound extensively used by cancer investigators and regulatory agencies worldwide. (See Chapter 2 for a more complete description.) Group 1 carcinogens are accepted as carcinogenic to humans and are specific as to site. Carcinogens in Group 2A are possibly carcinogenic to humans, and those in Group 2B have insufficient evidence for carcinogenicity in humans but may be carcinogenic in animals. The U.S. Environmental Protection Agency supplements IARC's list and adds many suspected carcinogens for purposes of regulation. The California Department of Health has emerged in recent years as another authoritative body, in that it maintains a list of known and suspected carcinogens that is widely used by other agencies.

Occupational carcinogens vary greatly in their potency. Bis-chloromethyl ether (BCME, used in the nuclear industry in preparing ion-exchange columns to refine fuel-grade uranium) is a highly potent carcinogen that induced oat cell carcinoma of the lung in a high percentage of workers exposed to the chemical. The dust of hard woods, on the other hand, is a low-level carcinogenic exposure resulting in carcinoma of the nasal cavity and sinuses, but although this type of cancer is devastating in its effects, the risk is still small in absolute terms. In some industries and occupations, such as rubber tire making and firefighting, respectively, there is an elevation in cancer risk, but the specific carcinogen is not known and may be multiple. In some settings, such as shift work (see Chapter 13), the induction of cancer is thought to be indirect and not based on the mechanisms of chemical carcinogenesis described in Chapter 2.

The "classic" occupational cancers are those reflecting exposure pathways or susceptible organs and include:

- Bronchogenic (lung) carcinoma
- Skin (squamous, basal cell, melanoma)

- Genitourinary cancers (chiefly bladder)
- Leukemia (acute myelogenous leukemia)
- Mesothelioma of the pleura

Lung cancer due to occupational exposures must be detected against a relatively high background rate in the general population and confounding with cigarette smoking. The minimum plausible latency is usually considered to be between fifteen and twenty years, but the latency period is shortened with more intense exposure and in studies of BCME workers averaged about ten years, which is probably close to a biological limit. Lung cancer is associated with many occupational carcinogens, including asbestos, silica, PAHs, vinyl chloride, arsenic, nickel subsulfide, hexavalent chromium, beryllium, radon daughters and other α-emitting radionuclides, and sulfuric acid mist (presumably from chronic irritation).

Smoking is the major confounding cause of lung cancer and presents another complication in that cigarette smoking has an interactive (synergistic) effect with exposure to many lung carcinogens, including asbestos, silica, BCME, and radon daughters and probably others carcinogens as long as they do not duplicate the dominant mechanism of cigarette smoking. (Polycyclic aromatic hydrocarbons, for example, are part of and probably contribute heavily to the carcinogenicity of cigarette smoke; the combined effect in that case would probably be simply additive.) The interactive effect is itself exposure-related and would act most strongly when both cigarette smoking and occupational exposures were high.

Occupational causes of cancer may cause any common histological type of lung cancer (epithelial cell, adenocarcinoma, small cell, large cell) and at any degree of differentiation and so, with one minor and one partial exception, histology cannot be used to evaluate potential causes. The minor exception, minor because it is unlikely to be seen today, is that BCME is almost exclusively found with oat cell carcinoma. The partial exception is adenocarcinoma, which although elevated following exposure to asbestos and other occupational carcinogens, is the characteristic cell type of lung cancer when it appears in nonsmokers (which occurs at about a tenth or less of the rate among smokers). It would be difficult to argue that lung cancer in a nonsmoker was spontaneous and unrelated to exposure if it were of a different cell type. However, the risk of adenocarcinoma of the lung is certainly elevated by occupational carcinogens such as asbestos, so one cannot argue that because a cancer is an adenocarcinoma it is unlikely to be occupational in origin.

Skin cancer arising from occupational exposures may involve direct contact with a carcinogen (for example, PAHs on skin), effects on the skin from permeation by circulating carcinogens (such as arsenic and inhaled PAHs), and photosensitization to ultraviolet radiation (a factor in intense exposure to PAHs). Occupations involving exposure to PAHs, such as roofing, combine all these elements of risk. Occupational skin cancer due to chemical exposure or ultraviolet radiation is squamous cell or basal cell, which is called Bowen's disease if it is in situ and associated with arsenic. Mineral oils and ionizing radiation are also known to induce skin cancer. Melanoma is associated with ultraviolet radiation and is unlikely to be caused by chemical carcinogens.

Bladder cancer is associated with occupational exposure because filterable carcinogens concentrate in the urine and expose the bladder epithelium for prolonged periods. The transitional epithelium of the bladder appears to be somewhat prone to initiation, and malignant tumors of the bladder have an unusually short latency period for a solid tumor. Latency as short as seven years was reported among aniline dye manufacturers in the early twentieth century under conditions of very high exposure. Bladder cancer has been associated with a number of chemical dyes that have since been withdrawn, except for benzidine, and with polycyclic aromatic hydrocarbons and arsenic. Bladder cancer is known to be elevated among workers in the rubber industry and among firefighters.

Leukemia is induced by ionizing radiation and alkylating agents. Exposure to benzene is associated acute myelogenous leukemia, and the weight of evidence suggests that this association is highly specific.

Mesothelioma is described below as an asbestos-associated cancer. Cancers at other sites may be associated with occupational exposure as well and a comprehensive list is outside the scope of this book.

Asbestos and Cancer

Asbestos is historically and quantitatively the single most important occupational carcinogen. The two characteristic cancers associated with asbestos are bronchogenic carcinoma of the lung and pleural mesothelioma. There is strong evidence that other cancers are associated with asbestos exposure, however, including cancer of the larynx, peritoneal mesothelioma, and, less strongly, colon cancer. Ingestion of expectorated fibers, lymphatic drainage, and macrophage migration to the peritoneum are thought to be plausible delivery mechanisms bringing the fibers to other target organs.

Lung Cancer

Individuals with asbestosis are at high risk of developing lung cancer, but persons exposed to asbestos may certainly develop lung cancer without having asbestosis. Radiological findings of asbestosis are not necessary to conclude that the risk is elevated in an injured worker or claimant. There is some evidence that chrysotile may be somewhat less potent than amphiboles in inducing lung cancer, mostly because fibers may be dissolved over time in the lung, but there is no doubt that chrysotile induces lung cancer. Asbestos exposure is highly interactive (synergistic) with cigarette smoking in causing bronchogenic carcinoma. (Some investigators disagree with each of the points in this paragraph, but the evidence does not support their position.)

The risk of lung cancer is associated with asbestos exposure, and a higher risk is associated with prolonged exposure. Lung cancer requires much less exposure to asbestos than does asbestosis but more than mesothelioma. The latency period between exposure and detection of the malignancy is on the order of two or three decades. In evaluating a possible occupational association with a patient's malignancy, a complete and accurate history of the patient's employment and the specific jobs performed is critical. Asbestos and smoking together raise an individuals' risk of cancer much more than the sum of either alone, to as much as 100 times that for nonsmokers in heavily exposed, smoking populations. The interaction is proportional to exposure to each agent. Current cases of lung cancer in asbestos-exposed workers reflect distant exposure at much higher levels and also the higher proportion of smokers and consumption of cigarettes in the past. However, current exposure to asbestos in construction and asbestos tear-out work that is noncompliant with occupational standards, a common situation, is high enough to place contemporary workers at risk for lung cancer.

Lung cancer associated with asbestos is not different in its clinical features from lung cancer from smoking cigarettes. It does carry a somewhat worse prognosis than lung cancer in the general population (which of course is usually caused by smoking) and is generally fatal within five years. Cancers in the lung, with a few exceptions, grow for long periods undetected before they become large enough to be seen on x-ray or grow into an airway and shed cells that can be detected. (Figure 17.25 illustrates an advanced lung cancer against a background of asbestosis.) There have been many trials to evaluate the potential benefits of screening for early detection and treatment. So far, they have succeeded in identifying the cancer earlier, but none has successfully demonstrated a benefit in reducing mortality. The net effect is that the injured worker simply knows about the cancer earlier. At the time of this writing, the findings of a major trial performed in Canada using helical HRCT were about to be released.

Mesothelioma

Pleural mesothelioma is a particularly aggressive and presently incurable malignancy that is closely associated with asbestos exposure. The five-year survival is essentially nil, despite numerous clinical trials. There are promising new avenues for early detection of this sarcoma through screening, such as circulating levels of a phosphoprotein marker called osteopontin, which may make

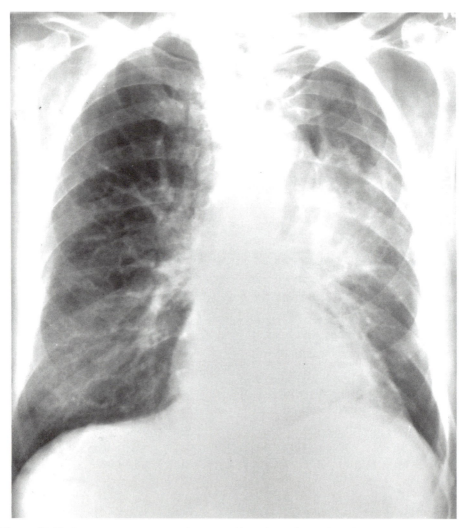

Figure 17.25. Lung cancer in a sixty-five-year-old smoking shipyard worker exposed to asbestos while installing lagging (insulation). Presented with recurrent laryngeal nerve palsy and hoarseness; lesion was a poorly differentiated squamous cell carcinoma. (Reproduced with permission of the American Academy of Family Practice.)

earlier intervention practical. At present, however, the prognosis is dismal.

Mesothelioma is specific to exposure to asbestos and similar asbestiform fibrous silicates (such as fibrous zeolites). The mechanism is probably highly nonspecific because it can be induced experimentally in animals by implanting almost any fiber in the pleural space, including cotton threads. Asbestos fibers are carried to the pleural space by lymphatic channels. Although there appears to be a familial predisposition to the cancer, it has been controversial whether it ever occurs in the absence of exposure to asbestos or other fibrous silicates.

Pleural mesothelioma is rare in the general population, but is frequently found in populations exposed to high levels of asbestos. Current cases in developed countries mostly reflect exposure in the distant past, when levels were much higher, but because of the often long latency of mesothelioma, developed countries are currently at or near a peak incidence of the disease. Developing countries, on the other hand, are seeing dramatic increases in rates of mesothelioma due to more recent imports and use of asbestos and will see the peak of their epidemic in coming years. (This has sometimes been called the "second wave" of asbestos-related cancer.) Peritoneal mesothelioma, a rarer but equally insidious disease that declares itself late and may progressively encase abdominal structures in a fibrous tumor mass, likely results from migration of asbestos fibers to the peritoneal space.

Mesothelioma often results from remarkably modest and short periods of exposure. Although it normally has an unusually long latency period of several decades, the latency is quite variable and can be short in the case of early exposure. It is not associated with smoking.

Pleural mesothelioma usually presents as a pleural effusion, characteristically but not always bloody, and a thickened, irregular pleural peel that invades the lung and chest wall (Figure 17.26). The tissue diagnosis is often difficult because these tumors have a highly variable morphology and large blocks of tissue may be needed to differentiate mesothelioma from a poorly differentiated adenocarcinoma. There are different tissue types of mesothelioma, but identification of them is not clinically useful.

The pleural peel is not in any way related to pleural plaques. Mesothelioma should not be confused with either pleural plaques, which are only markers of past exposure to asbestos and signify no additional risk for malignancy in themselves, or benign pleural effusions associated with asbestos.

Mesotheliomas occur spontaneously in the general population, but they are quite rare and many investigators believe that all cases reflect some past exposure to asbestos. Community residents have developed

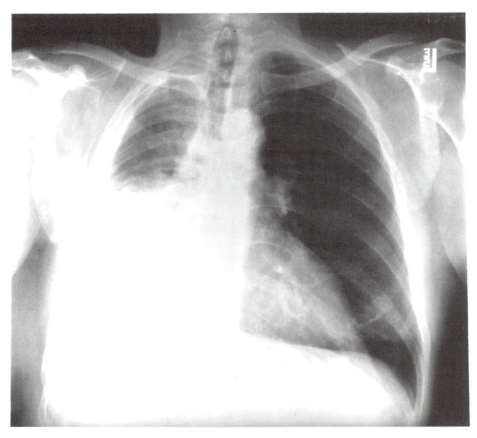

Figure 17.26. Pleural mesothelioma in a sixty-six-year-old nonsmoking retired shipyard maintenance supervisor. After thirty-seven years of employment, during which his exposure to asbestos was not intensive, he retired; two years later he became short of breath while carrying a suitcase and was found to have a massive pleural effusion.

the disease after playing on asbestos tailings as children. There have been clusters of mesotheliomas in families living near sites where asbestos was used or in which a family member was employed in an occupation involving exposure to asbestos and wore his work clothes home, an example of passive exposure.

The amphibole asbestos fibers appear to be most potent in inducing mesotheliomas, particularly crocidolite. The evidence suggests that chrysotile is weak in this regard but certainly not inactive.

REPRODUCTION AND DEVELOPMENT

Reproductive health effects interfere with the ability to conceive and carry a fetus to term. Developmental health effects result in a malformed fetus and present as birth defects. Issues involving reproduction and development are highly visible and often controversial because they evoke emotional responses. They often appear to be more complicated than they are. Most reproductive and developmental hazards have been discovered in animal studies.

The principles of reproductive and developmental toxicology are outlined in Chapter 2. Both generally occur as a result of moderate levels of toxicity; highly toxic exposures would be lethal to the mother and fetus. Reproductive health effects occur against a background of normal fetal loss and the reality that probably less than half of all conceptions continue to a normal delivery. Birth defects occur against a background of 2–3 percent, much higher than most people believe. In general terms, the male reproductive tract is much more susceptible to toxicity than the female. Exposure to an active teratogen (agent that causes birth defects) during gestation must occur at a certain time in organogenesis to cause developmental defects.

Most concern over reproductive hazards arises from the need for protection rather than from clinical problems that require an investigation into cause. Relatively few patients present for evaluation of infertility suspected to be due to occupational or environmental exposures. Relatively few occupational exposures have been found in practice to cause reproductive toxicity (which usually results in infertility) or developmental toxicity, although certain historical examples (the long-withdrawn pesticide dibromochloropropane, DBCP, and the drug thalidomide, for example) are much discussed models. The principal occupational management problem for reproductive hazards involves risk during pregnancy. The principal environmental issue is the emerging risk of endocrine-disrupting agents, mostly in consumer products and possibly water (which is clearly the major medium for ecological effects). The principal issue with respect to developmental risk at present is associated with pharmaceuticals, not occupational or environmental exposures, although research continues.

OEM physicians frequently find themselves managing issues involving worker protection from reproductive hazards, especially during a worker's pregnancy and often in response to a concerned supervisor. In contemporary North America, these concerns are particularly associated with healthcare institutions, where there is a history of inadequately controlled reproductive hazards (specifically cytotoxic drugs, ethylene oxide, and waste anesthetic gases) and where the workforce is mostly women. The management of women workers during pregnancy is a highly sensitive issue, but the basic rule is that the workplace should be safe enough for them as for all workers. If a job is not safe enough for a woman in pregnancy, it is an unsafe job for anybody and requires attention to hazard control. If there is an unsafe working condition that is an intrinsic part of the job, then guidelines for exclusion or accommodation should apply to all workers (of either sex and with a range of possibility temporary or permanent disabilities) and not solely to women during pregnancy. If the question is whether a pregnant worker can do the usual job, it is simply a question of fitness for duty: matching the job requirements to the worker's capacity to do the job and identifying a reasonable accommodation if there is a remediable gap. Pregnancy is not a disease or an injury, of course, but a normal condition associated with temporary impairment. The extent to which that impairment imposes a disability interfering with performance on the job or safety on the job depends on identifying and monitoring the condition with an emphasis on capacity—what the pregnant worker can do and finding an accommodation for what the worker cannot do.

The guiding principle, enshrined in U.S. law through the precedent of cases such as *Johnson Controls*, is that enforcing different standards for pregnant workers is discriminatory. Employers are obligated to provide a safe workplace for all workers without regard to sex, pregnancy, or anticipated pregnancy, and occupational hazards should be regulated to ensure safety for all. It is not acceptable to have different sets of standards and to treat pregnant women differently. It is of course prudent to ensure that during pregnancy there is no risk of an inadvertent or uncontrolled exposure.

The interest of workers is that there be no loss of income due to reassignment to a less well-paying job and at the same time that there be no risk to the worker.

As a practical matter, the most common exposures of reproductive concern in the workplace are associated with healthcare and have historically been a risk to women health workers such as nurses, central sterile supply workers, and radiology technicians. These hazards include anesthetic gases, cytotoxic drugs, cytomegalovirus infection, rubella, ethylene oxide, and ionizing radiation. Improvements in hospital and healthcare protection in the 1980s controlled these exposures after a series of alarming revelations regarding the risk of miscarriage among nurses and central sterile supply technicians. Beyond healthcare settings, a slowly increasing number of workplace exposures are suspected of having adverse effects on male or female fertility, birth outcome, fetal development, and congenital abnormalities. Particular occupations, including firefighters and welders, appear to have elevated rates of infertility. A somewhat smaller number show a suggestion of increased miscarriages, historically including oncology nurses. Documented outbreaks of birth defects due to occupational and environmental teratogens are very rare. Attributing an adverse reproductive outcome to a particular exposure is further complicated by exposure in daily life to potentially fetotoxic agents, such as some therapeutic drugs, cigarette smoke, and alcohol.

Many suspected reproductive and developmental hazards have been ruled out. Contrary to allegations in the 1980s, there is no risk from exposure to video display terminals, for example.

Physical hazards, specifically heat, vibration, pressure, and ionizing radiation, probably represent a greater management problem in practice than chemical hazards. Hyperthermia is potentially teratogenic and so excessive heat should be avoided during pregnancy. Total body vibration is poorly studied but may represent a risk factor for premature delivery and should be avoided. Decompression illness after diving, following work in hyperbaric atmospheric pressure followed by depressurization, represent a risk to pregnant women and especially the fetus due to gas embolism and diving should not be undertaken during pregnancy. Ionizing radiation is, of course, a major hazard to the fetus.

Ergonomic issues can generally be managed with easy accommodations during pregnancy. Moderate physical exertion is not any more of an issue during pregnancy than before it, but heavy exertion should probably be curtailed in the last few weeks before delivery. Heavy lifting has been studied and found not be a risk factor for adverse birth outcomes and so would not be contraindicated if the woman is accustomed to it and feels able to do the work. Many women find prolonged standing to be a problem during pregnancy, particularly if they are experiencing bloating, retaining fluid, or have developed varices. However, pregnancies are different and the management of accommodations during pregnancy should be worked out between the woman and her employer, not by a rigid standard. Employers may offer reassignment or pregnancy leave, but the worker, once informed, should make the decision about tolerable work conditions.

SYSTEMIC TOXICITY

The principles of clinical toxicology are outlined in Chapter 2. The toxicity of several common agents is presented in Chapter 10. This section highlights a few selected but important situations involving systemic toxicity. Confined-space incidents and "man down" situations are usually discussed in terms of safety and prevention, which in the workplace falls into the domain of the safety officer. However, an understanding of these situations is most important for the OEM physician when he or she encounters a patient with such a history or is called in an emergency.

Confined-Space Incidents

Confined-space incidents occur in enclosed areas not usually occupied by workers where gas accumulates or oxygen levels diminish, creating a hazardous atmosphere. There may also be mechanical hazards, electrical hazards, and obstacles to entry and exit. By definition, confined spaces are hard to ventilate, and workers caught in them may find it difficult to escape and especially to turn around in a narrow crawl space or to climb out on a ladder if access is overhead. Likewise, access may be difficult for rescuers. Common confined spaces include empty tanks, utility rooms, holds on board ships, wells, cisterns, refinery vessels, reaction chambers, and pits.

Within a confined space, toxic gases such as hydrogen sulfide may accumulate to high concentration without ventilation. Flammable or explosive gases may accumulate, for example, from solvents used to clean the inside of a tank. Relatively inert gases may be used to purge vessels (especially if they have held hydrocarbons or other potentially explosive gases), displacing oxygen. Welding inside the confined space may produce oxides of nitrogen and deplete oxygen levels. Oxidation or other chemical reactions may consume and deplete oxygen in the confined space. Gases and vapors that are heavier than air may accumulate in tanks that are open at the top, below decks in ships, in storage chambers, and in subsurface depressions, such as pits, holes, and trenches. Carbon monoxide, hydrogen sulfide, and hydrocarbon vapors may collect in such spaces, with lethal results, when emission sources are near the entrance to a confined space and can funnel in by gravity or air movement. A particular problem in agricultural and rural areas has been hydrogen sulfide toxicity in liquid manure collection pits and septic tanks. Heat and cold stress are potential hazards in some situations.

A typical scenario has a worker entering a confined space due to ignorance, impatience, or a false report of safety and then collapsing. A second worker, on observing or discovering the collapse of the first usually attempts a rescue unprotected by breathing apparatus, only to succumb. These incidents are often fatal and almost invariably come in twos (and sometimes threes or more) because of ill-advised heroic rescue attempts. They are a major cause of "man down" events (as described below).

Any setting in which a confined-space entry may occur requires that the workers be trained, that proper protective equipment be available, and that procedures are in place to prevent unauthorized entry and solo work in confined spaces. OSHA has confined-space standards for general industry, construction, and shipyards that must be followed in the United States.

Employers in industries in which this is a problem should have confined-space entry policies requiring certification of workers who are trained to work safely in confined spaces and who are issued a permit to enter the specific space. The confined space should be tagged and locked down at all other times. Entry should occur only after the atmosphere has been tested for oxygen level, combustible gases, and finally toxic gases that may plausibly be present, in that order (because direct-reading instruments for combustible gases require oxygen in the atmosphere for reliable readings). An oxygen level of 20 percent is required for safe entry; lower levels, whether or not they are high enough to sustain life, are associated with impaired judgment, impaired hand-eye coordination, and strength, making work unacceptably dangerous and impairing the worker's ability to escape.

Confined spaces should always be ventilated when work is being done, providing both air supply and exhaust channels. Supplied-air respirators should be used by workers entering the confined space if there is any question about the safety of the atmosphere and whether it might change (for example, if there is a leak of gas or a connection with a sewer that could result in entry of sewer gas). Air purifying respirators should never be used in confined spaces where the atmosphere presents a potential hazard of oxygen depletion or where the hazard could possibly exceed the protection factor of the respirator. Self-contained breathing apparatus, ropes, and harnesses should be immediately at hand near the confined space at all times for use in rescue efforts. Only trained personnel should be allowed to enter confined spaces, always using the "buddy system" of working with a competent companion capable of alarm and rescue actions who stays outside and is in constant contact with the worker inside the space.

"Man Down"

In industry, the usual term for a worker who appears to be unconscious and to have suddenly collapsed is "man down," a historical phrase borrowed from the military and emergency services which should be considered gender neutral. "Man down" situations should always be considered to be life threatening until proven otherwise.

As the term implies, "man down" calls involve a worker (or visitor) who has collapsed and cannot get up.

Rescue is primary, but the rescuer himself (it is almost always a man) must be protected (see Chapter 14) before attempting to remove the unconscious worker to safety from a confined space and, if there is any possibility of continued exposure, must be equipped with a supplied-air respirator. These incidents usually result in multiple casualties because of ill-advised attempts at heroic rescue.

CPR should obviously be initiated immediately if the patient is apneic and pulseless and the usual clinical measures pursued, including an immediate blood glucose determination. If there is a possibility of cyanide exposure, the rescuer and first responders must protect themselves from exposure due to contamination. The OEM physician should consider the usual causes of syncope and the possibility of a toxic or other occupational cause in the context of that specific workplace.

The cause may be obvious, such as a sour gas well blowout (hydrogen sulfide), an air compressor too close to a source of combustion supplying an air line (carbon monoxide), or anoxia in a confined space (oxygen deficiency), but sometimes it is not. In the absence of trauma or electrocution, the cause of a "man down" is most likely to be a health event, such as an arrhythmia, myocardial infarction, or overwhelming toxic exposure (see Chapter 9) Hypoglycemia in an insulin-dependent diabetic is possible but is most likely to have occurred before, and brittle diabetics usually wear alert bracelets. Vasovagal syncope, which might occur in an acutely stressful condition, with prolonged standing in place, or with heat stress, would be unusual in a healthy worker under normal circumstances.

Certain causes of loss of consciousness can usually be ruled out quickly: Seizures are usually obvious. Orthostatic hypotension corrects itself when the head reaches the level of the heart and the patient will normally revive quickly; it is unlikely in the workplace except among nonacclimated workers exposed to heat stress.

The most likely occupational exposures that could be responsible for this relatively uncommon pattern of collapse are asphyxiants (gases that displace oxygen in a confined-space situation as above), tissue asphyxiants (chemicals interfering with oxygen delivery and cytochrome metabolism), cardiotoxic agents, and anesthetic-acting vapors.

True "asphyxiants" are any gases, usually relatively inert, that displace an atmosphere containing oxygen, including hydrocarbons, chlorofluorocarbons, carbon dioxide, and the true inert gases, including nitrogen. This situation almost invariably occurs in the context of a confined-space incident. The problem is not one of toxicity but oxygen deprivation.

Tissue asphyxiants are agents that interfere with oxygen delivery or energy metabolism by inhibition of cytochrome oxidase or hemoglobin. There are four gases of significance as tissue asphyxiants, forming a spectrum as to their degree of toxicity to cytochrome and hemoglobin on the one hand and their degree of irritation to tissue, principally mucosa, and bronchial epithelium on the other. These are, in order, carbon monoxide (potently competing with oxygen for binding to hemoglobin, not at all irritating), cyanide (potent inhibitor of cytochrome oxidase, irritating), hydrogen sulfide (weakly inhibiting cytochrome oxidase, highly irritating and a cause of sudden loss of consciousness), and azide (weakly inhibiting of cytochrome oxidase, very irritating, and a cause of sudden hypotension). Carbon monoxide, cyanide, and to a lesser degree hydrogen sulfide act in different ways by interfering directly with oxidative metabolism at the cellular level. They are discussed more fully in Chapter 10. Cyanide contamination may place rescuers, first responders, and other healthcare providers at risk during unprotected mouth-to-mouth resuscitation and while handling contaminated vomitus. Hydrogen sulfide has the effect of a sudden, complete loss of consciousness, popularly called a "knockdown," which is rapidly reversible if exposure ceases, and has other effects associated with eye irritation, apnea, and mucosal irritation.

Azide is an important preservative in biotechnology and biological research and the critical component of the explosive charge used in automobile air bags. Its toxicity appears to be mostly unrelated to its weak inhibition of cytochrome and results from its potent effects on vasodilation. Like many other nitrogenous compounds, such as nitroglycerin, azide causes rapid venous capacitance dilation and a drop in smooth muscle tone in the walls of arterial and venous blood vessels, abruptly reducing both preload and afterload and precipitating acute hypotension and syncope. Once the person collapses and he or she is prone or supine, the pressure gradient between the heart and the brain equalizes and cerebral perfusion resumes; recovery may take place relatively quickly except for a residual headache and lightheadedness. The result is not quite so abrupt and may be preceded by a pounding headache due to vasodilation.

Cardiotoxic agents that can cause abrupt collapse act by inducing arrhythmia, including ventricular tachycardia or fibrillation. These are chiefly the chlorinated hydrocarbons, including chloroflurocarbons and chlorinated solvents.

Hydrocarbon vapors, especially solvents, may induce narcosis, like anesthetic gases. This effect requires exposure at high concentrations and occurs in confined spaces.

Arsine Toxicity

Arsine (AsH_3), and its germanium counterpart germane (GeH_4), are gases used mostly in semiconductor manufacturing. They may cause acute massive hemolysis and rhabdomyolysis due to their affinity for oxidized hemoglobin and myoglobin. Respiratory distress syndrome, acute renal failure, and marrow toxicity may occur simultaneously and almost instantaneously. In nonfatal cases, hemoglobinuria, hepatomegaly, and a drastically reduced red cell count occur. If the victim survives, complications are numerous, and treatment may require exchange transfusions, hemodialysis, and intensive supportive care. Blood or urinary arsenic is a useful aid to diagnosis and a means of following progress in arsine poisoning, but the diagnosis must be made immediately and clinically. Arsine toxicity has occurred historically in the semiconductor and smelting industries.

OCCUPATIONAL NEUROLOGY

Neurological conditions associated with acute toxic exposures are discussed elsewhere, with respect to the causal agent.

Three neurological conditions in occupational medicine are featured in this section: toxic encephalopathies, Parkinsonism disorders, and toxic peripheral neuropathies. Treatment of toxic neuropathies has been limited in the past to facilitating spontaneous recovery by removing from the patient further toxic exposure (and reducing body burden of heavy metals by chelation, if necessary) and nutritional supplementation (specifically using vitamin B_6, which unfortunately can also induce a neuritis at high levels of consumption).

Toxic Encephalopathy

High levels of exposure to variety of agents are capable of causing central nervous system toxicity. Some of these effects are discrete, as in the case of manganese. Encephalopathy is a general condition manifested as behavioral disturbance, changes in mood, cognitive impairment, and diminished short-term memory. Unfortunately, the term "toxic encephalopathy" has been appropriated and trivialized by some advocates associated with the "environmental sensitivity" movement, but it properly means a condition of gross functional impairment in the brain associated with toxic and metabolic causes. Toxic encephalopathy is a medical emergency requiring immediate diagnosis and intervention.

Lead has been the most common cause of toxic encephalopathy, historically, in occupational medicine. Lead encephalopathy in adults occurs at blood lead levels above 100 μg/dl and in children at levels around 80 μg/dl, which are catastrophically high (see Chapter 10). In children, lead encephalopathy is associated with projectile vomiting, irritability, hyperactivity, ataxia, visual changes, seizures, and a peculiar passive state that has been characterized as wakeful lethargy; it progresses to coma and has a very poor prognosis, fatal in 25 percent of the cases, and with residual neurobehavioral impairment in most survivors. Whether cognitive impairment of this severity occurs in adults, short of massive exposure, is controversial, but chronic lead exposure in adults is associated with impairment in attention, short-term memory, and psychomotor skills, as well as irrational behavior, labile effect, irritability, and apathy. Lead encephalopathy is a true medical emergency, whether in the adult or child and is treated by a combination of BAL and CaNa2-EDTA (never EDTA alone, because of the risk of inducing fatal hypocalcemia), but the need for this is rare. Because cerebral edema is part of lead encephalopathy, lumbar puncture is contraindicated. The edema is treated with mannitol (and other hyperosmotic treatment), steroids, and hyperventilation if required. Fluid management is necessary because cerebral edema may result in the syndrome of inappropriate ADH, and seizures are treated with benzodiazepines.

Tetraethyl lead, the additive in leaded gasoline, was the most potent exposure historically associated with severe lead encephalopathy and was responsible for an outbreak of fatal and disabling encephalopathic cases at the Ethyl Corporation in the 1920s, which presaged the hazards of leaded gasoline.

Among its other effects, arsenic may also cause a syndrome of malaise, labile affect, and neurobehavioral effects and is also recognized for neurocognitive effects in children at much lower levels.

The encephalopathic effects of mercury are dramatic and fortunately uncommon: extreme emotional lability, personality change (often characterized as pathological shyness), cognitive dysfunction, attention deficit, and irritability. The syndrome of mercury-induced encephalopathy, also called "mercurial erethism," is familiar in the expression "mad as a hatter" and in the characterization of the hatter character in Lewis Carroll's *Alice in Wonderland*; hat makers in the seventeenth and eighteenth centuries were at risk of mercury intoxication from contact with mercurials used as antifungal agents on the felt cloth used to make hats. Metallic mercury can be absorbed by the inhalation route, since it is a volatile substance, in quantities sufficient to cause toxicity (Chapter 10). The greatest concern over inhalation of mercury has been in the exposure of dental assistants, research laboratory personnel, and instrument and measurement equipment workers, all of whom may work with mercury under circumstances in which spills and prolonged exposure is possible. Organic mercury compounds are even more toxic, a severe outbreak of methylmercury poisoning from the consumption of food and water contaminated by a chloralkali plant on Minimata Bay, in Japan, received worldwide attention. The methylated, organic derivative of mercury is more easily absorbed by the body and is much more toxic; it is this form that is present in river and lake sediments in which mercury has been discharged into the environment.

Organic derivatives of tin, particularly the marine antifouling paint additives triethyl tin and trimethyl tin, are potent central neurotoxins. In animals and in the few human cases studied, trimethyl tin produced behavioral and affective changes, short-term memory loss, and hearing impairment. The limbic system appears to be particularly affected.

Among organic compounds, carbon disulfide (CS_2) is associated with a severe and characteristic encephalopathic condition, which includes the usual features but also, and sometimes in isolation, an induced thought disorder manifested by paranoid ideation, manic behavior, and suicide. With the introduction of improved containment and worker protection in the rayon industry and the reduction in use of CS_2 as a fumigant, the syndrome is rare today.

Solvent exposure may produce encephalopathic changes; toluene and trichloroethylene are most often implicated as single agents, but exposure to multiple solvents is usual and the problem is difficult to study. Many investigators believe that effects are not limited to these two specific agents. The specific neurotoxicology of the solvents is discussed in Chapter 10.

Organophosphate pesticides are associated with encephalopathic changes acutely, as described in Chapter 10. Many clinicians have suggested that persistent changes may follow recovery from acute exposure, manifested by labile affect, attention deficit, anxiety, memory deficits, headaches, and irritability, but this has not been confirmed.

Movement Disorders

Manganese produces a syndrome closely resembling Parkinson's disease, with an extrapyramidal motor disorder associated with injury to basal ganglia and the characteristic mask-like facies. Exposure is by inhalation. Figure 17.27 presents a woman who was exposed while working as an investigator conducting research on manganese compounds at a metallurgical research institute in China and who subsequently developed a florid condition identical to idiopathic Parkinson's disease. The disease is also found among welders who have welded on ferromanganese alloys. Prognosis is poor as the toxicity is irreversible.

Parkinsonism is also associated with intense solvent exposure and possibly pesticide exposure, but the specific solvents and pesticides that may be responsible are not clear. A related neurological condition known as "subacute combined system atrophy" or degeneration (not to be confused with combined degeneration of the cord, which occurs as a result of vitamin B_{12} deficiency) is an autonomic disorder characterized by orthostatic hypotension, and dementia may also be associated with occupational exposure to solvents and possibly pesticides.

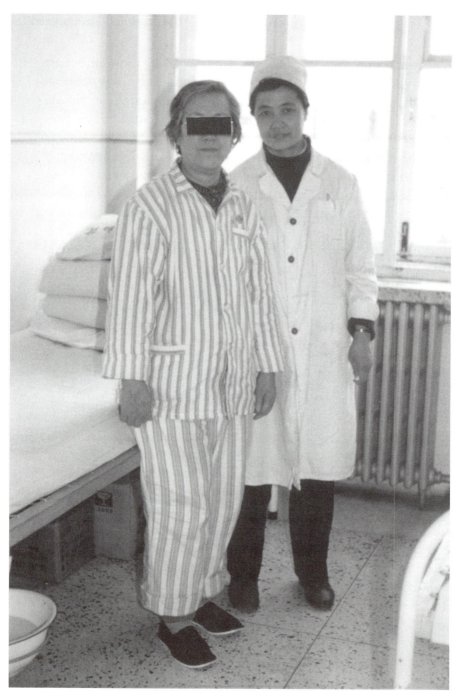

Figure 17.27. Parkinson's disease–like neurological condition in a Chinese metallurgical research scientist heavily exposed to manganese. Ferromanganese alloys are extensively used for rails, and most cases in China are seen in railroad welders.

Toxic Peripheral Neuropathy

Peripheral neuropathies may be predominantly or purely motor, sensory, or mixed. Motor neuropathies present as palsies, muscle weakness, and atrophy and diminished tendon reflexes. Sensory neuropathies usually present as dysesthesias, often of a burning quality, and numbness to pain and vibration, usually in a "stocking-glove" distribution. Neuropathies affecting autonomic nerves may result in characteristic malfunction of sphincter activity, orthostatic hypotension, and dystrophic changes over the skin. Nerve conduction studies, assessing conduction velocity and amplitude of response, are useful confirmatory tests for neuropathies affecting accessible nerves. Electromyography is less often helpful.

It is difficult to be sure that a peripheral neuropathy is due to an occupational cause in a particular case. The disorder occurs most often in association with diabetes, as a result of alcohol abuse, and idiopathically. Peripheral neuropathies are side effects of common drugs, including isoniazid, penicillin, phenytoin, furadantoin, and metranidazole, and with several antineoplastic drugs, including vincristine, adriamycin, procarbazine, and 5-fluorouracil. Consumption of excessive quantities of vitamin B_6 may cause a neuropathy. There are numerous other less common causes of peripheral neuropathy, among them porphyria, amyloidosis, hereditary conditions, collagen vascular disorders, and as a systemic effect of cancer.

Usually, there is a history of exposure to a known neurotoxic agent over a period of months or years, with gradual onset of the neuropathic symptoms. (An exception is Vacor, a neurotoxic p-nitrophenylurea rodenticide that resembles streptozotocin and may cause symptoms of peripheral neuropathy, diabetes and dysautonomia within days.) In the case of pesticides, exposure to the organophosphate pesticides may precede within two weeks of the onset of a primarily motor neuropathy.

Metals, especially lead, have been the most common cause of toxic peripheral neuropathy in occupational settings historically (see Chapter 10). Lead characteristically causes a "dying-back" motor axonopathy affecting the muscles of the forearm innervated by the radial nerve. The resulting extensor nerve palsy and unopposed flexor action causes the condition known as "wrist drop," seriously impairing use of the hands. Mercury is associated with tremor and motor disorders. Thallium also causes motor neuropathy, but toxicity is usually obvious because of patchy hair loss. Bismuth and arsenic may cause sensory neuropathies. Copper, zinc, gold, silver, and tin may cause mixed sensory or motor neuropathies, but these are rare.

The classical historical causes of peripheral neuropathy among organic chemicals have disappeared from the workplace: n-hexane and methyl-n-butyl ketone, both of which are metabolized to the highly neurotoxic product 2,5-hexanedione (see Chapter 10). The so-called γ-diketones form a pyrrole in the cell that eventually cross-links neural filaments in the axon, resulting in axonal swelling, a "dying-back axonopathy," myelin swelling, and a progressive neuropathy that continues after exposure ceases, a phenomenon called "coasting."

Other solvents, including trichloroethylene, benzene, carbon tetrachloride, and carbon disulfide, have been associated with peripheral neuropathy, but these are rare in the contemporary workplace. Exposure to tetrachloroethane (perchloroethane) has also been suggested as a contributing exposure potentiating neurotoxicity from other solvents. 1-bromopropane, a solvent introduced to replace ozone-depleting chlorinated solvents, has been associated with a severe neuropathy characterized by pain and spastic paraparesis.

Organophosphate esters may cause an acute or a delayed neurotoxicity, as described in Chapter 10 for organophosphate pesticides. Tri-ortho-cresyl phosphate was an important neurotoxin historically, responsible for a major outbreak of "ginger jake" motor paralysis during Prohibition, when flavor extracts adulterated with the substance were consumed in large quantity for their alcohol content. Some organophosphate pesticides may cause axonal changes and motor paralysis of the lower extremities as a long-term sequela: leptophos, mipafox, and trichlorphon in particular. The effect appears to result from inhibition of a specific esterase other than the acetylcholinesterase at the post-synoptic junction or neuromuscular junction responsible for the acute effects. This "neuropathy target esterase" is of unknown function. The organophosphate-induced delayed neuropathy syndrome consists of proximal weakness of limbs and the muscles of respiration, leading to a condition resembling Guillain-Barré syndrome and sometimes requiring assisted ventilation. Onset is usually within one to three weeks of exposure. Another distinct but less well defined delayed neuropathy has been described as having onset twenty-four to ninety-six hours after exposure.

A specifically autonomic syndrome has been associated with dimethylaminoproprionitrile (DMAPN), a catalyst formerly used in polyurethane manufacturing. DMAPN affects sacral nerves selectively, causing urinary retention and impotence. The identification of this devastating disorder was a particularly elegant example of astute clinical observation leading to identification of a hazard.

Acrylamide, the monomer of polyacrylamide gel preparations, is a potent neurotoxic agent that also produces a "dying back axonopathy" and induces a combined sensory and autonomic neuropathy with dermatitis and muscle wasting. Some immediate central effects have been reported with acute exposure, including ataxia and delirium. Fortunately, both the chronic and the acute condition appear to be reversible.

OCCUPATIONAL INFECTIONS

Compared to other areas of medicine, OEM deals less often with infectious agents and disease and more often with chemical hazards. However, infectious agents and disease and the risk of exposure to pathogens is an important part of OEM practice and are distinguished from encounters with infectious disease elsewhere in medicine mainly by context, not recognition or medical management.

Infectious agents and disease are part of the training of every qualified physician, and information on them is readily obtainable through the usual medical information sources. The diagnosis and treatment of infectious disease is the same in OEM as in clinical medicine otherwise. Therefore, this section will not go into detail on the individual infectious diseases encountered in OEM. Rather, it will discuss the context in which they are encountered and the broad management issues of each, apart from diagnosis and treatment.

The contexts in which infectious disease are managed in occupational medicine are:

- Management of pathogens and infectious hazards in the workplace
- Infectious disease arising out of work as a result of biological hazards specific to the workplace
- Infectious disease arising out of work due to location and activity that is not specific to the workplace
- Community-acquired infectious disease and its implications for the workplace
- Accommodation and adjustment issues for workers with chronic disease
- Travel and the risk of acquired infection

The latter two topics are discussed elsewhere in this book.

All of these examples are important for some infectious agents, such as HIV, which serves, unfortunately, as an excellent context for illustrating the issues. HIV/AIDS is a specific risk in the healthcare workplace with specific procedures for primary prevention (for example, preventing needle-stick wounds) and secondary prevention (antiretroviral prophylaxis when there is a high risk that infection may have occurred) in the workplace. It is fortunately uncommon among healthcare workers but critical to identify early when it does occur. HIV/AIDS is related to work in indirect ways as well, as demonstrated by the high prevalence among truck drivers and miners in southern Africa, where the risk reflects transmission patterns due to geographic distribution and lifestyle. It is as or more likely to occur due to exposure outside the workplace, and the risk is proportionate to the prevalence in the relevant general population; once a worker in a sensitive occupation, such as a healthcare worker, is infected, this information has implications for work capacity, although fewer than for more communicable infections. There may be accommodation issues for individuals with HIV/AIDS undergoing treatment and also work adjustment issues with respect to access to healthcare and maintaining an antiretroviral regimen. Travel to areas with a high prevalence of HIV/AIDS presents an opportunity for increased risk depending on personal behavior, the management of which may involve highly sensitive discussions with the travelling worker (who is often a technical expert, senior manager, or executive and who may often resist intrusive counseling by the physician with respect to sexual behavior). Promotion and even provision of protection (such as condoms) may be required when risk-taking behavior is unlikely to change. Another scenario in which HIV/AIDS may be a travel risk is when medical care is provided under conditions of questionable sterilization or when transfusions are required in high-risk areas. Travelers may need to carry their own sterile supplies, such as needles, to avoid infection during emergency care in high-risk areas. Because vehicular accidents are more common and more likely to result in serious injury in less economically developed countries, as a rule, the risk of HIV infection for some travelers may be driven more by traffic and transportation choices than another factor. Finally, there remain situations in which HIV positivity is a factor in immigration and visa eligibility. HIV/AIDS therefore well illustrates the range of occupational management issues for infectious disease.

Hepatitis B, which is more readily transmissible, reflects the same issues.

Infectious Hazards in the Workplace

In Chapter 2, chemical agents were described as having an exposure-response relationship that, at a certain threshold level or case definition, results in a certain frequency or risk of toxicity. The exposure-response relationship was a gradient, resulting in degrees of toxicity. Other disease types, such as cancer, were described as "stochastic," in that they occur with a certain frequency at any given level of exposure to a carcinogen but the disease itself is the same. Infectious agents, which propagate after an initial innoculum, follow stochastic dynamics. This means that the key to controlling infectious disease in the workplace is not so much to reduce the level of exposure, although this is desirable, but to eliminate the opportunity to come into contact with the pathogen altogether. Hospitals and healthcare institutions provide the most convenient example because they are high-risk environments and also familiar to every physician.

Infectious agents are encountered in many settings, but the single most hazardous employment sector overall for infectious disease is healthcare. This is not surprising, since the hospital and clinic bring to one place all manner of patients and medical conditions in close interaction. Whether on the ward or in the waiting room, patients with communicable diseases may encounter each other and health-care workers, who may or may not carry communicable diseases of their own (such as staphylococcus colonization in their nares), with the potential for transmission. This occurs under conditions dense enough to accelerate transmission in the population as a whole for the more communicable diseases. Healthcare settings are therefore rich environments for disease transmission as well as for the selection of resistant strains by passage through hosts who are being treated. However, healthcare occupations have acquired a false perception of being "clean" because of their environment, and so for many years, until very recently, healthcare lagged as a sector in worker protection. For many years the primary infectious threat in hospitals was hepatitis B, yet even the protean and potentially severe manifestations of that disease was insufficient to motivate adoption of universal precautions. The threats, in sequence, of transmission of HIV, multi-drug-resistant tuberculosis, the SARS agent (not known at the time to be a coronavirus), avian and other potentially pandemic influenzas ("novel influenza A H1N1" being the one circulating at the time of this writing), and methicillin-resistant staphylococcus dramatically changed attitudes in the healthcare sector. They also broadened concern over hazard protection from an emphasis on hand washing and needlestick injury, to the inhalation route to housekeeping, to rigorous control of all routes of exposure today. OEM physicians with responsibility for healthcare institutions, and especially hospital employee health services, are cautioned to benchmark programs, policies, and performance against both best practices in the healthcare sector and also general industry, where attitudes are different and often more proactive.

Because of the stochastic dynamics of transmission, the objective of infection control in the hospital workplace, used here as an example for workplaces at high risk, is the approach of multiple barriers. Exposure to a chemical hazard is reduced by the protection factor of each control measure (such as isolation, ventilation, engineering controls, personal protective equipment, and administrative or behavioral controls), and risk is reduced proportional to the reduction of exposure and stays reduced as long as the control measures are in effective operation. Infectious agents present a different problem. A lapse in protection against a communicable agent may reduce the probability of transmission, but once protection is breached the agent can propagate or may spread by person-to-person transmission. Isolation of infectious cases, negative air pressure in infectious disease wards and isolation units, universal precautions (which are not described here because they should be intimately familiar to all practicing physicians), antibiotic prophylaxis (for staphylococcal carriers), and meticulous hand washing each provide protection that, although potentially incomplete, reduce the risk in different ways. If a pathogen is not "intercepted" and so blocked by one barrier, it is likely to be blocked by the next. In this context the many modalities for hazard control (which run the gamut of control measures discussed in Chapter 14) are not redundant or duplicative but sequential. Unfortunately many of these control measures depend on individual behavior, making compliance with often complicated procedures the limiting factor for the entire chain of protective measures. A break in any step creates a gap that may result in transmission and spreading, undermining the whole of the infection control effort. The goal is to reduce the cumulative probability of transmission (a function of the product of individual protection factors of each control measure and their failure rates) to level far below the probability that a single case would ever occur in the protected population.

Infectious Hazards in the Workplace

There are many microbial hazards specific or even unique to certain occupations. The specific workplace hazards are associated with infections in the occupation, such as orf (a spirochetal disease) in sheep handling, leptospirosis among sugar cane workers, anthrax (usually cutaneous) among workers who handle unsterilized cattle hides, and brucellosis among large-animal veterinarians. These hazards are concentrated in occupations that involve animal handling, agriculture, microbiological laboratory services, healthcare, and behaviors that may lead to the exchange of body fluids (obviously rare in the workplace, with the exception of sex workers).

Other than healthcare, most infectious hazards are particular to the occupation and are relatively unlikely to be encountered in a general OEM practice. A somewhat broader range of infections may be encountered among animal handlers with an opportunity to encounter "zoonoses" (diseases carried by animals that can affect human beings). They are more likely to be seen in an infectious disease consultation. Sexually transmitted infections among sex workers are not unique as a hazard to those workers but are not usually managed by OEM physicians and because of social approbation may not come to medical attention early. There are special clinics and healthcare providers for sex workers, but they are not in occupational health centers. For example, there is a clinic in Los Angeles dedicated to the health of performers in the adult film industry; it emphasizes prevention of HIV/AIDS.

Most, but certainly not all, microbial hazards are well known within their industries, and guidance for the OEM physician is usually readily available through the usual sources of medical and occupational health information. For that reason, no attempt will be made to list the numerous possibilities here. *Couturier's Occupational and Environmental Infectious Diseases* covers the field exhaustively.

Work-Related Infectious Disease

Infectious diseases that are endemic to a particular location or setting within which work is performed constitute a much greater challenge for OEM physicians than unique infectious hazards in the workplace, outside of healthcare. Much of occupational medicine as it is practiced today arose from the need to control tuberculosis in the workplace at a time when it was highly prevalent in the community. The basic principles of pre-employment evaluations (before pre-placement evaluations replaced them) and periodic health surveillance were worked out to screen workers for the disease and to prevent transmission within the workplace, using the limited tools of the day.

Today the single largest health challenge associated with location and workplace setting is control of malaria, the most prevalent infectious disease in the world. Employers with operations that involve outdoor work in malaria-endemic areas, such as heavy construction and oilfield work, face a constant battle with the disease in their workers and the risk to business travelers. Of the four species of malaria that affect humans, falciparum malaria is most likely to be lethal or disabling, especially the cerebral form. It is geographically dispersed throughout sub-Saharan Africa and southeast Asia, including New Guinea. (The others are vivax, which predominates in southern Asia and north-central South America, ovale, and malariae, both less common, and found in a patchy distribution where other malaria is endemic.) Measures for malaria prevention include local mosquito control (with the controversial issue of the proposed reintroduction of low-level treatment with DDT for this purpose), pesticide-impregnated mosquito netting, chemoprophylaxis (with particular reference to the high frequency of unacceptable side effects of mefloquine and the relative underutilization of doxycycline), mosquito-resistant clothing, and mosquito repellant (DEET).

Guidelines on the use of these modalities (always in combination) and current recommendations for malaria prevention should always be sought from the most up-to-date authoritative sources, such as Web sites of the Centers for Disease Control and Prevention and the World Health Organization, in preference to textbooks and other sources that are much less often updated.

A particularly hazardous situation occurs when workers invade unfamiliar ecosystems and encounter zoonotic (animal-borne) pathogens with a previously restricted range. An extreme example of occupational infection due to location occurred during the building of the Panama Canal. In the nineteenth century a pioneering French effort failed due to the high attack rate and mortality among workers of yellow fever, which had originally been introduced to the Americas from Africa and had become established in the rain forest. The success of the subsequent American effort was largely credited to mission-specific public health research, leading to the recognition of the role of the *Anopheles* mosquito in transmission, followed by practical and effective measures for mosquito abatement. A more recent, catastrophic example may be the emergence of HIV, the most significant among retroviruses that may have emerged in this manner, from primate hosts in Africa to disseminate into a global epidemic.

Community-Acquired Infection

Although demonstrating nothing like the mortality and social impact of malaria and HIV, common infections circulating in the community naturally appear in the workplace as well and profoundly affect job performance. Absence and presenteeism (reduced productivity in a worker who is present but not functioning well) is highest from upper respiratory disorders and influenza, which are both very common disorders and easily transmitted in the workplace. Because of their frequency and transmissibility, they are the most important community-acquired illnesses introduced into the workplace and so will be used as examples.

As a general preventive measure, the most important intervention to prevent upper respiratory tract infections is clearly hand washing. Outside of healthcare, however, few industries promote this or make it a central theme in health promotion programs.

Control of upper respiratory disorders in the workplace requires measures to prevent the ill worker from introducing and transmitting the disease. This may be achieved by policies encouraging the worker to stay home during an acute illness. From the employer's point of view this may seem to be a mixed message, in that absence is being encouraged, but the risk of mass presenteeism caused by many workers struggling through the day with symptoms outweighs the temporary absence of one employee who may transmit the disease. Another approach to employers who are equipped for it is remote work from home, sometimes called "telecommuting," if the employee is well enough and doing office or creative work. This is not popular among managers, who are usually concerned that it will set a precedent for other employees wishing to work from home at other times and for their own reasons and because productivity is seen as more difficult to measure than for work at the office.

Work at home may also be an emergency measure in the event of widespread epidemic and transmissible disease, as proposed for pandemic influenza. This strategy, combined with canceling nonessential meetings or gatherings, discouraging employees from assembling into groups, and limiting face-to-face interactions is known as "social distancing" and is a prominent element in pandemic control contingency planning.

Immunization programs for employees have grown in popularity in recent years as their impact on workforce absence during influenza outbreaks has been demonstrated. This is a service that benefits individual workers and their families as well as the workforce overall and the community, while maintaining productivity and reducing costs. Compliance rates for employees vary, of course, and at least in hospital settings it is disturbing to note that the lowest compliance rates are generally found among nurses and physicians. This demonstrates that awareness and cognitive knowledge do not automatically translate into health-conscious behavior.

RESOURCES

Ad Hoc Committee [on Update of 1986 Criteria for the Diagnosis of Nonmalignant Asbestos-Related Disease: Guidotti TL, Miller A, Christiani D, Wagner G, Balmes J, Harber P, Brodkin CA, Rom W, Hillerdal G, Harbut M, Green FHY]. Diagnosis and initial management of nonmalignant diseases related to asbestos. *Am J Respir Crit Care Med.* 2004;170:691–715. (Source of Figures 17.14, 17.15, 17.16, and 17.17.)

Craighead JE. *Pathology of Environmental and Occupational Disease.* St Louis: Mosby; 1995.

Harber P, Schenker M, Balmes J. *Occupational and Environmental Respiratory Diseases.* St Louis: Mosby; 1995.

Quint J, Beckett WS, Campleman L, Sutton P, Prudhomme J, Flaherty J, Harrison R, Cowan B, Kreutzer R. Primary prevention of occupational asthma: identifying and controlling exposures to asthma-causing agents. *Am J Ind Med.* 2008;51:477–491.

Sataloff RT, Sataloff J. *Occupational Hearing Loss.* 3rd ed. Boca Raton, FL: Taylor and Francis; 2006.

Sullivan JB Jr, Krieger GR. *Clinical Environmental Health and Toxic Exposures.* Philadelphia: Lippincott Williams & Wilkins; 2001.

Wright WE, ed. *Couturier's Occupational and Environmental Infectious Diseases.* Beverley Farms, MA: OEM Press; 2008.

NOTEWORTHY READINGS

Adams R. *Occupational Dermatology.* New York: Grune and Stratton; 1982.

Adams R. Occupational skin disease. *Occup Med.* 1986;1(2):199–356.

Blanc P, et al. An experimental model of metal fume fever. *Ann Intern Med.* 1991;114:930–936.

Brain JD, Beck BD, Warren AJ, Shaileh RA. *Variations in Susceptibility to Inhaled Pollutants.* Baltimore: The Johns Hopkins University Press; 1988.

Brooks SM, Kalica AR. NHLBI Workshop summary: strategies for elucidating the relationship between occupational exposures and chronic air-flow obstruction. *Am Rev Respir Dis.* 1987;135:268–273.

Brooks SM, Weiss MA, Bernstein IL. Reactive airways dysfunction syndrome (RADS): persistent asthma syndrome after high level irritant exposures. *Chest.* 1985;88:376–384.

Chan-Yeung M. Occupational asthma. *Chest.* 1990;95(suppl 5):148S–161S.

Chan-Yeung M, Lam S. Occupational asthma. *Am Rev Respir Dis.* 1986;133: 686–703.

Cockcroft DW. Occupational asthma. *Ann Allergy.* 1990;65:169–175.

Cordasco E Sr, Demeter SI, Zenz C. *Environmental Respiratory Diseases.* New York: Van Nostrand; 1995.

Cullen MR. Clinical surveillance and management of occupational asthma: tertiary prevention by the primary OEM physician. *Chest.* 1990;98(suppl 5): 196S–201S.

Enright PL, Hyatt RE. *Office Spirometry.* Philadelphia: Lea and Febiger; 1987.

Guidotti TL, Abraham JL. Occupational lung diseases. *Am Fam Phys.* 1984;29:169–176. (Source for Figures 17.7, 17.10, 17.23, and 17.25.)

Guidotti TL, Miller A, Christiani DC, Wagner G, Blames J, Harber P, Brodkin CA, Rom W, Hillerdal G, Harbut M, Green FHY. Nonmalignant asbestos-related disease: diagnosis and early management. *Clin Pulm Med.* 2007;14(2):82–92. [Contains material following up on the revised ATS criteria.]

Guidotti TL, Novak RE. Hearing conservation and occupational exposure to noise. *Am Fam Phys* 1983;28(4):181–186. (Source for Figure 17.24.)

Hogan DJ, Dannaker CJ, Maibach HI. The prognosis of contact dermatitis. *J Am Acad Dermatol.* 1990;23:300–307.

King TE, Jr. Bronchiolitis obliterans. *Lung.* 1989;167:69–93.

Kusaka Y, Hering KG, Parker JE. *International Classification of HRCT for Occupational and Environmental Respiratory Diseases.* Berlin: Springer; 2005.

Maibach HI, ed. *Occupational and Industrial Dermatology.* Chicago: Year Book: 1987. [Classic. Now hard to find.]

Mathias CG. Prevention of occupational contact dermatitis. *J Am Acad Dermatol.* 1990;23:742–748.

Mazurek JM, Wood JM. Asbestosis-related years of potential life lost before age 65 years: United States, 1968–2005. *MMWR.* December 12, 2008;57(49): 1321–1325.

Morgan WKC, Seaton A. *Occupational Lung Diseases.* 2nd ed. Philadelphia: WB Saunders; 1984.

Perrin B, et al. Reassessment of the temporal patterns of bronchial obstruction after exposure to occupational sensitizing agents. *J Allerg Clin Immunol.* 1991;87: 630–639.

Salvaggio JE. The impact of allergy and immunology on our expanding industrial environment. *J Allerg Clin Immunol.* 1990;85:689–699.

Weaver JH. Monitoring hearing loss at United Airlines. *Occup Saf Health.* 1981;50: 35–39, 41.

Weill H, Turner-Warwick M. *Occupational Lung Diseases: Research Approaches and Methods.* New York: Marcel Dekker; 1981.

18 CAPACITY FOR WORK

This chapter deals with several important topics in occupational medicine that are connected in that they relate to the capacity of the worker to do the assigned work. These topics are:

- Disability rights
- Fitness for duty
- Certification of illness and medical leave
- Family and medical leave
- Absence
- Presenteeism
- Functional capacity evaluation
- Impairment and disability assessment
- Accommodation
- Drug screening

DISABILITY RIGHTS AND THE AMERICANS WITH DISABILITIES ACT

Disability rights, as a movement, has deep roots in American, Canadian, and British law and society. The emphasis initially was on human custodial treatment, then in the eighteenth century on education and institutionalization into a separate society, then on "overcoming a handicap" and participating in mainstream life. As technology and medical treatment improved, assistive devices and rehabilitation supported the inclusion of disabled people as full participants in society. The achievements of exceptional athletes and the example of disabled veterans also demonstrated that a rigid distinction between the disabled and the whole is spurious. Capacity is a continuum, and disability is a mismatch in a particular context. Disability that has meaning with respect to work may mean little in terms of a social or family role. Modeled on the civil rights movement, disability rights advocates in the United States first demanded more responsive services and then broadened the issue to removing barriers to participation, culminating in 1990 with legislation that provided employment rights. Since then, a major theme of the disability rights movement has been parity with respect to mental health care and recognition of nonvisible disabilities.

In the United States, the Americans with Disabilities Act (ADA) of 1990 changed the landscape at the time with respect to perceptions of disability and work capacity. ADA has been a pervasive influence in shaping what is perceived to be appropriate with respect to work requirements and individual capacity. Occupational and environmental medicine (OEM) physicians with any part of their practice in the United States are advised to become intimately familiar with ADA, which was amended in 2008. (Canadian employment law is equal to or more stringent than ADA because of the antidiscrimination provisions in the basic law of the Charter of Human Rights and Freedoms, which overrides other legislation, the Canadian Human Rights Act of 1977, which applies to federally regulated enterprises, and the provincial human rights codes, which apply to everything else. The major practical difference for employers is that human rights violations in Canada are heard by tribunals rather than being litigated in court. The British counterpart is the Disability Discrimination Act of 1995.)

With ADA, the emphasis shifted to the design of the job, identification of its essential requirements, and identification of reasonable accommodations that may be used to meet those requirements when a worker has a limited disability. ADA applies only in the United States but its provisions are consistent with Canadian law and precedent, and it represents a convenient framework for reviewing the fundamental principles of disability and work capacity.

Although ADA is written as a series of restrictions and prohibitions, it is actually legislation oriented to positive change that asserts a right of the disabled to fairness in hiring. It creates a framework within which the disabled applicant for a job can compete for jobs that he or she could perform and shapes the characteristics of the job to the capacity of the individual, within reasonable limits. Once hired, the worker who is able to demonstrate good work performance is promoted and treated on an equal basis with nondisabled workers. By requiring accommodation, so that persons who are able overall to do the job but need assistive devices or work modifications to do a part of their duties, ADA shifted the emphasis from finding a hire who fits perfectly into the slot to shaping the workplace with flexibility to fit the worker. This opens up employment prospects to many more people who can do the work. It also has a transformative effect on the workplace, because an adaptable workplace is generally a safer and more flexible workplace.

ADA prohibits discrimination in recruitment, hiring, advancement and promotions, job-related training, compensation, social activities, and employment benefits, including workers' compensation coverage and benefits, on the basis of disability. In order to ensure that discrimination will not take place in the hiring process, ADA restricts questions that can be asked about an applicant's disability before a job offer is made and does not permit medical evaluations before a job offer is extended. ADA requires employers to make a "reasonable accommodation" for new hires who have limited disabilities, short of the point that accommodation would result in "undue hardship" for the employer.

Medical evaluation may only be conducted after a job offer, must be matched to the work requirements of the specific position, must be given consistently to all workers who are candidates for such a position, and must be kept confidential. The purpose of the medical evaluation is to determine whether the selected worker, who is already deemed qualified and has been offered the job, can do the job and do it safely, not whether they are in good health or at risk for a future health problem. No medical question may be asked of job applicants before an offer of employment has been made. Employers may ask current employees questions about their health and impairment only when there is a visible, concrete reason to believe that the worker cannot perform the job or poses a risk to self or others due to the condition.

Key words in ADA include a "covered entity," which is generally an employer engaged in interstate commerce that has fifteen or more employees but may include employment agencies, labor organizations, trades, and joint labor-management committees. A "qualified individual" is a person who has a disability, visible or not. Drug abuse is excluded as a qualification. "Disability," for purposes of the Act, is a "physical or mental impairment that substantially limits a major life activity." What qualifies as a major life activity is decided by the Equal Employment Opportunity Commission. This provision led to a number of court challenges that confused interpretation of ADA, but in 2008 the Act was amended to clarify that major life activities are to be construed broadly, that "substantially limits" means "significantly or severely restricts," and that a limitation does not disappear from consideration because a disabled worker manages in daily life with ameliorative measures, such as eyeglasses or a walker.

Other American legislation that may affect occupational health is the Architectural Barriers Act, which requires that federal facilities comply with standards for physical accessibility, the Rehabilitation Act, which prohibits discrimination on the basis of disability with respect to employment and participation in federally sponsored programs, and the Air Carrier Access Act, which prohibits discrimination in scheduled air transportation serving airports in the United States and applies to accessibility to aircraft and assistance in boarding.

With respect to the broader world of environmental barriers and disability, ADA provides for barrier-free access in public accommodations and prohibits discrimination in services on the basis of disability by businesses that serve the public and on the part of state and local governments. Another title prohibits discrimination and requires accessibility in public transit and requires provision of "paratransit" (special services for the disabled who cannot manage public transit) where feasible. The Fair Housing Act, as amended in 1988, prohibits discrimination in housing on many grounds, including disability, and may require owners to provide access for persons with disabilities (in new multifamily housing with four or more units), to allow reasonable accommodations (such as allowing the tenant to modify doors to the width of wheelchairs, at the tenant's expense), and making reasonable exceptions in policies that exclude persons with disabilities (such as allowing guide dogs despite a policy of no pets). The Telecommunications Act, as amended in 1996, requires manufacturers and service providers to provide equipment and services that can be used by persons with disabilities. A title of ADA also requires "common carriers" (telecommunications utilities) to provide services accessible to the deaf.

FITNESS FOR DUTY

The OEM physician conducts, reviews, and designs fitness-for-duty (FFD) evaluations and in many cases supervises the FFD evaluations conducted by other physicians. FFD evaluations are a family of medical services that are specific to occupational medicine and involve (1) assuring that the worker or new hire is physically able to do the work assigned, (2) assuring that the worker or new hire can do so without presenting a safety risk to themselves or others, and (3) identifying any gap between the specific requirements of the job and the individual capacity of the worker and determining the accommodation that may be required in any essential function that might enable the worker to do the job despite an impairment. These evaluations must be applied universally and cannot be conducted selectively on certain applicants and not others. They must be directly related to the specific job requirements and conducted by persons who are familiar with both the working conditions in that workplace and the limitations of currently available evaluation procedures. They must be kept completely confidential, and only judgments regarding fitness for duty, not diagnoses, should be communicated to management by the physician conducting the evaluation, unless the worker gives approval.

Fitness for duty implies that the worker has the capacity to do the essential duties of the assigned job and is not impaired in such a way that essential functions are impossible to perform. It implies no more than this and certainly does not require that the worker have no medical condition, nor does it imply a judgment regarding future capacity to function. Fitness for duty is a critical evaluation for OEM physicians to make and a major part of OEM practice.

Fitness for duty is often referred to as "fitness to work," especially in the older literature. The terminology has changed because fitness to work implied a level of health or capacity for work in general, not limited to a specific job. Fitness for duty suggests fitness for a specific set of requirements that go with the job.

Historically, employers generally required their employees, especially new hires, to undergo medical evaluation (usually consisting of a general physical examination and basic laboratory tests, sometimes including a chest film) in order to determine whether they were healthy. These medical evaluations were often repeated on an annual basis as periodic health surveillance. The requirements for the "medical" or the "employment physical" were similar to a standard medical examination and bore little or no relationship to the job duties. The breakthrough in thinking about fitness for duty came in the realization, underlying ADA, that disability is not a condition of the individual but a mismatch between the specific capacity of the individual and the specific, essential requirements of the job and that a disability in one setting may be irrelevant in another. In most cases, a relatively limited disability may also be easily overcome in the setting in which it is significant by a simple accommodation (for example, amplification for the hearing impaired). ADA provided a legal framework that realized a change in attitudes and culture regarding the disabled that had been evolving for decades. ADA focused on the essential duties of the job and turned the pre-placement evaluation into a structured analysis of the work assignment rather than an arbitrary test of the worker.

The primary objective of an FFD evaluation is to create a fair match in which the employee is fairly evaluated for his or her capacity to perform the assigned job in a technically satisfactory manner while the employer's rights are protected by ensuring that the individual will be able to perform the job as required and will not pose a safety threat to themselves or others. The FFD evaluation also has secondary benefits. It documents the employee's health status objectively so that future claims of injury may be dealt with on the basis of fact rather than supposition. It establishes a point of comparison so that should the employer fail to provide a healthy workplace, the lapse can be detected through medical monitoring and corrected accordingly. FFD evaluations cannot be used to speculate on future disability or prognosis and do not in any case accurately predict sickness absence in the future for an individual worker.

Designing the FFD Evaluation

The FFD evaluation must be identical for all applicants for a given job description, matched against explicit job performance criteria, and treated confidentially.

Table 18.1 presents an example of how not to do it, a typical example of a regressive FFD evaluation of the type popular in the 1970s, incorporating irrelevant medical tests. It is presented here because such protocols are still in use and some employers still ask for them. They should be recognized by the OEM physician as an inappropriate service.

Table 18.1. An Inappropriate "Pre-employment" Protocol

This pre-placement evaluation is typical of those in use in the 1970s. They are sometimes still encountered and reflect poorly on the employers who request them.

Medical history (may contain numerous irrelevant questions)
Physical examination (may include inappropriate and intrusive examinations)
Complete blood count
Blood biochemistry
Urinalysis
Chest x-ray
Low-back x-ray★
Electrocardiogram
Stool guaiac for occult blood★★

★ Unethical because of excessive radiation exposure and low predictive value.
★★ Often included as a personal health benefit.

A major limitation on FFD evaluations is the sensitivity and specificity of medical screening tests. (See Chapter 5.) The tests that physicians use for FFD evaluations are adapted from clinical tests used by physicians to assess people with illnesses. They were originally designed to assist in making a diagnosis in a person who presents to the physician as clearly ill. They are seldom very sensitive or specific for disease and are mostly irrelevant to work capacity.

When one applies these tests to a group of patients who are being investigated because they are likely to have the disease in question, the lack of specificity presents relatively little difficulty in determining predictive value. Knowing that an individual has a high likelihood of having the disease or impairment in the first place, the physician uses the test for guidance in selecting among alternative diagnoses that are highly probable (see Chapter 5). However, most groups of workers are relatively healthy and have a low prevalence of the conditions medical examination is testing for (historically, mostly tuberculosis and obvious clinical disease). FFD evaluations therefore have an inherent problem with low predictive values of the screening tests used. It is not reasonable for an individual to be excluded from a well-paying job solely on the basis of a screening test with low predictive value.

Some tests are contraindicated because they carry an unacceptable hazard, as in the case of low-back x-rays. Low back x-rays do not accurately predict who will and who will not later develop back pain and carry an unacceptable radiation hazard; they are unethical for use in FFD evaluation. Even studies that withstand scrutiny are not terribly helpful in practice. Chest films are no longer useful because of the low prevalence of lung disease in the population today. Other tests are clearly irrelevant to work capacity: pelvic examinations were sometimes required for pre-employment medical examinations in the 1970s.

The findings obtained in a FFD evaluation must be compared against a set of criteria that are specific for the job assignment. For this reason FFD evaluations must be job specific, and requests to perform a FFD evaluation should always contain either a description of the job and the activities it requires or a set of validated health and performance criteria from an analysis of the tasks required by the job.

Formulation of specific performance standards and the derivation of medical criteria require a formal "job description." The job description is as detailed a description of the job as is required to identify the health and performance standards that should apply. The point of an FFD evaluation is to match an understanding of the job and the health requirements it entails with an understanding of the worker's capabilities and health, by comparing the health findings obtained from the evaluation to the working conditions as abstracted in a set of health standards for the job supplied to the examining physician. The physician is expected to be able to render a medical opinion regarding the fitness of that worker to work at a specific job.

An adequate job description useful to support an appropriate FFD evaluation should include at least the following:

- A description of the job function and performance requirements
- Location of work (i.e., special or hazardous work environment)

- Hours of work
- Occupational safety hazards
- Occupational health hazards
- Special or unusual requirements of the job
- Psychosocial demands of the job

Table 18.2 provides an illustration of an acceptable job description. This description was developed by the personnel office of a large public employer in California. The criteria for fitness for duty are implicit and can be easily inferred by a knowledgeable physician.

The description can then be used to decide on an appropriate FFD evaluation. The work mentioned above has resulted in sets of health standards that more or less dictate what tests should be conducted.

Obviously, there can be no justification for FFD evaluations for jobs that have no exceptional responsibilities or duties. There is no reasonable justification for performing elaborate medical evaluations on office workers or individuals whose jobs have no special physical requirements.

Table 18.2. Essential Features of the Pre-placement Evaluation

1. Scheduled *after* a job offer has been made, never a requirement for hire.
2. Contingency for job offer to be final, not for eligibility for employment. "Pre-placement" is *not* a synonym for "pre-employment."
3. Specific to work requirements of the assigned job.
4. May identify conditions that can be acceptable to employer with reasonable modifications in workplace.
5. Routinely administered, in a consistent manner, to all workers assigned to the job, not applied selectively to those with visible or declared disabilities.
6. Physician should never "approve" or "disapprove" employment. Qualification to be hired is a human resources decision, not a medical decision.

Whenever possible, the best evaluation procedure of all is to allow the employee to do the job on a trial or probationary basis and to assess performance, which is usually best evaluated by the immediate supervisor. If the individual can perform the job over a period of days and shows no sign of failing performance or a health problem, then the evidence of their capacity to do it should be clear. If the individual cannot do the job, however, this challenge test is much more sensitive than a clinical evaluation. The exceptions would be those jobs that present an unacceptable risk due to an intrinsic hazard or in which the safety of others may depend on the performance of the job by the worker (as in safety-sensitive positions). In these circumstances there is really no acceptable trial possible, and a test must be adopted.

Reporting Outcomes of FFD Evaluation

Once the FFD evaluation is completed and the physician has compared the findings of the medical evaluation with the health standards appropriate for that particular job, an opinion is rendered regarding the worker's fitness for duty.

There are three possible outcomes that the physician can report:

- Fit
- Unfit
- Fit subject to work modification [specify]

These outcomes are in all cases specific to the job under consideration, not a general statement of the worker's capabilities or ability to work in any job.

"Fit" means that the individual is able to work in the assigned job without restriction; is not likely to pose a threat to self or others in performing his or her duties; and is not likely to suffer adverse health consequences in performance of normal duties.

"Unfit" means that the individual is not able to work in the duties assigned and is not likely to be able to do so despite reasonable accommodation or work modifications.

"Fit subject to work modification" means that the worker would be able to return to work if the job or working conditions were modified to accommodate limited impairment, which may be temporary or permanent.

In the past, it has been common for physicians to use the term, "light duty" with respect to return-to-work determinations. Employers do not find these designations to be useful or practical, as discussed below in the relevant subsection. It is better to use the modern terminology "fit subject to work modification" and to specify the type of modification that is required. Whether the work modification can be accommodated then becomes a management decision, not a medical one.

When an evaluation is conducted by a physician outside the employer's occupational health service, the medical findings should not be reported to management or any representative of the employer other than the employer's occupational health service or a designated occupational health physician or nurse. Confidential information should never be sent to nonmedical personnel without the patient's explicit approval. The physician should not share confidential information on the employee with management. Only the medical evaluation regarding fitness for duty should be communicated to management.

Specific Types of FFD Evaluations

Fitness for duty involves the following types of evaluations:

- Pre-placement
- Return to work
- Performance-related (medical inquiries)
- Job change
- Safety-sensitive positions (including U.S. Department of Transportation)

Each will be discussed in turn.

Pre-placement Evaluations

Pre-placement evaluations are conducted to determine the suitability of an applicant for a job to which they would be assigned. The job offer is made contingent on one's being fit for the specific job. The essential features of a pre-placement evaluation are listed in Table 18.3. Because of the provisions of equal opportunity legislation, the pre-placement evaluation has replaced the "pre-employment" evaluation.

Pre-employment evaluations were general screens for health status that were conducted prior to a job offer. Before ADA, the applicant

Table 18.3. A Satisfactory Job Description

MAINTENANCE, HEATING AND AIR CONDITIONING MECHANIC

Definition

Under direction to perform skilled work in the repair and maintenance of heating, refrigeration and ventilation equipment; and to do related work as required.

Distinguishing Characteristics

The Lead Maintenance, Heating and Air Conditioning Mechanic is used to supervise the work of other skilled heating and air conditioning mechanics and perform skilled repair work personally.

Examples of Duties

Inspects, disassembles, repairs, maintains and services ventilation, air conditioning and heating systems and equipment; adjusts and installs valves, thermostats, fans and controllers; checks temperatures, pressures and differentials; lubricates, cleans and adjusts equipment; changes filters and strainers; flushes boilers, descales tubing, cuts and threads pipes; replaces valves, fans, motors, gaskets, filters and belts; uses various testing devices to locate defective parts; adjusts and installs switches, gauges, thermostats, valves, tubing and other parts as needed, makes pipe connections and general electrical repairs pertaining to equipment; schedules preventive maintenance; maintains logs and records on equipment repair or malfunctions; orders parts, maintains liaison with vendors; performs other maintenance tasks as assigned.

(Continued)

Table 18.3. (*Continued*)

License

Possession of an appropriate California operator's license issued by the State Department of Motor Vehicles.

Desirable Qualifications

Knowledge:

Tools, materials, methods and terminology used in the maintenance and repair of heating, air conditioning and ventilation equipment;

The proper operation of heating, air conditioning and ventilation equipment.

Skills:

Trades level skill in the maintenance and repair of heating, refrigeration and ventilation equipment;

Estimate the scope and cost of work assignments and select necessary tools, equipment and materials to complete the job;

Use required tools and equipment skillfully and safely;

Work from sketches, drawings and blueprints;

Keep work records;

Understand and carry out oral and written instructions;

Establish and maintain cooperative working relationships;

Read and write at the level necessary for successful job performance.

Training and Experience:

Any combination of training or experience that could likely provide the required knowledge and skills is qualifying. A typical way to obtain the knowledge and skills would be one year of journey level heating and air conditioning repair experience.

---

for a job was often required to pass a "physical" before being hired, which put the physician in an untenable position of gatekeeper, deciding who was employable, based on criteria of little relevance to the work to be performed. Often these medical evaluations had little or nothing to do with the specific job to which the applicant was to be assigned. In the 1970s it was not unusual for clerical personnel to be required to pass the same pre-employment medical evaluations as production workers.

Pre-employment evaluations reflected health issues held over from the early twentieth century. The employers were seeking to ensure that: (1) the new hire not introduce a communicable disease into the work-force, which was a holdover from the days in which tuberculosis was prevalent in the general population; (2) the new hire was sufficiently able to do physical labor, which became irrelevant to most jobs in the modern workplace and in any case is not well assessed by a medical evaluation; (3) the new hire was healthy and unlikely to be absent or to become ill on the job, which was a holdover from a time when morbidity in the general population was much higher; and (4) the work-force was strong enough to sustain productivity under pressure, which was a holdover from attitudes toward fitness in the military. Screening examinations in the military had provided a familiar but misleading model for fitness evaluation because the demands on the soldier and requirements for military readiness do not apply to most jobs in civilian life. It should not be necessary for a person to be in ideal health and free of disability to be hired to do a job he or she is able to perform.

By the end of the twentieth century, many employers had dropped pre-employment evaluations because they were not cost effective and many physicians were questioning the increasingly questionable rationale for them. After ADA, pre-employment evaluations became legal liabilities because they implied that the decision to hire would be based on a medical screening test, as opposed to a pre-placement evaluation that evaluated capacity for the specific work assignment after the job offer was made and the worker was deemed otherwise qualified.

The difference between pre-placement and pre-employment evaluations is more than just a legality. In the former a medical evaluation was assumed to be a requirement for joining the organization and therefore constituted a barrier to entry. The concept of pre-employment evaluations put the physician in a position of "approving" or "disapproving" employment on the basis of often arbitrary medical screening processes.

A pre-placement evaluation, on the other hand, implies that the evaluation is specific to the working conditions and to health standards that are relevant to the job requirements. A pre-placement evaluation may identify conditions that are acceptable to the employer with reasonable and relatively inexpensive modifications in the workplace. This concept was missing, however, from the earlier concept of a pre-employment evaluation, which emphasized screening out any physical abnormality and often placed modestly impaired individuals, who could do the job very well with slight modifications, at a decided and unfair disadvantage. The modern pre-placement evaluation specifies the role of the physician in assessing fitness for duty for the specific job and establishes a more objective set of medical criteria to be followed.

Return to Work

"Return-to-work" (RTW) evaluations are conducted after a worker has been off the job for a prolonged period and is thought to be ready to return to work. Here, the goal is to ensure that a worker who has demonstrated an ability to perform the job in the past is sufficiently recovered to perform safely and reliably again. Many injuries or illnesses involve deconditioning, muscle atrophy, persistent fatigue, reduced exercise tolerance, or new conditions that may interfere with job performance. Simply being off work for more than a few weeks changes behavioral patterns and habits and makes it difficult to return to the pace and organization of work immediately. Whether the health problem was an occupational or personal injury or illness, the RTW evaluation ensures that functional capacity has been restored to the extent that the worker can resume performing the assigned job or identifies an accommodation that will allow phased reintegration into the workforce.

Ideally, an RTW evaluation is scheduled at the point when the worker is nearing or at end of a period of rehabilitation, or following a short illness or recovery from injury. Physical therapists are often asked to perform RTW evaluations at the end of a course of treatment, before discharging the patient. At that time gaps can be identified, for example in the limits on the number of repetitions of a hand action or fatigue in working a full day. Accommodations can be specified, such as an assistive device or partial work hours.

Returning the worker to the job as early as it is safe to do so helps to condition the worker physically, to restore the habits and structure of work, and to reintegrate the worker socially with the workplace. The employer should gain from early and safe return to work because it reduces costs associated with the total time off and restores an experienced employee.

The practical problem of RTW evaluations is that many employers will not accept workers who are "less than 100 percent" in work capacity. This is in part a reflection of an attitude on the part of management that they expect 100 percent from all employees, but it is also a response to perceived liability, because workers who are recovering from an injury are thought to be at greater risk of a second injury until they are fully healed. Employers may also be responding to practical issues of labor management. Temporarily assigning returning employees to jobs that are perceived as easier or lighter disrupts the organization of work and may create resentments among other workers who feel that they are expected to "carry" or "cover for" the recovering worker. Many unions are unenthusiastic about the practice because it disrupts seniority for the lighter jobs and is perceived as pushing the worker back before he or she is fully recovered.

The terms "light duty" and "partially fit" are often used as recommendations to employers for RTW determinations, often to encourage early return to work. The terms mean that the worker could return to work other than their usual job, as long as that work is not demanding given this impairment. Unfortunately, such a term is meaningless without a description of what the worker can or cannot do. It implies that the worker can be reassigned to other duties easily, which is often not the case in a highly structured and lean workplace. "Light duty" is a sloppy term and should be replaced with "modified duty with [specify restrictions or accommodation]." Many employers have a policy against any employee returning to the job until they are able to do their usual job safely with no special consideration in job assignment. The reasons for this include fears of re-injury and of legal liability if the employee cannot do the job safely. Light duty or alternative jobs simply may not be available in the workplace. Assignment of employees to other duties may also be constrained by contracts with unions or may complicate labor-management relations, since one groups of employees may complain if preferential treatment is being given to one worker.

RTW evaluations are similar in concept and design to pre-placement evaluations and are conducted in a similar manner, with equal attention to the requirements of the job assignment. The worker previously assigned to the job is assumed to know how to do it, and his or her own opinion about capacity to do the job is usually reliable.

Physicians sometimes find themselves under pressure to extend the leave period well beyond the time when the worker is fit to return to work. Physicians are often urged by the patient to let them stay off work, particularly if there is a holiday, weekend, or social event ahead. The pressure may be even greater if the physician also treats the patient's family, has many other patients who know the insistent patient, or has close ties with the community and will inevitably run across the patient and his or her close associates again and again. It may seem a small matter to bend on a seemingly administrative issue. However, such an act is neither good medicine nor good occupational health practice. It is very costly to the employer and further delays the return of the patient to a normal life, which is part of the recovery process. The patient should return to work when the patient becomes fit to work, definitely not before but also not long after.

Medical Inquiry and Performance-Related Evaluations

Performance-related FFD evaluations are medical evaluations triggered by the observation, usually by a supervisor, of a decline in job performance, unexplained and unexpected considering the worker's past performance. The essential features of this type of FFD evaluation are outlined in Table 18.4. These evaluations may be suggested by supervisors who detect failing or substandard performance in an individual with an otherwise good work record and who may be concerned that a health problem is interfering with the worker's ability to do the job. Under ADA, these are called "medical inquiries"

Table 18.4. Example of a Set of Health Standards Based on Criteria Derived from Analysis of the Specific Job (described in Table 18.3).

Critical features
    Working near operating equipment
    Bending, lifting, pulling
    Working in awkward or cramped quarters
    Hand tools

Critical exposures and work characteristics
    Ergonomic
    Vibration
    Solvents
    Noise

Health standards
    Hearing surveillance (audiogram)
    No medical condition precluding working alone
    No medical condition interfering with detailed, close-up work
    Musculoskeletal strength, flexibility, dexterity

and must be directly related to job requirements and "consistent with business necessity." Asking about medications, for example, is a highly sensitive medical inquiry.

The U.S. Equal Employment Opportunity Commission (EEOC) recognizes that not all questions about health are medical inquiries that are sensitive with respect to discrimination. Some questions are allowable based on visible evidence, direct relevance to work performance, and legitimate business reasons to know. These include the following:

- How are you feeling today?
- Can you perform your job?
- Are you using alcohol or taking illegal drugs?

Such questions are allowable if the employer "has a reasonable belief, based on objective evidence" that the employee has a condition (whether the disorder or medication required to treat it) that either impairs him or her from an essential job function or poses a direct threat to the safety or health of that employee or others.

Referral for a medical evaluation can often make the encounter with the worker tense and anxious and puts an additional responsibility on the physician to be sensitive to psychological factors and to identify problems such as substance abuse. Under ADA, the employer and the OEM physician who is involved must confine themselves to the particular issues of job performance and safety. Broader inquiries into the worker's personal health are not appropriate. Once the worker discloses an impairment, the medical inquiry is over except insofar as an accommodation can be recognized. There is no legitimate reason to know the details of a personal illness or to obtain the full medical history. As with all medical information, the findings in the medical inquiry must be kept strictly confidential but so must information regarding the accommodation.

The employer should have clear policies for when an FFD evaluation might be suggested or directed, and the OEM physician should have a protocol or plan for evaluation that conforms to fitness for duty for the work assignment and would be applied consistently to all employees in the same situation. The model of an independent medical evaluation (IME) should be followed (see Chapters 15 and 23), with the physician making it clear that his or her investigation is limited to assessing the reason for the decline in performance and not for purposes of treatment. Follow-up and therapeutic intervention should be done with the worker's personal physician, so as not to confuse the roles of objective evaluator and treating physician.

Performance-initiated FFD evaluations should be done in conjunction with the usual procedures for an employee assistance program, if one is available. This opens the possibility of intervention and rehabilitation. It is important to maintain a relationship with the worker-patient that is cordial and appropriate to a medical encounter rather than a personnel action. The physician should emphasize the role of the FFD evaluation in maintaining a balance between the obligations and rights of the employee and the employer.

Performance-based FFD evaluations offer the opportunity to identify a previously unsuspected problem and to find a solution that benefits both the worker and the employer. For example, if there is an on-site occupational health service or an on-site general medical facility, it may be possible for the OEM physician, occupational health nurse, or primary care provider in an embedded facility to monitor and help manage chronic medical conditions during the workday, such as brittle diabetes, asthma, and hypertension. These are opportunities for health gains in patient care and in managing employee wellness (see Chapter 19). The OEM physician should recognize that assuming direct-care responsibilities may make it more difficult to maintain objectivity in evaluating work capacity, and the arrangement should be governed by an explicit policy or by a written contract between the worker/patient and the physician. There should be agreement on all sides that the OEM physician will take on this role, it should be limited to the time that the worker is physically present at the facility, and care should be directed by the worker's personal physician with the OEM physician in a supportive role. Such arrangements are likely to become more common as on-site medical clinics become more common in large retail and employer facilities. Such arrangements obviously must be voluntary on the part of the worker, who may not wish to share personal medical information with another physician.

On the other hand, performance-based FFD evaluations are easily abused. Performance-initiated FFD evaluations should never be a covert form of discipline, but in the past they have often been used by supervisors and human resources departments to find a way to remove unwanted or troublesome employees. Requiring a medical evaluation may also be used as a threat by management to prompt the resignation of an employee who does not wish a health condition or a drug or alcohol problem to be revealed. The OEM physician should be aware of this and avoid getting in the middle by asserting professional independence and going by the book. Employees missing a certain number of days of work should not be automatically sent for review to the physician. The physician should never, ever be expected to give the employee "a good talking to." The OEM physician is not an enforcer and is not there to do the work of the human resources department. Being used in this way discredits the physician and undermines trust in the professionalism of the occupational health service on the part of both the employee and the employer.

Given the many sensitivities and pitfalls associated with ADA violations, restraint is advised. The OEM physician, when asked, should advise the employer that it may not be in the employer's best interest to make a medical inquiry, especially if an accommodation can be made without knowing more about the worker's condition. The employer does not need to know the diagnosis or details of a worker's impairment and is better protected when management does not have this information. Policies and mechanisms to ensure confidentiality must be in place. There should always be a legitimate business reason or a medical inquiry is not appropriate.

It would be very wise to consult legal counsel experienced in ADA and EEOC case law before making any medical inquiry. Case law involving ADA and the EEOC is developing rapidly compared to other areas of law.

Job Change–Initiated FFD Evaluations

FFD evaluations initiated by a change in work assignment alone are rare but by the logic of ADA should not be. If a worker moves from one job with a given set of requirements and demands another job with very different requirements, an FFD evaluation ought to be provided just as if it were a pre-placement evaluation for a new hire. To do otherwise is to contradict the relationship between the initial evaluation and work requirements. However, there is no logical contradiction if the work requirements of the second job are incorporated into the evaluation of the first job or are less stringent.

The most common exception to this is that new jobs requiring the worker to use personal respiratory protection when they have not done so before always require an evaluation, as described in

Chapter 14. The evaluation incorporates tests for capacity to use respirators, which is an essential part of such jobs.

Safety-Sensitive Positions

Safety-sensitive jobs still require rigorous FFD evaluation. They are required in cases in which the physiological demands of the job are extreme or the consequences of inability to perform the job are intolerable. For example, the fitness and medical criteria for airline pilots are quite rigid. Deviations from them immediately ground the pilot. Similarly stringent FFD evaluations are required for divers, police, firefighters, and transportation workers in safety-sensitive jobs (such as drivers, railroad engineers, air traffic controllers, and marine pilots—merchant marine seafarers have a FFD that is less rigorous). In each case, the FFD evaluations are designed to protect the individual worker but also the public and other workers from harm. The FFD evaluations and the individual programs of which they are a part are highly specific and detailed, and it is beyond the scope of this book to provide more than a few examples. The most important in practice are those related to surface transportation and to aviation. Any OEM physician conducting these evaluations must train and achieve certification to do so.

Most OEM physicians, even in Canada, will at some time have some contact with the special evaluations of the U.S. Department of Transportation (DOT). (The United States Coast Guard, formerly part of DOT but now part of the Department of Homeland Security, handles FFD of mariners.) Many will qualify in order to conduct them, as they are one of most common services OEM physicians provide.

The Federal Motor Carrier Safety Administration (FMCSA) of DOT requires medical certification for up to two years of truck and bus drivers ("commercial drivers"), with exclusionary criteria for disabling conditions that may result in inability to control the vehicle. The Commercial Drivers Medical Examination (CDME), for example, requires visual acuity of 20/40 on the Snellen chart (corrected) and color vision for traffic signals. There should be no hearing deficit at more than 40 dB at specified frequencies. The exclusions from certification include cardiovascular and respiratory disorders that carry a risk of loss of consciousness, insulin-dependent diabetes, epilepsy, current alcoholism, and a variety of conditions that would affect coordination and control of the extremities while driving. However, drivers who can demonstrate that the conditions are under control or have been successfully treated can apply for an exemption. Some of these conditions, when stable, require re-evaluation every year. Drug screening is mandatory, and a positive test excludes the applicant from driving. The certifying physician can make one of three decisions: certify, "time-limit" (certify for less than two years), or disqualify. There are many nuances in the CDME and much conferring among physicians who do this work to achieve consistency and fairness.

Obviously, the decision in a DOT is critical to the driver's future and the public safety. The essential evaluation may require follow-up of specific medical problems, such as hypertension, and there is some room for interpretation. In order to facilitate fair and consistent evaluations, DOT recognizes certification by examination of "medical examiners" who have undergone a training program but does not limit itself to any one training program or certification program. Certified medical examiners are entered into the FMCSA National Registry of Certified Medical Examiners, which is accessible to drivers. FMCSA is advised by an advisory network of medical expert panels.

Another safety-sensitive FFD evaluation is the Aviation Medical Examiner program of the Federal Aviation Administration (FAA) in the United States. The FAA qualifies pilots by classes: First class is airline transport pilots. Second class is commercial pilots. Third class is private pilots. Like the CDME, the FAA has standards for vision and hearing and many disqualifying conditions, most relating to potential causes of sudden incapacity or misjudgment. In order to retain high standards and consistency, the FAA manages a training and certification program to qualify physicians as Aviation Medical Examiners. Transport Canada has a similar program for Canadian Aviation Medical Examiners.

Safety-sensitive jobs in the private sector must be identified in advance. Medical qualifications must be justified as essential to the position, and a periodic medical evaluation must be a requirement of the job. An example would be mine rescue personnel, who operate at maximum levels of exertion during an emergency and must therefore train vigorously. Their own lives as well as the lives of those they are trying to rescue depend on their capacity to work in unpredictable extreme conditions. Such a position would justify stringent medical evaluation on a regular basis.

CERTIFICATION OF PERSONAL HEALTH PROBLEMS

Assessing a worker's ability to work as a result of personal health problems is usually a function of clinicians in the community, in the form of the familiar "note from the doctor." Certification of illness should be accepted as a medical function requiring conscientious management. This function places considerable responsibility on the physician, who has rarely had any training in how to do it and usually perceives it as a bother. The physician should never certify an illness that was not observed or sign a "blank check" when an employee presents claiming to have been ill for several days but not having sought medical attention. Unfortunately, this commitment is rarely taken seriously, and physicians continue to treat medical certification very casually.

Some employers ask the OEM physician to certify time off work as resulting from a medical or health condition. Certification of illness should either be performed with a knowledge of the employee's health problem or conducted as an FFD evaluation. In other words, the physician should not be placed in a position of having to write a note that states "certified off work because of influenza for last two weeks" but, more realistically, should be able to write "medically certified as fit to return to usual work after reported illness of two weeks." For the OEM physician, certification is actually an opportunity to conduct a less structured variation of the FFD evaluation.

For occupational physicians approving return to work and certifying time off work are a clear commitment to understanding the worker's personal health problems. If a worker's absence is likely to be prolonged or to be repeated, the physician should consult with management to see if work modification or accommodation could be introduced to facilitate recovery or if some medical management could be undertaken by the occupational health service to ease the transition back to usual employment.

In fairness to the practicing physician, patients frequently ask for certification or a "note from the doctor" after the fact or for complaints that are impossible to confirm or deny. There is no excuse, however, for knowingly acquiescing to a false certification or to pad the amount of time for reasons of personal convenience. One way to deal with this is to treat it as an implicit FFD evaluation rather than a certification of an illness the physician has not seen.

FAMILY AND MEDICAL LEAVE

In the United States, the Family and Medical Leave Act of 1993 (FMLA) sets the minimum allowable absence time that covered employers, generally those with more than fifty employees within seventy-five miles (not necessarily in one place), must provide if required to employees who qualify, generally those who have worked more than a year or a total of 1,250 hours. FMLA was under review by the U.S. Department of Labor at the time of this writing and may be amended by Congress in the near future, so readers are advised to seek current information.

Under FMLA, the employers with must grant eligible employees up to twelve work weeks of unpaid leave during any twelve-month period for the following purposes:

- Birth and care of a newborn child
- Placement with the employee of a son or daughter for adoption or foster care
- Care of an immediate family member (spouse, child, or parent) with a serious medical condition
- Medical leave when the employee is unable to work because of a serious health condition

Paid annual leave or sick leave may run concurrently with FMLA, providing the employee with income, or FMLA may be taken as unpaid leave with sick leave preserved. FMLA leave may be taken as a bloc or as intermittent leave for treatment. Employers are free to provide more generous policies and benefits, as long as the provisions of FMLA are present in full.

FMLA has functioned remarkably smoothly since it was introduced. Several problems have been noted with FMLA to date, notwithstanding the value of the act's provisions.

One problem has been that the burden of adapting to leave has fallen hardest on employers who work on tight schedules, with small numbers of skilled workers, in less flexible workplaces. That tends to describe many new start-ups or high-technology firms.

Another problem has been the definition of "serious health problem," which is sometimes disputed. For example, a qualified worker recently asked his employer for four days of medical leave under FMLA to obtain and to recover from intraocular lens placement for simple vision correction, not for cataract; this previously specialized procedure is coming to be used much like Lasik® for refraction. Although the case has not been arbitrated, it raises many questions. It would seem that this procedure would not be covered by FMLA because the underlying problem is not a "serious medical condition." Under FMLA, the employer has had the option of requiring the employee to get a second opinion from a physician of the employer's choosing, but could not name a physician who "contracts" with or regularly provides care for the employer; a third, mutually agreed-upon physician can break the tie. That provision excludes many OEM physicians. This is unfortunate because OEM physicians know about the workplace, possible accommodations, disability management, and fitness for duty and could assist in reentry.

A third major problem has been that time off for medical treatment is often not scheduled in advance with the employer, although routine medical appointments should be known well in advance. The employer then has to cover for unexpected absences.

The short duration of family leave provided by FMLA places a particular burden on nursing mothers who, after twelve weeks, must rely on employer policies regarding lactation breaks and the availability of suitable locations to express milk unless child care is on site and readily accessible. Breast feeding is a public health priority and a bond between mother and infant. Evidence suggests that exclusive breast feeding, optimally for six months, is associated with a reduced frequency of gastrointestinal disorders in the child in developed countries and reduced rates of Type I diabetes, and longer duration of breastfeeding appears to be associated with better health status for both mother and child. Breast feeding is associated with reduced infection rates and infant mortality in developing countries and in disadvantaged communities. However, return to work places nursing mothers who need to work but would prefer to nurse their child in a bind. This bind is only partially resolved by employer policies regarding lactation breaks and rooms.

FMLA has had a positive impact on worker's lives and has made employment more flexible and responsive to the demands of life. However, it must be noted that other countries, including Canada and members of the European Union, provide much more generous benefits for workers in need. In those countries, family and medical leave is part of the social contract between workers and employers. Seen from a global perspective, FMLA balances human needs against economic productivity in the United States, but it is nothing special.

ABSENCE

Absence from work is a difficult management problem in industry, since it introduces considerable uncertainty into the scheduling of work and of staff assignments, is an important cause of lost productivity, and is a very common precipitating cause of labor-management conflict and misunderstanding. Because absence from work is viewed very differently depending on one's cultural background, the issue is laden with prejudice, misperceptions, and hidden hostility. There is no other area of working life where expectations of the work ethic are more likely to conflict with notions regarding personal freedom and flexibility and where abuse so directly undermines the relationship between manager and worker.

Because absence triggers emotional responses and attempts to control unauthorized absence often makes matters worse, human resources personnel often persuade management to take a more "objective" approach by treating the problem as one of validation and documentation. Much of the total absence experience in industry is because of sickness and even more is claimed to be sickness. From management's point of view, therefore, it may be only logical that absence be dealt with through medical means by requiring employee screening to identify workers likely to be frequently absent, medical certification of claimed illness, and investigation of individual cases. Some go so far as to expect their occupational health service, if they have one in-house, to monitor absence directly as a principal responsibility. Unfortunately, such responsibilities work no better than other tactics and have the potential to destroy the effectiveness of the occupational health service overall by turning it into the attendance enforcer.

Absence Management

The transfer of responsibility for absence monitoring and control from the personnel or human resources department to the occupational health service converts an administrative problem into a medical and programmatic nightmare. It succeeds in getting the human resources department off the hook but presents the occupational health service with a fundamental inconsistency that workers are quick to see and some managers are quick to exploit further. When workers view the occupational health service as the means by which management reviews their attendance and singles them out for discipline, cooperation and goodwill promptly evaporate and are seldom if ever regained. The physician in such a position becomes labeled as just another management functionary, and medical judgments from the occupational health service are viewed as untrustworthy and prejudicial to the worker. Having taken the occupational health service this far down the road, insensitive managers may then press even further for the physician to become a "team player" siding with management for violations of confidentiality.

Although the occupational health service should never accept monitoring and control of absence as an operational responsibility, there are many ways in which the occupational health service can have a positive effect on the absence experience of an employer to the mutual benefit of employer and worker. These include evaluating employees who are referred either voluntarily or individually by their supervisors for frequent or prolonged absence due to apparent health problems. This evaluation is an extension of the medical inquiry concept. A private, confidential interview and, if the worker allows, examination may uncover a treatable illness, may suggest a means by which the patient could be treated at work conveniently and without disruption to the work schedule, may suggest a minor modification in the work environment or in responsibilities that would allow the worker to stay on the job, or may identify a worker with emotional or substance dependency problems that might benefit from referral to an employee assistance programs.

In all such cases, the emphasis should be on fitness for duty and the well-being of the worker, not on policing compliance with the policy on sick leave. The occupational physician is primarily concerned with work-related health problems, but a question of at least as great of significance in practice is the assessment of a patient's ability to work in the presence of a personal health problem. There are circumstances in which a personal health problem is optimally managed and monitored at the worksite, as has been shown for hypertension, or in which the occasional attention of the OEM physician may prevent loss of work time and improve the quality of life for the worker, as in the management of brittle diabetes. Such individual patient management at the worksite should be considered complementary to the management of the worker's personal physician, providing the patient/worker with the best opportunity to remain on the job while insuring that health care needs are met.

Health promotion programs in the workplace may reduce absence in various ways.

Absence Monitoring

There are only two ways to keep track of absence: to record attendance at work or to record incidents of absence, assuming attendance unless notified otherwise. One is the time clock and the other keeps track more or less by voluntary notification or observation by supervisors.

For a variety of reasons that have as much to do with assumptions regarding social class and behavior as with flexibility in work, attendance recording is normally used for blue-collar and manual labor occupations and some office workers in automated or data-entry jobs in which wages are calculated by the hour and productivity is measured by quantitative standards or on a group basis. The implicit assumption is that without close tracking, the worker would not reliably show up to do the work and would abuse sick leave.

Absence recording, on the other hand, is usual for professional, white-collar, and most office workers who are paid on a salary basis and whose productivity is judged primarily by standards of individual performance. At higher levels of responsibility, the freedom to take time off whenever one's schedule permits is tantamount to an executive perquisite, but the socialization process of executives is such that while the option is provided, it is not expected to be used, let alone abused.

Absence is usually measured in terms of days, since this is the most convenient and universal unit to record. There are other measurements, however. Hours or shifts lost both reflect loss of productivity more directly, although it should be kept in mind that presence at the worksite may represent the opportunity to be productive better than actual productivity. For example, a worker in an academic or creative field may find inspiration at any time on or off the job and may spend relatively little time actually producing a tangible product but that product may have high value, while an office worker with ambiguous or poorly defined responsibilities in a large and complex organization may sit at a desk daily for years with no substantial output. For most jobs, however, time put into the task bears some relationship to productivity.

The frequency of "spells" (the term of art used in the older literature), or identifiable episodes of absence, may reveal a pattern suggestive of a medical cause. For example, binge drinkers not uncommonly lose a day or so preceding or following weekends or holidays. Their pattern of absence may be frequent but not necessarily excessive in terms of lost days. The severity of the problem may not be reflected in the numerical count of lost work days. An individual with a severe, chronic illness may lose many days, but only have a few episodes of illness per year.

Once counted, absences can be compared and monitored by the calculation of summary measures, each with their own limitations:

- Frequency rates reflect the number of episodes of absence per year, for a person or the average for a group; they may include all episodes of absence, short-term absence only, or only absence lasting more than a few days depending on the purpose for which the statistic will be used.

- Severity rates are based on the number of days (or shifts or hours) lost per year, either for an individual worker or the average for a group; these are sometimes expressed as the percentage of total working time lost due to absence.

- Prevalence rates are calculations of the percentage of employees absent on a particular day; unlike the other two types of measurements, prevalence rates cannot be calculated for individuals and are not meaningful beyond one point in time, but they are useful in making estimates or evaluations of manpower needs and are commonly used in departments of human resources. (A common benchmark for general industry is 2 to 3 percent.)

In practice, employers who track absence use many different systems to calculate and to express absence, and there is little consistency among companies or between private corporations and public agencies except for the crude measurement of days lost. Comparisons among organizations are difficult, and no absolute standards exist by which to compare an employee's experience with others in their industry or community. One should not confuse measures of absence with epidemiologic measures of the frequency of illness such as morbidity, incidence, point prevalence, and period prevalence, each of which has precisely defined meanings. Absence measurement is just that and cannot be readily converted into measurements of morbidity without additional information, which are rarely available in practice.

Absence rates vary greatly from place to place, employer to employer, industry to industry, and with socioeconomic factors such as the state of the economy and available sick leave benefits. There is no generally accepted "normal" absence rate that can be used as a standard of comparison. In general, however, absence rates have slowly risen over the last thirty years; this is true throughout the developed world.

Absence can be categorized in many ways, but the most satisfactory, simple system recognizes five basic categories:

- Sickness absence, defined as absence attributed to incapacity due to illness or injury that is not work related.
- Personal leave, defined as absence for personal reasons having nothing directly to do with incapacity.
- "Time-lost" occupational injuries or, much less commonly, illnesses. By definition, these are reportable under workers' compensation and are therefore closely monitored.
- Pregnancy and child-care leave. By its nature, this is planned and preauthorized under the employer's policy, which is regulated by the Family and Medical Leave Act in the United States.
- Leave to care for a dependent.

- Bereavement.
- Partial absence (late arrival, early departure, temporary absence).

Each of these has further subcategories and nuances of measurement, as suggested in Table 18.5. Sickness absence and personal leave will be discussed in greater detail. These categories are useful on an aggregate basis for administrative purposes, in keeping track of reasons for absence. It is not appropriate to track these patterns for individuals.

A further problem with monitoring absence is that it is often to the worker's or the employer's benefit to misclassify absence. A worker may call in sick rather than take allowed vacation time in

Table 18.5. Classification of Absence

- Sickness absence (up to maximum allowed by sick leave policy)
  - Certified (by physician)
  - Uncertified (up to 3–5 days usually permitted), or "self-certified"
  - Prior authorization (e.g., for a physician's appointment)
- Personal leave (with or without pay, with or without authorization)
  - Personal business
  - Family illness
  - Bereavement
  - Jury duty
- Occupational injuries and illness ("time lost")
- Family and medical leave
  - Antenatal and confinement
  - Postpartum and early child care
  - Paternal
  - Medical problem in family
  - Self-care
  - Care of dependent adult
- Partial absence
  - Late arrival
  - Early departure
  - Prolonged absence from post

order to preserve paid sick leave or to take the day at a more convenient or spontaneous time. An employer may count a real illness that is inadequately documented against an employee's vacation time in order to avoid paying wages for the time off. Abuses of the system occur in every industry and in almost every workplace; a perfect system has yet to be devised.

The primary classification problem from the point of view of industry is differentiating sickness absence from unauthorized personal leave. This is typically done by requiring a physician's "certification" of the illness, as discussed in the previous section. Certification is intended to be a check on the employee's declaration of illness, but leads to its own problems and complications.

Historically, women are absent from work, on average, at about twice the rate of men if pregnancy is not counted. The reason is not that women use health services more often than men, although this is true, but that women generally have had greater domestic responsibilities and have been more likely to be employed in lower-status occupations in which time keeping is rigidly enforced and hours are inflexible. Women do not seem to have more severe illnesses on average than men and are less likely to work in hazardous occupations.

Smokers are, in general, absent more often with minor illnesses than nonsmokers. Abusers of alcohol not infrequently are absent sporadically, often on days following weekends and holidays and often without communication or notice. Despite these general trends, there is no accurate way of predicting absence for individual workers. Those with chronic illnesses are not uncommonly among the most reliable because they are committed and have learned to adapt. Normal, healthy workers may be absent for reasons having little to do with health or other characteristics that can be assessed in advance. The only predictor of absence in the individual case is the worker's individual history of absence. Even then, a person's pattern can often change, either for the better or for the worse.

Control of absence has been a major challenge to human resource managers in all industries. Few universally successful strategies have been identified, but a few observations have emerged. Personal leave, including unauthorized personal leave masquerading as sickness absence, may be reduced by introducing flexible hours or permitting a certain number of days off per month or year to attend to personal business, subject to prior notification. This reduces the disruption caused by the need to attend to pressing personal errands or appointments during regular working hours and reduces the incentive to claim paid sick days. Institution of a sensible sick leave policy removes abuses engendered by the desire of some workers to "get back" what they may feel is owed them. A policy of requiring medical certification only after three days absence, as long as the worker phones to inform the supervisor daily, shows some degree of trust while minimizing the opportunity for flagrant abuse. The most effective control measure, however, seems to be an overall improvement in attitude and relations between labor and management. Absence is often affected by personal attitudes toward the employer, personal identification with the performance work and objectives of the group, and personal attitudes of self-respect. A general sense of personal satisfaction and of identification with the success and objectives of the employer may remove the temptation for abuse while motivating workers who are only somewhat inconvenienced by minor complaints to come to work.

Absence is determined in some part by attitude. Persons who have similar levels of illness and discomfort may vary considerably in their adoption of "sick" behavior, with one stoically carrying on and another taking to bed. Some of this difference is cultural, some is due to family attitudes and upbringing, and some is due to circumstances such as other stresses in the worker's life and individual patterns of strength and weakness. There are always a few individuals in any large group who are immature and who seize on any inconvenience as an excuse to avoid work; such people are a small minority, however. The majority see work as a responsibility to be met with varying degrees of commitment and use their working environment as an opportunity to make friends, to engage in social interaction, and to develop a social support system. Such workers may even come to work when they should stay home, out of identification with their group.

Finally, the alert physician whether in a corporate setting or in community-based practice, may spot a pattern in absence from work that leads to the identification of a health problem. One should be particularly alert to the following:

- Alcohol or substance abuse
- Depression
- Incomplete recovery, followed by subsequent absence or re-injury
- Covert illness, such as dementia, associated with inability to do or sustain the work
- Stress and emotional distress, whether personal or job-related, as in the case of "burnout"
- Abuse of sick leave, which may predict poor compliance or lack of cooperation

Control of absence is not a medical responsibility. Ultimately it is a performance issue that must be dealt with by human resources. The physician should never be placed in a position of monitoring absence or of being the "police" for attendance on the part of worker. Adopting this function puts the physician in an adversarial relationship with workers and interferes fatally with the worker's perception of the physician's perceived objectivity and fairness. The physician can, however, support the worker with a health issue and point the way to a reasonable solution.

The occupational physician can play a constructive role in evaluating individuals with repeated, unexplained, or suspicious absences for health problems that may require treatment, work modification, or close monitoring at work. Repeated spells of absence should be considered as possible indicators of a serious health problem. In cases in which repeated absence or failing performance indicates a problem, the physician may play a positive role by detecting the health problem before its effects are irreversible, before it interferes with the life and well-being of the employee and deprives the employer of a valuable worker.

FUNCTIONAL CAPACITY EVALUATION

"Functional capacity evaluation" (or "assessment," sometimes called "physical capacities evaluation") is a comprehensive approach that arose in the 1980s from vocational and occupational rehabilitation and which incorporates insights from biomechanics, kinesiology, and exercise physiology. A typical functional capacity evaluation would test up to twenty different physical characteristics (such as the maximal strength of a worker, flexibility, agility, stamina, range of motion, hand-eye coordination, and so forth) and compare them against norms for the population and requirements of the assigned job. The objective is usually to profile the entire range of capabilities of a new applicant or of an injured worker before return to work.

Functional capacity evaluations have their highest application in assessing the maximal performance characteristics of the body. This makes the approach useful in situations in which it is useful to measure peak performance, such as athletics, military training, mine rescue, or research, or in public safety occupations in which peak or strained performance must be sustained in extreme conditions, most obviously firefighting. It could also be useful in determining what a person with multiple or interacting impairments can do, regardless of job assignment.

Work capacity varies greatly from person to person. The objective of functional capacity evaluation is to determine how much a person can do. The requirements of the job, however, are consistent for everyone, both in principle and in law under ADA. The capacity to do more than is required for the job is actually irrelevant to work performance and to fair selection under ADA. It would therefore be discriminatory to exclude one applicant from a job assignment just because another applicant could do more, when both could do the job quite adequately.

Functional capacity evaluations have many pitfalls. Because proprietary functional capacity evaluations are comprehensive protocols, not job-specific simulations, they generate a lot of data that are irrelevant to the employment relationship and which employers collect at considerable risk, because they must then be able to demonstrate that although it was collected, most of the data were not in fact used in making decisions about employment and job assignment. EEOC (which interprets ADA) would almost certainly consider it a violation if an applicant were excluded on the basis of a modality that could not be demonstrated to be directly relevant to a specific job requirement or excluded solely on the basis of poor performance on any modality compared to population norms rather than some validated performance standard.

Some employers have sought to get around ADA by using functional capacity evaluation as a screening tool to demonstrate ability to do the work before a job offer is made. This is possible because under ADA, as interpreted by the EEOC, a test of job-related skill, such as agility, was not a "medical inquiry" or "medical examination." However, the inclusion of any test that monitored the worker-applicant's response to the job-related activity, such as blood pressure determination after exertion, or the use of medical equipment made the entire process a "pre-offer" medical examination in violation of ADA. This is a particularly risky skirting of the law if the person conducting or interpreting the test is a health professional.

If a functional capacity evaluation is required as a post-offer evaluation, they may replace or supplement a medical examination, but the same problem of relevance applies. If modalities of the test are not directly related to the requirements of the job and do not reflect a legitimate business interest, then they should not be taken into consideration. This makes most of the functional capacity evaluation a rather expensive irrelevancy.

The physical measurements of a functional capacity evaluation are made in order to ensure a match between the capacity of the worker and the job requirements. Many tests of physical capacity are not necessary for a particular job, and therefore exclusion of an applicant based on inadequate performance on those irrelevant measurements in a functional capacity evaluation would be in violation of ADA. Most jobs in the modern economy do not require such finely tuned matching in any case. The most practical way to tell if a worker can do the job is simply to have him or her do it.

Another problem is the limited duration of functional capacity evaluations. Many work requirements show training effects: increased skill, improved hand-eye coordination, muscle strength. Evaluating a modality in one sitting cannot capture the training effect. Single-session tests are also irrelevant to the risk of repetitive movement.

Notwithstanding their many limitations, comprehensive functional capacity evaluation may be useful in certain specific applications:

- To evaluate ability and maximal effort in sports medicine, and to document training effects
- To evaluate the capabilities of a patient with severe, multiple, or subtle impairment (for example after recovering from multiple trauma or brain injury) to determine what they can do physically
- To validate a level of impairment where there are many inter-related factors involved
- To resolve a dispute over degree of impairment in which more than one body part and modality are involved
- To evaluate capacity to function under extreme conditions in the military.

When the term "functional capacity testing" is used today by a naïve speaker, he or she often really means impairment assessment.

IMPAIRMENT AND DISABILITY ASSESSMENT

"Impairment assessment" is a medical determination and quantification of the loss of function that limits the activities of a disabled person. Disability is a determination based in part on the impairment assessment that interprets the implications of the impairment for participation in activities of life and work. Disability reflects not only the degree of mental and physical impairment but employability, loss of future income, education, retraining prospects, and the job market.

Impairment is the complement of functional capacity. "Impairment assessment" focuses on identifying and quantifying deficiencies in function as objectively as possible. If functional capacity evaluation, as an ideal, would describe everything that a person can do, impairment assessment as an ideal would describe in precise terms what a person cannot do that they normally should be able to do. Impairment assessment also measures the degree to which a person falls short of a standard, which may be either the population norm, their personal baseline, or what is required for a specific task. The measurement can be translated into a "rating" (in workers' compensation terminology) that can be used to compare apples and oranges: degrees of impairment of the one part of the body with an unlike other part, such as hands compared to the brain. This rating has applications in disability evaluation and compensation.

Impairment assessment is most heavily used in workers' compensation and disability programs, and the vocabulary of impairment assessment reflects its origins. However, impairment assessment has more general utility than is commonly recognized. For example, it could be used more than it is now to guide accommodation, to quantify the gap between the level of function that is required and the level of function possible, in personal injury cases to quantify damages, and to study the patterns by level of disability in populations.

When complete objectivity is not achievable, impairment assessment seeks to be at least consistent. Many contributing factors to impairment are not objectively quantifiable, including pain, shortness of breath, and fatigue. Others may be measurable, but the scale may not reflect functionality: for example, the last few degrees of range of motion of the thumb are much more important to the functionality of grip incrementally than the sweep of the range up to the end.

The objective of impairment assessment is to determine what the person cannot do and to measure the deviation from "normal" or intact function or decrements from the pre-existing situation when there was already an impairment in the first place. The impairment evaluation is then used in workers' compensation of "disability evaluation" to take the next step of matching the impairment against requirements of the job. This comparison leads to a determination of disability. Disability, however, is a term that applies to the implications of the impairment for activities of living, social functioning, earning an income, and pursuing one's usual occupation. It is a description of the effect of impairment, determined by a complex derivation that takes more factors into account than impairment.

The comparison or standard against which function is compared can be the person's own baseline (which is usually not documented before an injury), normal physiology, norms statistically derived from large populations (in which case the selection of the reference population becomes an issue), or functional requirements of universally required activities of daily living (benchmarked against a threshold for disability and a gradation of increasing significance with progressive loss of function). Ideally, the two most useful standards would be loss of function compared to the individual's own baseline, which would provide an indication of compensable loss, and the threshold for disability, which would establish the significance of impairment. In practice, impairment is usually measured against normal physiology by the use of guidelines, of which the most important are the *AMA Guidelines for the Evaluation of Permanent Impairment* for workers' compensation and *Disability Evaluation Under Social Security* (the "Blue Book") for the Social Security Administration. (There is no counterpart for the Canada Pension Plan.)

Definitions and Concepts

Definitions are not settled for three essential terms: impairment, disability, and handicap. In general, in North America, "impairment" means a physical or mental limitation on activity, "disability" means the implications of the impairment to the degree that it interferes with social expectations and employment, and "handicap" refers to the gap between what the person can do and what is required.

Different systems within different countries use the same words differently, and it is important to understand what is actually meant, because there is a tension between two opposing points of view. On the one hand is the view, which underlies ADA, that impairment is a characteristic of the person, subject to mitigation by medical means or rehabilitation, and that the disability is that which remains after treatment and rehabilitation and which defines that person's interaction with the world. On the other hand is the view adopted by most other economically developed countries that impairment and disability primarily reflect barriers to participating in work, social, and family life, and that when a person cannot participate fully because of reduced physical or mental capacity, it is the barriers that should be lowered. This is reflected in a set of subsidiary definitions worked out by the World Health Organization (WHO), which holds that impairments, disability or activity limitations, and barriers to participation are all dimensions of the interaction between the body and the environment, including the social environment: "Impairments are interactions affecting the body; activity limitations are interactions affecting individual's actions or behavior; participation restrictions are interactions affecting person's experience of life."

There are many formal definitions of impairment, the most important of which derive from the disability movement (especially arising out of the United Nations Decade of Disabled Persons, 1983–1992), WHO (especially the International Classification of Functioning, Disabilities and Health, 2001, known as ICF), imputed definitions implicit in ADA (and the earlier Rehabilitation Act of 1973), the Social Security Administration, Canada Pension Plan, state and provincial workers' compensation acts, and in various authoritative guides such as the *AMA Guides to the Evaluation of Permanent Impairment*. The United Nations Decade of Disabled Persons adopted definitions of impairment, disability, and handicap in 1983 that have proven very influential: Impairment is "any loss or abnormality of psychological, or anatomical structure or function. An impairment [is] any loss or deviation of physiological, neurological or anatomical structure or function of an organ or body part (organ and body dimension), a physiological disorder or injury." ADA does not differentiate disability and impairment in functional terms but treats disability as arising from impairment and so implicitly defines it as a permanent derangement of function. Essentially all defining bodies agree but do not make explicit in their definitions that certain "normal" states that may impose limits for a period are not true impairments, for example, pregnancy, childhood, and advanced age. A synthesis of the various definitions would yield something like the following: Impairment is a loss of capacity, arising from an abnormality in structure or a derangement in physiological function that is clearly identifiable as a deviation either from normal or from that person's own baseline and which imposes a new limit on activity.

A comparable definition of disability would take into account the implications for the person's social role. In the United States, disability is generally perceived as a characteristic that attaches to the person and differentiates them from "normal" society. In Canada, Europe, and the United Nations system, disability is a stage or quality of life, representing the interaction between the person and the physical and social environment. The older WHO definition (1980) was "a disability reflect[ing] any limitation or lack of ability that a person experiences in performing an activity in the manner or within the range considered normal for a person, in other words, a limitation in learning, speaking, walking or some other activity (individual dimension)." The current WHO definition of people with disabilities holds that "[p]ersons with disabilities include those who have long-term physical, mental, intellectual, or sensory impairments which in interaction with various barriers may hinder their full and effective participation in society on an equal basis with others." The United Nations adopted the Convention on the Rights of Persons with Disabilities in January 2009 and it is currently undergoing ratification by member states. In effect, it has redefined disability as arising from the environment, not from the person's capacity to function.

The ADA, on the other hand, does not distinguish between impairment and disability, which is a serious conceptual drawback of the legislation. The current (2008 amended) ADA definition of disability is "a physical or mental impairment that substantially limits one or more major life activities of such individual; a record of such an impairment; or being regarded as having such an impairment." A comparable synthetic definition, given that the American and the international views are very different, might therefore read something like "disability is reduced capacity, imposed by an impairment, to manage the barriers and challenges within society, the family, employment, or as required for the pursuit of employment prospects, such that the person is impeded in performing normal activities and duties and the normal activities of daily living (taking into account the person's age)."

"Handicap" is out of fashion as a term, and its meaning has been conflated with disability. This is unfortunate because historically the term means something quite different and useful. Handicap refers to a seventeenth-century game ("hand i' the cap") that involved placing bets against unequal odds; the term later was applied to horseracing and golf to refer to adjustment of the gap between unequal players. This is a very useful concept: It recognizes a differential between expectation and capacity to perform that, if remedied, gives all players equal opportunity. Use of the term as a synonym for disability came much later, at the beginning of the twentieth century. (The story that it refers to a beggar holding a "cap in hand" is not true.)

Most formal definitions of handicap, however, equate it with disability and therefore obscure an important distinction between functional impairment and its significance in the real world. The Disability Decade definition from 1983 was "Handicap [is a] disadvantage for a given individual, resulting from an impairment or disability, that limits or prevents the fulfillment of a role that is normal, depending on age, sex, social and cultural factors, for that individual." The WHO (1980) definition is "Handicap [is] loss or limitation of opportunities to take part in the life of the community on an equal level with others; encounter a person with disability and social, physical environment...an inability to accomplish something one might want to do. The term emphasizes the focus on shortcomings in the environment and in many tasks and activities, [for example: in] education, occupation, information or communication (social dimension)." It would be very useful to go back to the older definition, perhaps as follows: A handicap is a quantification or description of the gap between real and expected performance or between capacity and requirements to perform activities important to social, family, and employment roles and activities of daily life. A handicap can be overcome by accommodations or adaptations that bridge the gap.

Impairment can be temporary or permanent. In workers' compensation, impairment is not assessed until it is permanent (common term of art are "at permanence" or "maximum medical improvement," which is abbreviated MMI). American usage of "impairment" and "disability" assumes that the condition is permanent, as does ADA, so the terms "temporary impairment" and "temporary disability" are rarely seen. International usage makes no such assumption and considers that anyone may pass through periods of temporary impairment or disability, if only and preferably through advancing age, and that every living person has at a minimum experienced the dependency of infancy. International, and especially European, usage therefore recognizes "temporary disability" as a life stage and uses the term much more often.

It often happens that a person has a pre-existing condition that may be asymptomatic, symptomatic but not to a level of impairment, or stable at some level of impairment. A common example is asthma. When a work-related factor (an injury or exposure) makes the asymptomatic condition temporarily symptomatic or makes the symptomatic condition temporarily worse, this is called "exacerbation." If a worker with pre-existing asthma encounters a trigger at work (such as an allergen or heavy dust), he or she may experience an exacerbation of asthma, with bronchospasm, cough and other evidence of airway inflammation lasting for days or at most a few weeks. If a worker with pre-existing asthma encounters an exposure that decompensates the disorder and leads to a permanent change in level of function, this is called an "aggravation." If a worker with preexisting asthma encounters an irritating chemical exposure, the worker may experience a more severe worsening of the condition and symptoms that might lead to a permanent condition with worsened symptoms. This would move the disorder to a new baseline of reduced function. This could be classified as a "second injury." The difference in impairment and disability between exacerbation and aggravation is that the former is temporary and the latter is permanent, but the medical difference is that exacerbation is a short-term perturbation in a stable condition and aggravation destabilizes the condition and moves it to a new and unfavorable level. A second injury would be a more discreet event that added new impairment to the existing impairment.

In Canada, for a person to qualify for Canada Pension Plan (CPP) disability benefits, the impairment must cause a disability that is "severe" (meaning the person is incapable, in the sense of not fit or able, of pursuing, in the sense of actively working in, any "substantial gainful employment," not just the former job) and "prolonged" (of indefinite duration and likely to keep the claimant from work for at least twelve months). This is different from most other social insurance systems, in that to qualify the applicant cannot be capable of any work for which he or she is otherwise suited, but the disability does not have to be permanent. Benefits are "all or nothing" (i.e., no partial benefits) and not tied to financial need, because the amount is based on contributions to the system. As a consequence, the process required for CPP is streamlined and focused on reviewing the medical information provided by the physician rather than having the physician conduct an impairment assessment.

Impairment Assessment Outside Workers' Compensation

The OEM physician is often called upon, because of skills developed in workers' compensation cases, to evaluate impairment for other benefit or insurance programs, which provide income replacement after disability that does not arise from work. These programs may have a complicated relationship with workers' compensation in individual cases. Such programs include the following:

- Social Security Administration (SSA) disability insurance
- Canada Pension Plan (CPP) disability benefits
- State temporary disability plans
- Long-term disability insurance

SSA and CPP are social insurance programs designed to prevent catastrophic loss of income. They require demonstration of eligibility, applying a set of criteria that assess whether the applicant is working; if not, whether the applicant has the capacity to perform the activities required to work; if so, at what level; and given that level whether employment is likely to be available. SSA and CPP determinations are highly individualized, taking into account age, education, training prospects, and the local job market for any jobs (not the applicant's previous job). Thus, the outcome may be very different for two applicants with identical impairments. Social insurance programs are predicated on employability and therefore recognize disability as present or absent, not rated by degrees of impairment, as in workers' compensation. Social insurance programs assume that the disability is long term, if not permanent, but require periodic re-evaluation to determine whether there has been improvement and if so whether the recipient's functional status is such that benefits can be terminated.

Some states, such as California, provide temporary disability benefits. They are designed to support the income a person may lose because of either a period of illness or recovery from an injury that is not work related.

Long-term disability insurance (LTD) is commercial insurance against permanent disability that does not arise from work. LTD usually is based on incapacity to work, either at the worker's usual occupation or at any occupation. Policies are increasingly stipulating the latter and must be read carefully to determine eligibility criteria.

These programs exclude disability arising from work-related injury or illness. They are therefore, in a sense, complementary to workers' compensation, and between the two a disabled individual with significant limitations should be covered. The reality, however, is that the systems do not coordinate well. An LTD carrier may determine that an injury was work related after it is denied by workers' compensation, or the reverse. When this occurs, the injured person may face a considerable struggle.

Assessing Impairment in Workers' Compensation

All OEM physicians, however, will at some time evaluate patients in one or more workers' compensation system, so the workers' compensation system will be emphasized in this subsection. Most workers' compensations use or at least acknowledge the authority of the *AMA Guides to the Evaluation of Permanent Impairment* (*AMA Guides*), and so frequent reference will be made to that resource. Some states, notably California, use their own guidelines, but a recent evaluation of the California guides showed that it performed less well that the *AMA Guides* in consistency of use and precision. As the *AMA Guides* improve since the sixth edition, it is likely that states will fall into line in recognizing its authority.

A key threshold in the spectrum of disability and therefore the source of important benchmarks in impairment assessment is the capacity to perform "activities of daily living" (ADLs). ADLs have been defined and delineated mostly through research in nursing and occupational therapy, and there are numerous evaluation scales and instruments. Basic ADLs include bathing, dressing and undressing, eating, transferring from bed to chair and back, continence, using a toilet, and walking. Obviously losing the capacity to do any one of these is profoundly disabling. Instrumental ADLs are a higher level of functioning associated with independent living, including light housekeeping, preparing meals, using a telephone, managing individual transactions involving money and counting change, shopping, and taking medication. A higher level of activities are more directly related to work capacity and involve the capacity to communicate, mobility in the community, a broader spectrum of physical activity, sensory functions, general use of the hand, and other functions. It is this level that the *AMA Guides* addresses.

Ideally, functional loss would be correlated with an objective, ergonomic standard for the ability to participate in life and work activities. For example, the grip strength required in the thumb might be correlated to the minimum required to take care of oneself and to do different types of work. However, that degree of accuracy is unachievable in practice. It is less important that impairment evaluation be accurate than that it be precise, that is reproducible and consistent. (See Chapter 4 for a discussion of the difference between accuracy and precision.) References such as the *AMA Guides* are arbitrary in the sense of the choices that are made for representing impairment but represent a reasonable consensus by which different cases can be evaluated on the same scale and with consistency.

Impairment assessment for workers' compensation is based on "anatomic loss," which is reflected in structural derangement (often called "deviation" in this context) and "functional loss." Although anatomic loss also involves loss of the function of that body part, the term "functional loss" here means a derangement that affects physiological function rather than the physical integrity of the body. An anatomic loss might be a reduced range of motion for the thumb or abduction at the shoulder and underlies assessment of the musculoskeletal system, which is the most commonly evaluated system because injuries are more numerous than diseases. A functional loss might be reduced pulmonary function or impaired sensation as with a neuropathy. Certain types of functional loss are much more difficult to assess, particularly pain (subjective) and asthma (episodic, with many symptoms, such as cough, that are transient and not easily measured). (The term "function" is used from this point on in its usual meaning.)

The tests that are used to measure impairment are mostly the standard, noninvasive tools of medicine. Some special devices have been invented for the purpose of impairment assessment but have not achieved widespread use. For example, an "inclinometer," which acted much like a carpenter's level to measure angles from horizontal, was recommended by the *AMA Guides* for a time. However, the familiar but less exact goniometer was always more commonly used.

The theory of impairment assessment, as applied in the *AMA Guides,* rests on the notion of the "whole person" (formerly "total person"), defined as having no impairment (no structural or functional derangement) and no limitations on activities of daily living or employment. This ideal person is given a rating of 0 percent impairment of the whole person. "Total impairment" refers to an individual with 100 percent impairment of the whole person who is not dead but is impaired to the point of being unable to perform basic activities required of work and daily living. Total impairment may arise from one major impairment, such as cognitive dysfunction due to brain damage, or to the aggregate effects of many partial impairments. Between the two extremes of 0 and 100 percent impairment of the whole person is a spectrum of "partial impairment."

Partial impairment is rated on the basis of percentage points reflecting loss of function. Most "organ system" or systemic categories of impairment are rated directly as percentage impairment of the whole person, often by classes of impairment. The system for respiratory disorders, for example, reflects a range within classes of impairment based on criteria for pulmonary function tests, developed by the American Thoracic Society. The system for cardiovascular disease includes a range of impairment within the functional classes defined by the American Heart Association.

The system is slightly different for the musculoskeletal system, which is anatomically based. Each body part is assigned a nominal percentage of the whole person. For example, an upper extremity is deemed to be 60 percent of the whole person, which is not unreasonable when one considers how difficult it is to participate in the activities of life and work with only one arm but at the same time how one might be able to adjust. The loss of function is then assigned a percentage specific to that body part. For example, if the upper extremity could not be used through atrophy or ankylosis, the loss of function for the upper extremity would be 100 percent. Another impairment of the shoulder might result in 50 percent impairment of the upper extremity. An impairment of the hand and wrist might result in 30 percent impairment. These impairments of the body part are then applied to the percentage of the whole person in order to derive the percentages of the whole body. In the example given of the upper extremity, which is 60 percent of the whole person, a 50 percent impairment of the upper extremity would yield 30 percent impairment of the whole person, and 30 percent impairment of the upper extremity would yield 18 percent impairment of the whole person.

There are often multiple impairments, either of different measurements on the same body part (such as strength and range of motion) or different body parts (such as the upper extremity and the lower extremity). Because 100 percent is an upper bound of impairment of the whole person and because multiple impairments tend to reduce to a more general pattern of impairment, they cannot be simply added. The *AMA Guides* uses a "combining table" that combines the values without adding them arithmetically. For example, the 18 percent impairment of the upper extremity combined with a 30 percent disability would yield a disability of 43 percent, still high but not as high as 48 percent.

"Second injuries" are subsequent injuries after the first to the same body part that lead to cumulative impairment. The principle is to measure the impairment after the second injury is at permanence and then subtract the impairment that was documented from the first injury. The difference is the impairment attributable to the second injury. Second injuries have important implications for compensation management.

The individual protocols place appropriately greater weight on functional limitation than on anatomic derangement. For example, the impairment ratings for the thumb are not linear over adduction, that is, across the entire sweep of the thumb over the palm. The rating goes up exponentially as the thumb approaches neutral position. This is because the thumb is needed to grip, and this function is much more important than full adduction.

The *AMA Guides* place great weight on activities and functions that are important in activities of life and work. They address that part of the spectrum of impairment that reflects the capacity to do work and are therefore most useful at lower levels of impairment. Other instruments would be needed to evaluate degrees of severe disability, for example for nursing or assisted-care services.

The *AMA Guides* have gone through many editions. Many states require the most current edition (currently the sixth), but some states require the fourth because the fifth was widely perceived as a failed product and inter-rater reliability was poor. The sixth edition has moved strongly in the direction of compatibility with the ICF and incorporation of modern insights into functional capacity and is also easier to use. The *AMA Guides* are still complicated and require training to use.

Two organizations provide comprehensive training in impairment assessment and use of the *AMA Guides*. The American Academy of Disability Evaluating Physicians (AADEP) is a membership organization, consisting of a variety of specialists, that offers comprehensive training in the form of continuing education and certifies practitioners by examination (Certification of Evaluation in Disability and Impairment Rating, CEDIR). AADEP is particularly strong in Texas, where the state workers' compensation system uses a "designated doctor" system of referrals for impairment assessment and has relied on AADEP training. The American Board of Independent Medical Examiners (ABIME) is organized as an autonomous body providing training courses in all aspects of independent medical evaluation but emphasizing impairment assessment. It certifies practitioners by examination for its own credential (Certified Independent Medical Examiner, CIME). (ABIME is not a medical specialty board recognized by the American Board of Medical Specialties.) ABIME may be more widely recognized, has made inroads in some other countries, and is more prominent in occupational medicine. AADEP and ABIME have certified comparable numbers of physicians and are equally respected. In Canada, the Canadian Society of Medical Evaluators is a membership organization that certifies on the basis of submitted examples of impairment assessments.

ACCOMMODATION

Returning to the early, still useful definition of handicap, bridging the gap between what a disabled person can do and what is required can be viewed either as equipping the worker to make up for a limitation in function or lowering the barriers to allow participation in an activity. The means to do this is "accommodation," which is simply working out a plan or modification that allows a worker with a disability to do the work.

As the working population ages, accommodation may become less a specific intervention for a person with disabilities than a factor in workplace design for safety and productivity for all workers. Accommodation, by definition, is specific to the individual. Every disabled person's disability is unique to their own combination of work capacity, skills, impairment, and personal adaptations to the impairment. However, many disabled persons have similar needs, and tools, workplaces, and equipment can be designed in the first instance to accommodate workers with or without disabilities. This concept of "universal design" has become increasingly influential in design and engineering as it has become apparent that many accommodations for disabled persons are also easier and more efficient for persons without disabilities. Good ergonomic design, which is at the root of universal design, also reduces injury risk. For example, scissors are particularly difficult for people with hand disabilities or arthritis to use. Scissors designed with flared handles and with the blades at an angle to the handle instead of straight are much easier to use for workers who are disabled but also for those who are not, and these designs greatly reduce fatigue with repeated use. They are also likely to reduce the risk of repetitive strain injury. Universal design may make accommodation unnecessary for many, perhaps most, situations in which it would otherwise be required while at the same time allowing greater productivity and reducing barriers to employment as workers age.

"Accommodation" is a term that predated ADA, but its meaning as a means to bridge the gap between disability and job requirements has been redefined and fixed by ADA, which requires "reasonable accommodation" to a qualified person with a disability in order to meet the essential requirements of the job. Accommodation is usually considered in the context of new hires and qualified applicants for the job assignment. Accommodation may also be required for return to work (RTW), when a recovering injured worker returns to modified duty, either in job-related activities or shorter working hours. In this context, most modified duty for RTW is temporary and bridges the gap created by temporary impairment. Sometimes, however, a worker who has a new permanent impairment will require a permanent accommodation.

An accommodation may be any of the following:

- An assistive device, such as large screen for the vision impaired, an amplification system for the hearing impaired, or ergonomic tools that are easier to grasp and use (particularly scissors)
- Companion animals, specifically guide dogs for the blind, which would be considered an accommodation modifying a policy against pets at work because guide dogs are not kept as pets
- Workplace modification, such as a wheelchair-friendly workstation or enhanced illumination
- Rebalancing job assignments so that the person with the disability can do those parts within their capacity and other workers can do the rest
- Restructuring work organization so that medical and rehabilitation appointments can be kept without disruption, responsive leave policies, and modified work hours, if needed
- Modification of equipment, such as ergonomic adaptations and interventions for persons who do not have full use of their hands
- Removing barriers to access to the workplace, such as reserved parking spaces for the disabled or use of a different entry point
- Removing barriers to access at the workplace, such as placing files in lower drawers for easier access to persons in wheelchairs,

providing Braille labels beside elevator buttons, or ensuring that there are no barriers to washrooms

- Adjustment of examinations and evaluations, as for a worker with a cognitive impairment who may require more time to finish a test (but a timed test might be acceptable if it addresses a specific work requirement, for example, the ability to read and act on messages rapidly, and is given to all applicants)

- Training materials and policies for co-workers to help them understand the implications of disability

- A dedicated assistant, such as an amanuensis to take dictation for a worker who cannot physically write, a sign-language interpreter for a worker who is deaf, a page-turner for someone who cannot use their hands, a travel assistant for required business trips, or a reader for a worker who is blind

- Communications devices, such as Text Telephone (TTY) and Braille devices

"Reassignment to a vacant position" is an accommodation mentioned in ADA that would apply to current employees. Reassignment to another, vacant position should not be considered unless it has not been possible to make a reasonable accommodation to the employee. The new position should be equivalent in terms of responsibility, pay, and status if at all possible. An employer is allowed to reassign a worker with a disability to a lower-status position if accommodation would impose an undue hardship, but this is likely to cause problems and to raise suspicion that it is being done to encourage the worker to leave (as a form of "constructive dismissal"). Legal guidance from an expert on ADA and employment law is advised for any employer considering this option.

Facilities for employees, such as health centers, cafeterias, lounges, and fitness centers also fall under ADA, and similar accommodations are required to allow persons with disability to use the facilities.

Employers are not required under ADA to supply medical or prosthetic devices that are required for activities of daily living. For example, employers would not be expected to provide eyeglasses for a person with vision impairment, unless they were somehow specific to requirements of the work. Employers are not expected to provide amenities (such as air fresheners), conveniences (such as an office refrigerator), or personal products (such as tissues) that are not provided to employees without disabilities.

ADA requires reasonable accommodation, defining "reasonable" as that which does not cause undue hardship. "Undue hardship" might include excessive cost, an investment disproportionate to the size of the facility and the number of people working there, or one causing detrimental impact on operations at the facility. An employer should consider alternative reasonable accommodations before concluding that an accommodation would impose an undue hardship; an accommodation does not have to be ideal.

The best accommodations are simple and sustainable and are designed in partnership with the employee, who is the best expert on his or her specific disability. Most accommodations under ADA cost little or nothing. It costs little to reassign work. Whenever possible, commercial "off-the-shelf solutions" are preferred because they are less expensive than custom-built devices and are supported by the manufacturer. Tailored, jerry-rigged, or custom solutions are more likely to be expensive, take more effort to design, are less likely to be successful, and quite possibly may cause hard feelings if they fail after the effort has been expended in good faith.

Most employers do not object to minor modifications in the workplace, but they often do not know how to make these modifications. Fortunately employers in the United States and Canada have access to assistance in the form of the Job Accommodation Network (JAN), a project of the President's Committee on Employment of the Handicapped. JAN is coordinated out of an office on the campus of West Virginia University that serves as a clearinghouse for ideas and suggestions regarding work modifications to accommodate the handicapped or the temporarily impaired. JAN has an extensive experience with workplace modifications, some of which are very simple to make and at low cost. They can be reached by calling 1-800-526-7234 (or 1-800-526-4698 inside West Virginia), a toll-free number. Their services are free of charge. Examples of the modifications they may recommend include use of a slightly different tool, a change in the seating arrangements, providing a different type of switching mechanism, a special chair, and installing lever handles rather than door knobs on doors for individuals who have trouble with grasp.

Accommodation requires recognition of the need by both employer and employee and cooperation between them to reach a practical, sustainable solution. Most employers are understandably reticent to raise the issue at the time of the job interview because it may be construed as a pre-employment medical inquiry, which is not allowed. Having the physician evaluate the need for accommodation as part of the pre-placement evaluation is the solution for applicants. For current workers, ADA allows employers to inquire about accommodations that may be needed if a problem is obvious and business related. Most large employers have policies that put the responsibility on the worker to request accommodation if it is needed. Sometimes workers may be reluctant to raise the issue with their immediate supervisor. The policy should state that the worker has the option of discussing accommodation with a representative of the employer's department of human resources.

DRUG SCREENING

Drug screening has become a major emphasis in occupational medicine in the United States. Not every OEM physician will be involved in drug screening, but all should understand it in principle because it is a common and critical service, particularly in certain important industries such as transportation.

Drug use is considered to be a voluntary form of work incapacity, one that has the potential to place the worker and others at risk, particularly when the worker is assigned to a "safety-sensitive" job, one in which incapacity may present a direct threat to the public or other workers. In the 1980s, there was also concern that high levels of drug use in the community were spilling over into the workplace, causing a serious risk to the public, encouraging drug abuse, and reducing national productivity. As a result, many employers introduced drug screening programs, and federal agencies began to require drug screening for safety-sensitive positions under federal jurisdiction. At first, there was great opposition to the institution of drug testing programs, on grounds of human rights, administrative complexity, legal liability, and ethical pitfalls. However, the initial high rates of screening appeared to validate the view that screening was necessary. Although detection rates are now much lower, drug screening is a permanent fixture of working life in many industries, particularly transportation, and has become driven by federal legislation, although many employers continue to be motivated by social attitudes regarding drug use among their employees.

Drug abuse follows regional trends. Drug use in the workplace was thought to be mostly an urban phenomenon when widespread drug screening began. Alcohol abuse is ubiquitous but is a particular problem in isolated and remote workplaces and in rural and far northern regions. For many years amphetamine usage occurred predominantly on the U.S. West Coast. However, the current methamphetamine epidemic in the American middle states and the rapid spread of heroin in rural areas has made the problem more geographically dispersed in North America. Drug abuse may have different implications in rural settings, for example, because of longer driving times, which increases the risk of motor vehicle incidents. Drug abuse also both reflects and contributes to local patterns of crime, domestic violence, mental health services, and outlets for more constructive community activity, especially for young people.

Drug screening is uncommon in Canada, except among subsidiaries of American companies, among oil companies, and by transportation companies that carry people and goods across the border into the United States, where they are subject to U.S. Department of Transportation regulations. In 1994, the Government of Canada decided not to pursue legislation empowering Canada Transport to require drug screening, as in the United States. Individual companies were free to establish their own programs within a set of guidelines established in 1988 by the Canadian Human Rights Commission, which requires that the testing be relevant to the essential requirements of the job (the term of art is "bona fide occupational requirement," BFOR), that there be a demonstrable need to ensure a drug-free workplace (safety being the obvious need), that testing meets that need, and that there be a system for referral and accommodation, such as an employee assistance program, for workers who test positive. There are also broad requirements for the protection of human rights and privacy. Random testing has been disallowed under case law, but testing on the basis of "reasonable grounds" for suspicion of impairment and pre-placement or pre-employment testing (ADA terminology does not necessarily apply in Canada, of course) have been upheld, with some exceptions. Few employers in the transportation sector have initiated drug screening programs, relying on the threat to drivers of criminal sanctions for operating vehicles while impaired. Employers that have drug screening programs incorporate alcohol by breath testing as well as drug screening in urine.

Medical Review Officer

The primary role of the physician in drug testing is documentation, so that the essential facts are recorded and the decision that is made will withstand scrutiny and future litigation. The U.S. Department of Transportation (DOT), by requiring urine drug testing for transportation workers, particularly commercial drivers, has created a demand for physicians with certified expertise in drug testing and interpretation. Positive screening tests must be confirmed and interpreted by a physician, the "medical review officer" (MRO); issues arising include cross-reactivity or confusion with prescription medication. Because of the potential for serious repercussions in the event of a false positive test, the system relies heavily on quality assurance mechanisms and certification of laboratories by the National Institute of Drug Abuse (NIDA). The system requires the MRO to contact the test-positive subject personally before reporting the result.

The knowledge and professional demeanor of the physician serving as MRO are critical, but the field is changing so rapidly that it is difficult to keep up as an individual without formal continuing education.

The preferred way for OEM physicians to prepare for service as an MRO is to take a two-day course offered twice yearly by the American College of Occupational and Environmental Medicine: the "Medical Review Officer Training Course." A formal certification examination is offered by the Medical Review Officer Certification Council, and independent, nonprofit certification body. The other major certification body is the American Academy of Medical Review Officers.

Although many occupational physicians perform MRO services as private consultants as part of their overall mix of services, it takes a great deal of organization and a high volume to base an entire practice on this service. The key is a committed system organized with employees who are extremely reliable in handling the paperwork. There have been several proposals to remove the requirement than an MRO be a physician, but DOT has kept this provision because of the need to have some professional accountability guaranteed and for a licensed practitioner to take responsibility in each case for medicolegal purposes.

In essence, drug testing as it is usually practiced is a structured forensic program for the detection of illegal drug use among current or potential employees. The tests are usually performed on urine for the detection of the five drugs identified by NIDA as the priority drugs of abuse among adults in the United States: opiates, cocaine, marijuana, amphetamines, and phencyclidine. Alcohol is conspicuous by its absence, but its use and even abuse in private is not against the law. When alcohol testing is performed at the discretion of the employer, it is by breath test with confirmation of positive results by blood test. The scheduling of such testing is typically on presentation for applying for a job and randomly thereafter among employees after hire, although few employers do routine alcohol testing. Semisynthetic opiates, such as oxycodone, are also absent, although they are common drugs of abuse. Discretionary testing by employers for these drugs does not seem to occur.

Most drug testing programs are set up in compliance with the mandatory programs required by the DOT and rely heavily on NIDA recommendations. In additions, employers may add their own discretionary programs, but these must be kept strictly separate from the federal programs, even to the point of using different urine samples. Drug testing must be handled carefully to prevent legal action for discrimination. Policies should be explicitly documented, and drug testing schedules (random or otherwise) should be equitable for all employees, not applied selectively or arbitrarily.

The initial emphasis in drug testing programs was punitive; the drug-using employee was an "offender" who got "caught." After several years of experience, the prevailing attitude has become more sympathetic to the employee, with an emphasis on early detection of a drug habit leading to referral to an employee assistance program (EAP, discussed in Chapter 19) and mandatory treatment. Some experts advise keeping mandatory treatment programs for drug test-positive employees separate (with separate records) from EAP services for employees in general, so as not to compromise or create a stigma for the EAP program.

Compliance with drug testing is made a condition of employment by the employer; refusal to test is insubordination and grounds for dismissal. Most employers provide EAP services and mandatory treatment for their drug test–positive employees once, and some provide a second chance; none tolerate repeated positive tests or accept positive tests among job applicants. Evidence that an employee has willfully tampered with a drug test is generally grounds for immediate dismissal.

The profile of the drug-using employee is not always predictable. Some high-producing employees have been demonstrated to get high on cocaine or methamphetamine, and a few managers have even managed impressive careers while on heroin.

The experience of drug testing programs has been changing. Rates of positive testing ran as high as 25 percent in some areas when testing was first introduced in the mid-1980s (which may also have reflected where they were first introduced). Rates now are typically around 1 percent (as they have been when attempted in Canada and in the U.S. military) or less. Conventional wisdom in the field is that "only stupid employees get caught," which is harsh but probably not far off.

Most employees who test positive eventually move on to other employers. It is said among some personnel managers that one effect of the program has also been to displace applications from drug-using job seekers away from employers that test and toward nearby employers that do not test. It is said that some employers that do not test have seen much more trouble with drug use among their new hires after major employers in the same community have instituted testing. As well, employers that require testing of employees of their subcontractors often find much higher rates of positive tests than among their own employees. Employers who have instituted drug testing often find that after the initial impact there are diminishing returns to committing further resources or intensifying the testing program. The deterrent effect of random testing seems to be early and all at once. The deterrent effect of pre-placement and nonrandom or openly announced drug testing is minimal, and it has been said, not altogether without cause, that these programs serve mainly to weed out the young, the confused, and the uncreative from the employer's workforce applicants.

Given the initial emphasis on the magnitude of the problem of drug use to the American economy, it is surprising that the institution of drug testing has had little or no effect on injury rates, health care costs, productivity, or other health or management outcomes.

Some OEM physicians find MRO work distasteful because it is intrusive into the private lives of workers. Others accept it as necessary in the public interest.

Technical Aspects of Drug Testing

Drug testing programs tend to parallel DOT regulations and the recommendations of NIDA, in part to provide a defensible position in the event of litigation.

The technical aspects of drug testing are complicated. Besides the laboratory procedures, which will not be dealt with in detail here, the procedures for obtaining the urine specimen (or "sample") and certifying that it has been guarded to prevent tampering are involved. One should always assume that the findings on the sample will be evidence in court.

Urine collection must be done in a highly structured manner, discouraging efforts to adulterate or dilute the sample. Collections are not usually observed directly unless the employee is being retested after a questionable initial sample that showed evidence of tampering; when this is necessary, it is usually done with mirrors in the toilet stall (and is no less distasteful to all concerned). A large underground business exists in drug-free urine and devices to deliver it into specimen jars while appearing to urinate. Since one effective means of lowering the probability of a positive test result by a subject who is borderline, having used drugs several days before, is to dilute the sample, it is important to prevent access to any source of water. Taping of the toilet tank and coloring of water in the toilet bowl by blue dye is standard practice. The temperature of the urine must be checked and must be within reasonable range of body temperature. The specific gravity is also checked for physiological plausibility.

The urine sample is split, and the second sample retained for retesting in the event of a legal need to do so. The sample, once obtained, must be kept in a strict "chain of custody" with supervision at every step and every transfer documented. In practice, this is accomplished by sealing the sample container, labeling it with a number (not with the employee's name), and following its path on a form in which anyone who handles it affixes his or her signature at the point of transfer. The actual procedure is spelled out in the paperwork at every step.

Testing of the sample is subject to the same factors of clinical epidemiology described in Chapter 5; modern drug testing techniques have high sensitivity and specificity and are usually performed in tandem. A positive radioimmunoassay, for example, will be followed by a combined analysis by gas chromatography and mass spectrometry

(GC/MS). This is expensive but necessary to provide accurate identification for legal purposes and to rule out cross-reactivity. For example, the Vicks® brand nasal inhaler contains the l-isomer of methamphetamine, which is not a psychoactive drug of abuse. Differentiating this from the illicit d-isomer required GC/MS until the introduction of monoclonal radioimmunoassay kits. Over-the-counter nasal decongestants that include ephedrine have also produced confusing cross-reactivity.

The technology of drug testing is increasingly sophisticated. A quantitative analysis may yield evidence of the presence of a drug; above a certain cutoff the test is considered positive. The cutoff is essentially zero detectable for most, but is usually set at 100 mg/l for cannabinoids (marijuana residues). Except for opiates, for which the quantity found is important in assessing the possibility of prescription medicine usage, laboratories report the test as positive or negative for the five drugs of concern.

Samples that are stored, even under refrigeration, may undergo degradation, and retesting may not replicate the initial concentration of drug residues quantitatively. This is a particular problem for marijuana and the cannabinoids.

Interpretation of positive drug tests requires a grounding in toxicokinetics and is beyond the scope of this section. However, a few points will illustrate the complexity of interpretation. Urine testing by conventional means does not detect the common drug residues after more than a few days, even for cannabinoids, which tend to be more persistent. Opiates may be interpreted by reference to the quantity found of codeine compared to morphine; if the ratio is more than an order of magnitude with a predominance of codeine, codeine administration is a plausible explanation for the positive test (except that very late in excretion and at low concentrations the ratio can equalize). Poppy seeds, baked on bread, rolls, or bagels or mixed in muffins are rarely responsible for positive tests; the subject may have been unaware of eating them. However, most positive tests are clearly positive and not so easily explained. Drug-using subjects quite commonly invoke such stories and explanations to cover their drug use.

Urine testing is accompanied at some facilities by plant searches and inspections of lockers, vehicles, and the personal property of workers. The legal implications of such searches should be reviewed with legal counsel before considering such programs.

Department of Transportation

The Department of Transportation (DOT) mandates drug testing for four million workers in the transportation industry covered by the Federal Highway Administration (mostly interstate truckers), the Federal Aviation Administration, and the Coast Guard, as well as workers on interstate pipelines. There is also an internal DOT testing program for the agency's own employees, mostly air traffic controllers; it is used by the agency as a model for development of national regulations.

Testing is required following accidents, with reasonable cause (to suspect the influence), pre-employment, and at random, and may also be performed on a periodic basis when these workers receive their medical evaluations. The DOT system emphasizes confidentiality (to the point of prohibiting identification of the employee to the laboratory except by number) and is exclusively for DOT purposes; no other tests can be performed on the sample. Information on medications being taken are obtained by the MRO only after a positive test is obtained and cannot be collected in advance as part of the drug test. Testing must be done at a NIDA-certified laboratory. On-site drug testing is not yet permitted.

All drug testing reports must be received by the MRO in hard copy, not orally in person nor by telephone; employers cannot receive reports directly. (Self-employed individuals may receive information about themselves.) Positive test results must be signed by the certifying laboratory scientist; negative tests do not need to be certified. Positive screening tests are confirmed by GC/MS. Medical interviews and interpretation to investigate positive tests can only be performed by licensed medical practitioners acting in the capacity of MROs. This investigation must take place before the test result is reported to the employer and may require tracking down the employee while maintaining confidentiality as to why. The employee, who frequently challenges the test result, may demand a retest of the original sample within seventy-two hours for (nonquantitative) confirmation. Employers are entitled to know which drug tested positive, but not how much was found.

DOT regulations require the employer to remove the test-positive employee from the critical safety function in which that person is serving, effectively suspending him or her from driving, flying, and piloting. Positive tests among aircraft pilots must also be reported to the Federal Aviation Administration, and a determination must be made whether or not the pilot is dependent on drugs. DOT regulations do not require referral to EAPs or mandatory treatment.

The paperwork required for DOT drug tests is extensive and legally precise. There are several tricky aspects to the current paperwork that could invalidate the test documentation if performed incorrectly.

Other Government Agencies

Mandatory drug testing is also required by the U.S. Nuclear Regulatory Commission for operators of nuclear power stations and other personnel handling critical radiation hazards. The paperwork protocol for testing differs from that of DOT. The Department of Defense has a drug-testing program for military recruits and may have programs for other personnel.

Some states have imposed drug testing regulations on intrastate drivers similar to the DOT regulations for interstate drivers. State legislation may change, and inquiries should be made locally before making assumptions.

In the occupational setting, prevention takes the form of worksite programs. Typically, occupational approaches to prevention are blended, as in matching noise control (hazard control) and hearing conservation programs (surveillance). New and more effective strategies for delivering preventive services have been developed in recent years that lend themselves to introduction in the workplace. However, the implementation of these strategies is often constrained by business considerations, distrust of management, questions about cost effectiveness, and the contradictory health messages and choices that are embedded in society as a whole.

RESOURCES

American Medical Association. *AMA Guides to the Evaluation of Permanent Impairment*. 6th ed. Chicago: American Medical Association; 2008.

Hartenbaum N, ed. *The DOT Medical Examination*. 3rd ed. Beverley Farms, MA: OEM Press: 2003.

Roelen CAM, Koopmans PC, Notenbomer A, Groothoff JW. Job satisfaction and sickness absence: a questionnaire survey. *Occup Med*. 2008;58(8):567–571.

Talmage JB, Melhorn JH. *A Physician's Guide to Return to Work*. Chicago: American Medical Association; 2005.

Taylor NAS, Groeller H. *Physiological Bases of Human Performance during Work and Exercise*. Edinburgh: Churchill Livingston, Elsevier; 2008.

Thomas VL, Gostin LO. The Americans with Disabilities Act: shattered aspirations and new hope. *JAMA*. 2009;301:95-97.

NOTEWORTHY READINGS

Anonymous. Workers' health—occupational or personal? *Lancet*. 1984;i:1390–1391.

Baker CC, Pocock SJ. Ethnic differences in certified sickness absence. *Brit J Indust Med*. 1982;39:277–282.

Carey TS, Hadler NM. The role of the primary physician in disability determination for social security insurance and workers' compensation. *Ann Intern Med*. 1986;104:706–710.

Cowell JWF. Guidelines for fitness-for-duty examinations. *Can Med Assn J*. 1986;135:985–988.

Cox RAF, Edwards FC, Palmer K. *Fitness for Work: The Medical Aspects*. Oxford: Oxford University Press; 2000.

DeHart RL, ed. Medication-induced performance decrements. *J Occup Med*. 1990;32(4):special issue.

EU-MAHDIE Working Group. Measuring Health and Disability in Europe: Supporting Policy Development. A European Coordination Action for Policy Support. 2006. Available at www.mhadie.it/getDocument.aspx?FileID=158.

Guidotti TL, Cowell JWF, Jamieson GG. *Occupational Health Services: A Practical Approach*. Chicago: American Medical Association; 1989.

Hartigan JA, Wigdor AK, eds. *Fairness in Employment Testing: Validity Generalization, Minority Issues, and the General Aptitude Test Battery.* Washington, DC: National Academy Press; 1989.

Himmelstein JS, Pransky GS, eds. Worker fitness and risk evaluations. *Occup Med: State of Art Rev.* 1988;3(2):169–364.

Holleman WL, Holleman MC. School and work release evaluations. *JAMA.* 1988;260(24):3629–3634.

de Kort WLAM, Post Uiterweer HW, van Dijk JH. Agreement on medical fitness for a job. *Scand J Work Environ Health.* 1992;18:246–251.

Leonardi M, Bickenbach J, Ustun TB, Kostanjsek N, Chatterji S, MHADIE Consortium. The definition of disability: what's in a name? *Lancet.* Oct 7, 2006;368:1219–1221.

McKeown KD, Furness JA. Sickness absence patterns of 5000 NHS staff employed within Northallerton and South West Durham Health Authorities. *J Soc Occup Med.* 1987;37:111–116.

Pransky GS, Dempsey PG. Practical aspects of functional capacity evaluations. *J Occup Rehab* 2004;14:217–229.

Reville RT, Seabury SA, Neuhauser FW, Burton JF Jr, Greenberg MD. *An Evaluation of California's Permanent Disability Rating System.* Santa Monica CA: RAND Institute for Civil Justice; 2005.

Shepherd RJ. Assessment of occupational fitness in the context of human rights legislation. *Can J Sports Sci.* 1990;15:89–95.

Social Security Administration. Disability Evaluation Under Social Security. SSA Pub No 64–039. September 2008. Available at http://www.ssa.gov/disability/professionals/bluebook.

Task Force on Health Surveillance of Workers. Health surveillance of workers. *Can J Pub Health.* 1986;77:91–99.

Taylor PJ. Occupational and regional associations of death, disablement, and sickness absence among Post Office staff 1972–75. *Brit J Indust Med.* 1976;33:230–235.

Taylor PJ, Burridge J. Trends in death, disablement, and sickness absence in the British Post Office since 1891. *Brit J Indust Med.* 1982;39:1–10.

Taylor PJ, Pocock SJ. Sickness absence—its measurement and control. In: Schilling RSF. *Occupational Health Practice.* London: Butterworths; 1981: 339–358.

19 WELLNESS AND HEALTH PROMOTION

Occupational and environmental medicine (OEM) is a specialty of preventive medicine. A fundamental concern of occupational and environmental medicine is to protect the health of workers by preventive action, most obviously by preventing or controlling exposure to hazards. This chapter deals with interventions that are intended, in general, to change individual health risk, mostly by changing personal behavior and lifestyle. These organized programs are variously called wellness, health promotion, and applied prevention. They apply the theories and insights of prevention science (see Chapter 8). The ideal is, whenever possible, to go further than disease prevention and to strive for achieving gains in individual health and fitness. Applied to disease management, this includes improving the health of people with chronic diseases (such as diabetes) and preventing complications.

On the occupational medicine side, much effort is devoted to organizing and administering programs intended to keep workers healthy, especially in large corporations. In recent years, wellness programs have become increasingly prominent in occupational medicine practice and have become an integral part of the OEM physician's responsibility. The essential idea behind wellness and health promotion programs is that there are health gains to be achieved by applying the resources, technology, and management available through large organizations to the objective of helping workers or community residents, as individuals or as groups, to enhance their health. This is also, of course, the fundamental idea behind managed care in another context.

On the environmental medicine side, wellness and health promotion (at least as expounded by the Ottawa Charter, as described below) are largely a matter of identifying and protecting the community against exposure to environmental hazards. However, community-based programs can also enhance health by promoting environmental interventions that are under the control of individuals, families, and communities, such as injury prevention or preventing childhood lead exposure. They overlap with other community-based health promotion, screening, general prevention, and public health programs. This topic will be addressed only to a limited extent in this set of volumes. The major emphasis will be on the traditional role of prevention in modifying individual health risk factors and of health promotion in seeking health gains.

In occupational and environmental medicine, physicians are called upon to advise on health protection, to partner with other health professionals in the prevention of exposure to hazards, to conduct periodic health evaluations and surveillance programs for exposure-related disorders, to support health promotion or wellness programs, and to advocate control of exposures to well below permissible exposure levels, an example of the "public health" approach.

HISTORICAL CONTEXT

Preventive medicine is as old as medicine, and its history, and that of environmental health protection, is beyond the scope of this chapter. The idea that the health of workers could be protected and improved by interventions and services delivered through the workplace is newer and has its roots in the social disruption that accompanied the work-related hazards introduced by technology and rapid economic growth in Europe and North America in the nineteenth century.

The idea of protecting the general (as opposed to occupational, or work-related) health of workers and their families has a long history going back to utopian and industrial reformers of the nineteenth century. During the Industrial Revolution, living conditions fell dramatically for the new working class in many (but not all) new industrial cities, and large numbers of immigrants strained charity and social services. The predominant social philosophy of the day was *laissez-faire* economics and "survival of the fittest" (sometimes called "social Darwinism" but in fact predating Darwin and the probable source of inspiration for his theory of natural selection). By this philosophy, workers had to expect to endure hardship. If the weak did not survive, the process of selection supposedly made society all the stronger. As a general rule, efforts to reform conditions of the working class took an ideological turn in Europe but kept to a less ideological, reformist path in the United Kingdom and the United States, although there were many exceptions. In Europe, the reaction against the threat of revolution in 1848 ultimately included many concessions and reforms, especially around 1880, when the ideological momentum for a political solution to workers' conditions was waning. By the end of the nineteenth century, it was revived again in Europe by Marxism.

Although conditions of the working class were a political issue during the nineteenth century, some employers, chief among them Robert Owen (1771–1858), who was widely influential in both Britain and the United States, genuinely felt a strong obligation to improve the lives of their employees and introduced reforms in working conditions, nutrition, and programs to discourage alcohol abuse. He established utopian communities for his workers that ultimately were unsustainable and failed. Owen later refined his political beliefs into a program of social action that is considered by many to be the forerunner of modern socialism, notwithstanding that he was a prominent and successful capitalist. Other employers, such as George Pullman, used their power as employers to coerce workers into what they considered to be healthy and responsible lifestyles.

Pullman, who invented and manufactured luxury sleeper cars on trains, founded a utopian community for his employees that became Pullman, Washington, in the 1880s, which later experienced a historic workers' strike against autocratic rules governing health, hygiene, and civil liberties. Underlying these ideas was the notion that working people could not take care of themselves and needed guidance from a paternalistic employer.

By today's standards, these measures were uncomfortably patronizing in tone, but they often, as in the case of Owen's reforms, represented dramatic improvements in the quality of life of working people compared to their less fortunate neighbors who worked for employers with then-conventional views. On the other hand, these experiences created distrust in the vision and motivation of employers. This distrust is still reflected in the skeptical attitude of organized labor toward health promotion programs.

One humanitarian response to deplorable working conditions in the nineteenth century was the "settlement movement" in the United States, which was particularly strong in Chicago. The settlement movement was led by Jane Addams, a formidable but class-conscious reformer who was concerned with raising living standards for the working poor. Addams was mentor to Alice Hamilton, the great occupational physician and toxicologist (see Chapter 1). Her goal with respect to health education and protection was to help new arrivals settle their families in decent living quarters, teach them to eat a balanced diet, and provide medical care for their children. The settlement movement undoubtedly did a lot of good, but what really changed the picture of working life in North America on a large scale was education and rising wages.

Modern concepts of workplace-centered health and wellness were developed by Harry Mock around 1907. Mock was a luminary in occupational medicine, also working in Chicago (see Chapter 1), In a seminal textbook, he argued that workers and employers benefit from health protection and that reducing health risks brought a more stable and productive civil society. He initiated educational programs, direct assistance to workers and their families, and programs to address the needs of vulnerable populations (specifically, working women and immigrant groups) at Sears Roebuck & Co., where he was medical director. The assumption was that a large company, with all its resources, efficiencies, and capital, could achieve health gains for its workers through organization, training, and economies of scale. The roots of managed care can be found in this concept, no less than the forms of prepaid care and closed healthcare delivery systems that had already been introduced by railroads and some other large employers.

Concepts of population health, although the term was not used then, came to public attention during both world wars when, at the beginning of each war, U.S. Army recruits were found to be in generally poor health. If presumably able-bodied young men were in such bad shape, the reasoning went, the health of the nation as a whole must have been dismal. This realization that the health of the population was linked to readiness caused concern and led to studies and reports, but options for action were limited during wartime. They became even more limited during the Depression.

During World War II, health insurance was introduced as an employment benefit so that employers could attract and retain skilled workers during the wartime labor shortage. At first, health insurance was inexpensive and there were few organized wellness programs, but interest on the part of government in health education grew following the war. Efforts by employers to build on the opportunities for health gains through worker-oriented programs were fought by organized medicine in the 1950s on the grounds that patients' personal physicians were responsible for their health and well-being, not employers, and as part of the battle against occupational health services on a corporate scale.

In the 1960s a movement took hold called "multiphasic screening" that provided a battery of physical and lab exams to employees on site on an annual basis, the results of which were then passed on to the employee's own physicians. Employers stopped paying for this when they realized that the findings were almost never acted upon, either because they were already known or because the employee's personal physician did not read the report.

The next phase (give or take a few fads) was worksite health promotion. This was a major movement in the late 1970s and through the 1980s. Employers put together educational programs, built fitness centers, changed the menus in cafeterias, and made other modifications that, in the end, were mostly used to advantage by health-conscious, younger workers and rarely by workers who needed them most. A rather large industry developed for the training and certification of fitness trainers, consultants for worksite health promotion, and evaluation methodologists. This resulted in a huge (and overly optimistic because of strong publication bias) literature on the evaluation of these programs. With the downsizing of corporate medical departments around 1980–1985, enthusiasm for these programs waned. Employers, in the end, dumped a lot of these programs in the 1990s but mostly kept the fitness programs because they were a popular employment benefit for headquarters staff. The reason they were dropped is that they were not cost-effective (other than as a competitive enticement for hard-to-find technical employees) and they were not used by the blue-collar workers who needed them most.

In the meantime, however, prevention science had been slowly developing new approaches and methods. More effective means of inventorying and evaluating health risks were developed in the form of "health risk appraisal" instruments. "Behavioral medicine" was a broad movement based loosely on "behaviorism" (a school of thought in psychology that emphasizes "operant conditioning," reinforcing learned behavior by rewarding or aversive response, and was most closely associated with the psychologist B.F. Skinner). Behavioral medicine began largely outside of mainstream medicine but demonstrated efficacy for a number of clinical modalities such as biofeedback, behavioral therapy for smoking cessation and weight loss, and deeper understanding of psychosomatic disorders. "Health psychology" was a closely related field emphasizing cognitive and emotional responses and their effect on mood and perceptions of health. New approaches to changing health-related behavior on the scale of communities were introduced, particularly "social marketing" (the use of marketing techniques to persuade people to change behavior). Improved methods for community surveys and the application of more advanced methods of epidemiology to community needs assessment were developed. By the late 1990s, when the field started to slow due to lack of support, prevention science had refined the "technology" available to preventive medicine to measure health needs and to design more effective interventions, both for individuals and communities.

In the mid-1990s, a new movement started called "corporate wellness." The name is deceiving, however, because the emphasis is not on prevention as much as case management. This movement is basically concerned with demand management, reducing healthcare expenditures, and managing managed care. It was developed earliest in those companies that were self-insured, because they were motivated to reduce costs and had ready access to data (with protection of confidentiality) on individual cases as well as group experience. The movement is also concerned with keeping employees with health problems on the job and productive, for the mutual benefit of both the employer and the worker.

Corporate wellness programs tended to be heavy handed in the early days. In the early 1990s, one major electronics manufacturer and a beer company both proposed to increase the employee contribution to healthcare premiums for employees who did not meet health targets on periodic health evaluations. A well-known manufacturer of candy proposed to fine its employees to recover the increased cost of health insurance for those who did not meet individual health goals and were not on medical treatment plans. These anecdotal reports raised great concern among employees and unnecessary resistance among unions, because of the perception of employer coercion, intrusiveness, discrimination, and compromised privacy.

The corporate wellness movement subsequently moved in another direction, emphasizing optimizing individualized care and managing individual chronic health conditions, such as diabetes, in order to improve quality of life for the worker and to reduce healthcare costs. This trend, poorly documented in the literature, is also led by self-insured employers and seeks to better manage the most expensive and potentially disabling conditions in the subset of employees at highest risk, most of whom are already under medical treatment and may need help complying with complicated medication regimens and monitoring their condition.

Most recently, as this is being written, wellness and health promotion programs are increasingly motivated by efforts to keep workers productive and on the job for as long as possible. There is a strong social argument to be made that prevention of disability plays a major role in economic security and sustainability. As the population gets older, more people will develop age-related disabilities and chronic illnesses. Unless preventable illness and disability are addressed with strong measures to prevent or delay their onset and progression, the burden of disease and disability will increase and interfere with the ability of more and more people to live vigorous and satisfying lives. The burden of disability and chronic illness will place a rapidly growing burden on the healthcare system and will become a progressively greater social problem if there is no large population growth. Specifically, as the number of people who are retired or cannot work due to disability increases, fewer productive workers contribute to the economic system that supports them, including Social Security, Canada Pension, and healthcare insurance for the aged and disabled (such as Medicare in the United States). This "dependency ratio" has moved and is moving steadily downward in the United States (see Table 19.1). In order to make up this gap, workers will have to become more productive and may (depending on productivity gains) need to work longer and well beyond traditional retirement ages of sixty or sixty-five in order to maintain both national economic stability and their personal income. Disability that interferes with work removes people at a younger age from active employment to dependency and so aggravates the problem.

Some demographers and economists believe that the aging-population aspect of this argument has been overstated, pointing to the British experience, in which labor market changes played a much more important role than aging in skewing the dependency ratio (the arguments are summarized in a book by Mullan, *The Imaginary*

Table 19.1. Dependency Ratio for Selected Years

Year	Dependency Ratio*	Historical Note
1950	18:1	Postwar boom period, productivity level low
1965	4:1	Marked increase in productivity per worker due to technology
2005	3:1	Current situation
2080	2:1	Projected to probable retirement age of young people entering workforce today

Source: Economic Policy Institute, EPI Issue Brief #208. Washington DC, 11 May 2008.

Time Bomb, 2000), and the observation that American society went through a much greater transition in the dependency ratio in the 1950s and 1960s, which coincided with a period of dramatically increased productivity per worker.

Concern over productivity led the Centers for Disease Control and Prevention, through the National Institute for Occupational Safety and Health (NIOSH), to convene conferences in 2004 and 2007 on wellness and working life that examined these issues. These raised concern among occupational health and safety professionals that NIOSH was being forced to divert energy and resources away from its traditional mission of investigating occupational hazards.

Periodic Health Evaluation

Periodic health evaluation is the scheduled, routine screening of an individual for health problems when no symptom or obvious health issue has triggered the encounter. Periodic health evaluation for purposes of mandated surveillance is discussed in Chapter 5. Periodic health evaluations for purposes of health maintenance have been extensively reviewed (most recently by Boulware et al. for the American College of Physicians, 2007) and have shown a benefit with improved delivery of preventive services and reduced concern over health. The periodic health evaluation allows these services to be packaged, programmed with rational periodicity, and incorporated into insurance plans. Piecemeal services do not, and useful preventive services are often omitted when healthcare is limited to occasional physician visits as needed.

Maintaining the health of employees is just as important a commitment of physicians as treating acute injuries and providing clinical care. An employee who is later found to have been unfit for his or her job assignment can be an expensive proposition in terms of liability, bad feelings, and lost productivity. The provision of pre-placement and periodic health evaluations is a responsibility not to be taken lightly. Routine examinations should never become an assembly line, where the doctor just goes through the motions. Physicians who are doing routine examinations should be rotated and the number that they do at any one time should be limited to ensure that they do not get tired, bored, or lose their mental sharpness.

Screening programs are secondary prevention programs organized as campaigns for the detection of treatable early illness. They can feature a single screening modality, such as mammography, or combine modalities into a program. Properly designed, they create opportunities for health education and may include a structured health questionnaire, sometimes called a "health risk assessment," that identifies serious health risks and may even calculate probabilities of future disease. Referral for follow-up of positive findings and subsequent care is essential in these programs, which are often sponsored by hospitals and healthcare institutions.

"Multiphasic health screening" was a general screening program for large groups of employees that involves a battery of selected, often automated tests given periodically, briefly described above. Multiphasic health screening was often provided for nonexecutive personnel in the form of a mobile screening center, often in a van, that would visit the employer's facilities in rotation once a year. Because numerous tests were performed in a battery on each participant, and one in twenty was likely to be abnormal, there were usually one or more abnormal or borderline for every participant. The predictive value of these tests were found to be very low (see Chapter 5), and when the results were sent to the employee's personal physician they were often ignored. As an approach, multiphasic health screening did not emphasize health education opportunities and instead served as a means of conducting screening tests more efficiently. Its effectiveness was often disappointing because the findings, although usually forwarded to the workers' own physician, were seldom actually used in the patient's personal healthcare. The approach is seldom used today.

"Health fairs" are events held at the worksite or in the community under the sponsorship, usually, of a major employer or healthcare institution. The health fair is an opportunity for participants to obtain a set of screening tests (such as body mass index, blood pressure determinations, urinalysis by dipstick, spirometry, vision checks, cataract, and inspection of skin lesions for cancer), but tests that require fasting or are difficult to interpret without controlled collection are not recommended, for example serum cholesterol or blood glucose tests. Often free influenza immunizations or other preventive services are offered as well. Although not common at health fairs, cooking demonstrations would be a logical addition and a natural attraction. The health fair is a good opportunity to provide basic health education through free seminars and general advice in a convenient, nonclinical setting, such as booths staffed by nurses and other trained health professionals. The health fair is usually staffed by a nurse with a physician on call or on site but not necessarily involved in every encounter. Some healthcare facilities offer basic health fairs once a year as a free service to employers, in part as a marketing promotion and in part to encourage workers to obtain their own and their family's care at the same facility. For example, UCLA sponsored what it called "HealthFest" on an annual basis for residents of west Los Angeles and their own employees, locating it in an accessible part of their medical center and providing free parking. Child care or entertainment for children is a key element for success of the community health fairs. Prizes and handouts add to the attraction. Health fairs offer timely and nonthreatening opportunities for health education and probably raise awareness of health issues among community members and workers, at least for a while, but their screening services share the same general drawbacks as multiphasic health screening, unless abnormal findings can be followed up by the sponsoring facility.

The annual periodic health evaluation (more familiarly known as the "annual physical") is now considered obsolete as a strategy for periodic health evaluation. Most screening tests are not required as often as once a year, especially in younger age groups. The physical examination in itself, even when combined with standard clinical laboratory tests, is now recognized as an inefficient means of detecting health risks or the earliest stages of most treatable disorders. However, the cachet enjoyed by the physical examination after years of promotion by the medical profession and its status as an employment benefit have made it difficult to deny to managers and service employees. Executive health evaluations are discussed below.

The "lifetime health monitoring program" (LHMP) is a phased program that prescribes different screening tests at different frequencies as one ages. The LHMP combines periodic health evaluation with health education and prevention-oriented interventions appropriate to the individual's stage of life and known risk factors. The LHMP has seldom been offered on a large scale in industry despite its advantages in cost, its efficiency, and its medical rationale. The approach was developed by Lester Breslow and Anne Somers and proposed in 1977 as a cost-effective alternative to the annual physical.

Since 1984, the authoritative guidance for preventive health services in the United States has been the U.S. Preventive Services Task Force (USPSTF), managed by the Agency for Healthcare Research and Quality (AHRQ), Department of Health and Homeland Security. The Task Force disseminates guidelines and updates for evidence-based clinical preventive services intended to assist physician practice in screening and preventing disease. These guidelines cover the spectrum of clinical preventive medicine. Some guidelines are controversial or counterintuitive. For example, USPSTF does not recommend screening for chronic obstructive pulmonary disease by spirometry in the latest guideline as of this writing (2008) because there is no net benefit in survival or quality of life over and above smoking cessation for smokers and there is a risk of overdiagnosis in "never smokers." Likewise, USPSTF considers the evidence available to support screening for prostate cancer to be insufficient to make a recommendation for men under seventy-five years of age and sufficient to recommend against it for men over age seventy-five. Because these recommendations are tightly reasoned, are updated periodically, and take into account many factors (among them risk of disease, probable outcome, performance of the screening test, efficacy of the intervention, and risk of adverse effects of treatment), the OEM physician is advised to access the most current guidelines directly from AHRQ and not to depend on printed publications. They are available by category or as a "pocket guide" and as an electronic, downloadable version for PDAs at http://www.ahrq.gov/clinic/uspstfix.htm. USPSTF also publishes guides in hard-copy, book form and articles on the rationale and evidence behind its recommendations.

Physician Compliance with Preventive Medicine Guidelines

The prevention-oriented services expected of a physician in a primary care setting are well established. Authoritative guidelines for providing these services are widely disseminated. It is therefore puzzling why physicians do not perform any better than they do in following these guidelines and providing these services of proven efficacy to their patients.

Physicians tend to think that they do better than they do in providing preventive services. There are few recent comprehensive studies of physician compliance with preventive medicine guidelines. Most of what is in the literature dates from the 1980s and 1990s and may not take into account omissions in documentation, but the data overall are not encouraging and probably have not improved much, especially in view of the increasing time demands on the physician.

There are many influences on a physician's practice of prevention. Unfortunately, most current compensation systems do not reward the provision of preventive services to any substantial degree likely to change physician's practice habits. On the contrary, prevention takes time, and physicians are seldom rewarded in quite the same way as they would be if they were to treat a critically ill patient who then recovers. The immediacy of the interaction and feedback is lacking in prevention. This removes the direct satisfaction that a physician may derive from doing well by his or her patient.

Many physicians still carry deep-seeded doubts about the efficacy of preventive services. The treatment of disease can be monitored against an expected outcome (recovery) in the individual patient, but preventive services, if they are successful, result in nothing happening. They can only be monitored on a population basis by demonstrating lower rates of adverse health outcomes, which requires large numbers. Physicians are more motivated to provide preventive services when there is rapid feedback on their performance, test results, and patient outcome.

Training helps to improve compliance with prevention guidelines, at least among family physicians. Also, individuals who trained relatively recently or who are members of professional organizations seem to do better in providing preventive services than those who are relatively isolated from the professional mainstream. OEM physicians, with the advantage of a practice that links individual and population health, are in an excellent position to provide and supervise effective prevention-oriented programs.

Executive Health Evaluations

The executive health evaluation (commonly and colloquially known as the "executive physical") is a periodic comprehensive medical evaluation for executive and other key personnel whose health is thought essential to the employer's future. In actual practice, the annual physical and particularly its executive version continue to be requested by both employees and employers because it is perceived as a perquisite or benefit of employment. One reason is that it provides a convenient opportunity for counseling, health education, and the individualization of health promotion activities. Employers see the executive health evaluation as a means of obtaining an early warning in the event that a company officer whose judgment is critical to the firm may become impaired or unable to carry out his or her duties.

Another reason for their continued popularity is that facilities that provide executive health evaluations are usually located in desirable locations (such as the Mayo Clinic in Scottsdale, AZ, or the Greenbrier Hotel in White Sulphur Springs, WV) and can be combined with short vacations, golf, and other amenities. Most executive health evaluations are very comprehensive and can be very intrusive, raising high expectations for privacy, which make a facility distant from the executive's home office appealing. While confidentiality may be respected throughout the organization, it must be visible to an executive who is used to discretion and deference and who is likely to make snap judgments.

Executive health programs require that the service be scheduled at the convenience of the executive rather than the healthcare provider and that time be managed effectively. In practice this usually means a health interview by questionnaire (usually online), administered before the appointment, and coordinated scheduling in advance of all tests during the visit, such as screening laboratory tests done early in the morning, and expedited access to any necessary diagnostic tests. The visit may be punctuated with breaks for conducting business, checking e-mail, and recreation. The service requires a business arrangement with an upscale hotel nearby that executives will find attractive and that has a full-service business center.

It is highly advisable to create a separate facility for executive health evaluations, preferably on a separate floor of a hospital or in a free-standing location. Combining executive health within general healthcare facility often does not work well. It is not unusual for other patients and for staff to resent the special treatment afforded to executives and for staff to undermine efforts to cultivate the executive service by allowing delays to occur and refusing to give executives priority over other patients. Also, the creation of a "two-tier" approach to delivering medical services leaves the institution open to criticism for appearing to be discriminating in favor of the affluent and against the needy. Finally, workers who may be directed to occupational health services in the institution may suspect that their cases will be prejudiced or treated less sympathetically because the institution has engaged in an apparently "cozy" relationship with their bosses. These problems can be largely overcome by insisting on as complete a separation as possible between the executive health service and the rest of the organization.

Such programs present an excellent opportunity to encourage sound health practices. The executive participants are likely to be more receptive to concepts of health promotion than they might be at home. Programs on stress reduction, smoking cessation, prevention of alcohol and drug abuse, health education, motivation, and exercise are very popular when combined with screening services. Lifestyle-oriented programs presenting healthier alternatives to the hard-driving executive workaholic stereotype are very attractive in today's more health-conscious society. Spouses of executives can be involved also. Many of these programs can be offered at extra cost or as part of an attractive package within the executive health service.

DOMAINS OF PREVENTION

OEM physicians are members of the preventive medicine and public health communities. The vocabulary of prevention and the nuances of the schools of thought in the field are confusing but important for OEM physicians to know. In part, this is because preventive medicine, like all technical fields, uses jargon as shorthand, and OEM physicians should have no barriers to communication with their colleagues. Jargon is also, as in any field, a means of rapidly sizing up a newcomer. Appropriate and unforced use of the right vocabulary sends a signal to one's colleagues that reassures them with respect to one's expertise. The inappropriate use of words sends a signal that the user is not prepared and may not be a serious professional and so may close opportunities for cooperation. The definitive guide to the vocabulary of preventive medicine, public health, and epidemiology is the *Dictionary of Epidemiology,* which has been edited for many years by John Last.

The essential first distinction is between "preventive" and "preventative." Preventive, by traditional usage, not dictionary definition, is the only acceptable word in verbal usage for all applications in this field. "Preventative," while a synonymous English word in the dictionary, is never used among preventive medicine specialists or prevention professionals. If an OEM physician refers to "preventative medicine," preventive medicine and public health experts who hear it will immediately discount his or her credibility. The effect is similar to hearing a surgeon refer to the "lar-nix" rather than the "larynx."

Colleagues outside preventive medicine often use terms such as "preventive medicine," "public health," "population medicine," and "community medicine" interchangeably. However, these terms do have formal definitions, and each of the fields they represent has developed its own culture, tradition, and history among its practitioners.

"Preventive medicine" is defined by Last as "the branch of medicine that is primarily concerned with preventing physical, mental, and emotional disease and injury, in contrast to treating the sick and injured." He notes further that prevention is often inseparable from treatment and cure, but that the emphasis of the discipline rests on applying many of the same sciences, skills, and attitudes shared by public health to clinical practice. "General preventive medicine" is defined by the American College of Preventive Medicine as "the specialty of preventive medicine which deals with health promotion and disease prevention in communities and in defined populations."

At one time, "general preventive medicine" was combined with public health in medical specialty boards, and at times they were treated separately. Preventive medicine practice includes population-level interventions as well as services to individuals, which may be educational (usually done by health professionals other than physicians), interventional (such as immunization), screening for disease, and the evaluation of individual risk, when an individual's entire health profile is considered. Public health, as described in Chapter 8, implies a population- or community-level commitment, such as traditional environmental health services or community-based health promotion programs that touch everybody, rather than individual-level services. Since the two approaches are closely intertwined and usually combined in public agencies, the labels can be considered to refer more to emphasis rather than mutually exclusive missions.

The domain of "clinical preventive medicine," as the term is currently used in the United States, corresponds more closely to the description made by Geoffrey Rose of "preventive medicine" (prevention for individuals and the "high-risk" strategy) compared to public health (prevention for populations and the "population" strategy). A definition of "clinical preventive medicine" was provided in 1982 by a major task force on curriculum development: "those personal health services, provided within the context of clinical medicine, the purpose of which is to maintain health and reduce the risk of disease and untimely death." The definition was seen by many practitioners to be outdated or limiting, and in 1989 a new consensus definition emerged, in which clinical medicine was "an integral part of preventive medicine concerned with the maintenance and promotion of health and the reduction of risk factors that result in injury and disease." Practitioners agree, however, that the domain of the specialty includes behavior modification, risk assessment and modification, health promotion, and health education, all with an individual and clinical emphasis.

"Public health," on the other hand, is defined (again by Last) as "the combination of sciences, skills, and beliefs that are directed to the maintenance and improvement of the health of all the people through collective and social action," and is noted to be oriented primarily to protecting the population concerned, rather than necessarily individuals within the population. An annotated dictionary produced by the U.S. federal government further emphasizes that "public health activities are generally those which are less amenable to being undertaken or less effective when undertaken on an individual basis, and do not typically include personal health services." In other words, public health interventions typically involve structural change, as in the formulation of policy and procedures, measures to reduce exposure to hazards, and the assessment of risk.

"Population health" is a relatively new term, emerging in the 1990s and defined in 2002 (Kindle and Stoddart) as "the health outcomes of a group of individuals, including the distribution of such outcomes within the group." It is not exactly synonymous with public health. It refers to the sum of influences on health from various social and physical factors (the "health field concept") and the health status of the community as a whole, including distributions, vulnerabilities, and pockets of ill health, as opposed to the health of individuals in the community. A similar usage has become popular in Canada, reflecting the name of a program introduced by the Canadian Institute for Advanced Research that covers studies relating population-based phenomena and social change to health outcomes, irrespective of whether they are targeted public health interventions. (The essential features of this model are presented in Figure 19.1.) "Population medicine" is an older term, also more extensively used in Canada. It was defined by Kerr White, a pioneering thinker in

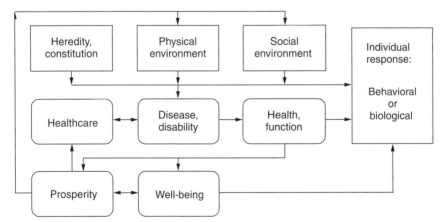

Figure 19.1. The "population health model," adapted from the Canadian Institute for Advanced Research.

health, and others, as the "application of these concepts and methods embodied in such largely quantitative disciplines as epidemiology, economics, demography, and statistics, and in such behavioral sciences as cultural anthropology, sociology, and social psychology." Population medicine is similar to its British predecessor "social medicine" in concerns and method, but tends to be more conservative in political tone and liberal (in the philosophical sense of individual-oriented) in orientation than social medicine, which was (and remains) vigorously, enthusiastically, and unabashedly left-wing.

"Community medicine" is much more difficult to define, because its meaning has been expanded in institutional rubrics. The term was used loosely in the 1960s and 1970s as a synonym for preventive medicine, public health, and primary care, with a considerable loss of precision. Its founders defined community medicine as "the academic discipline that deals with the identification and solution of the health problems of communities or human population groups." The emphasis among purists was always placed on provision of primary care and the elimination of obstacles to obtaining care. Although the ideas are closely related, this is not the same as mobilizing resources specifically to prevent disease and to maintain health in individuals or protecting the health of populations. Community medicine has been described as "a social movement" and "a method for accomplishing social ends." In practice, the approach used by its founders has been one of community needs assessment, analysis of social and cultural barriers to adequate health services, and provision of primary care in a culturally appropriate structure. The term is out of fashion, but the idea of building community-level health interventions around individual primary care continues in, among other initiatives, the World Health Organization's drive for primary care for all. The original concept of community medicine is now subsumed under the term "community-oriented primary care."

Public health may be seen as a collection of disciplines, embracing epidemiology, biostatistics, health services administration, environmental and occupational health, and behavioral sciences, all applied to the protection of populations with respect to health risk. Preventive medicine may be seen as embracing the same disciplines but emphasizing their clinical application to the individual case. Community medicine may be seen as a systematic approach to all health needs of a defined community. Population health and medicine may be interpreted as perceiving health as an outcome of particular interest given a universe of inputs, outputs, and social constructs. These are not so much four parallel and distinct disciplines as four different approaches transecting the same problem, and inevitably intersecting with one another. When these terms are used interchangeably, important meanings are obscured.

HEALTH PROMOTION

In the 1980s, a new strategy became popular for disease prevention and enhancement of health. This strategy was called health promotion and it assumed the proportions of a social movement toward improved health. The *American Journal of Health Promotion*, which became the leading vehicle for evaluation and scientific studies in health promotion, defined it in 1989 as "the science and art of helping people change their lifestyle to move toward a state of optimal health." The World Health Organization (WHO) formally defined it in 1986 as "the process of enabling people to increase control over and to improve their health." Health promotion was not just a repackaged version of clinical prevention, but a strategy emphasizing positive aspects of enhanced health. Instead of adopting the essentially negative approach of "health maintenance," which underlies the traditional strategies of preventive medicine, the authors of health promotion adopted a more positive approach of "health enhancement," conveying a new message to participants that not only can disease be prevented and decline arrested, but participants can improve their physical and mental well-being through activities borrowed from clinical medicine, physical fitness, and health education.

There were actually two movements that shared the same name and operated more or less in parallel but as different schools of thought:

- The American school of thought, as represented by Office of the U.S. Surgeon General and the Office of Disease Prevention and Health Promotion, emphasized disease prevention and fitness and the attainment of explicit goals in population health, codified in a series of goals for the United States that appeared at decadal intervals under the overall title "Healthy People." (The goals were generally not, in fact met.) The American school of thought has been highly prescriptive, presented largely as a series of rules or measures with which citizens or their physicians should comply.

• The WHO school of thought was embodied in the Ottawa Charter, a consensus document that emphasized social change that would support "healthy public policy," healthy consumer choices (for example, with respect to food), and individual decisions that lead to healthier life choices (for example, by widespread condom availability). The WHO school of thought has been more influential in the rest of the world.

Health promotion in Canada follows European and WHO models and particularly a commitment to social change, especially modeled on a series of innovations pioneered in the then-health department of the city of Toronto in the 1980s. There, the core concept of health promotion has been to create an environment of choice in which the individual is motivated to pick the healthy choice rather than the least expensive or the most expedient choices in their lives.

Health promotion as it is applied in the United States emphasizes individual initiative and compliance. Health promotion has had particular success in employer-sponsored worksite health promotion programs. Combined with aggressive marketing and backed by employers that recognized the short-term as well as the theoretical long-term advantages, health promotion quickly entered the workplace and became a popular, if unproven, employee benefit in the early 1980s. In recent years an increasing number of employers have introduced health promotion activities for their employees. This movement represents a new point of view complementary to the traditional approach of occupational health services. Health promotion programs based in the workplace or on employment sought to enhance the personal health of employees for the benefit of both employee and employer. Health promotion was one way in which OEM crossed the line from occupation-related disorders to involvement in non-occupational factors determining health.

Health promotion programs typically blend three approaches to employee health: health education, preventive medicine and health screening, and fitness programs.

The health education component is concerned with teaching employees the essentials of a healthy lifestyle, such as good health habits, sound nutrition, and the consequences of smoking, alcohol, and drug abuse. Beyond the informative aspect of health education, however, is attention to the psychological principles that motivate people to comply with sound health practices or to take unnecessary risks that jeopardize their health. Simple information transfer is not enough, which is why lectures on health seldom change behavior. Likewise approaches that may be appropriate to patient education are not always helpful in health education for well employees. A health education component within a workplace health promotion program must be designed with attention to the characteristics of the population of workers to be reached (age, sex, class, education, health status, language, etc.), the most important health problems in the community as perceived by the workers, the most important health problems actually present in the community, and the goals to be attained in changing health-related behavior. Programs that fail to address these basic concerns are usually ineffective. Meeting these needs usually requires professional consultation and is beyond the training and experience of most physicians.

The preventive medicine component is typically limited to screening for common disorders and risk factors and intervention activities that complement but do not substitute for personal health-care, such as smoking cessation. The emphasis in health promotion programs is on primary prevention to reduce disease incidence in the working population and secondary prevention, the early detection of disease and referral for care. Reducing risk factors for later health problems (such as reducing cholesterol levels of cardiovascular fitness training) is more easily accomplished in an integrated health promotion program. In such programs the group spirit, constant encouragement and feedback, and support network make compliance easier to achieve than on an individual education, preventive medicine, and physical conditioning.

Health education is an integral part of these programs. For community and employee-sponsored programs, health education opportunities may be passive dissemination of information, through newsletters or emails, or active, with discussion groups and employee feedback on topics workers would like covered. "Lunchtime listen and learn" seminars, with an invited speaker available over the lunchtime break, are particularly popular and can be shared among employers in the same building.

Physical conditioning is an important part of most health promotion programs for several reasons. Participation in fitness activities and sports programs provides a regularly scheduled opportunity for conditioning with encouragement and the sense of belonging to a group, both of which make compliance more likely. Fitness programs within worksite health promotion are discussed below.

The concept of health promotion is a powerful one because it places a positive emphasis on enhanced well-being as a social expectation. As a strategy, health promotion gives the momentum to the proponents of sound health-related behaviors and to the advocates of constructive social change. It gives the individual participant a sense of belonging to a larger community of health-conscious peers. One would expect this strategy to be more effective than trying to persuade people to cease practicing unhealthy habits that they may enjoy or that give them a sense of comfort. As nominally healthful behaviors become a social norm, increasing pressure is placed on those who do not comply for reasons of personal choice or the appropriateness of the recommended behavior to their needs and abilities. This is evident in contemporary social attitudes toward smoking and obesity, for example, which suggest that the health messages of the previous decade were internalized into both individual thinking and the culture.

"Corporate culture" programs are highly sophisticated campaigns that link the employers' image and identification with health and vitality. The emphasis is on energy, optimism, productivity, and teamwork. These campaigns weave health promotion elements throughout, including fitness programs, fundraising for health-related appeals, heart healthy cafeteria menus, and positive thinking.

Whatever the model of health promotion program, there are certain implicit principles that should be followed. Effective programs are easily accessible to employees, both geographically and culturally. They are adaptable to individual needs and emphasize personal responsibility and empowerment. They may contribute to a positive corporate culture and image, but they are not extensions of human resources departments or ways of monitoring employee behavior outside of work hours. It is never acceptable to break confidentiality with personal health information. Employees who choose not to participate in designated activities such as fitness programs should not be coerced or made to feel that they are letting down "the team." For this reason it is not appropriate to combine health promotion programs with athletic competition.

Worksite Health Promotion Programs

Employer-sponsored health promotion programs may be community-based, such as the provision of discounted gym memberships, or worksite-based. Worksite health promotion began in the 1970s and became a major movement in the 1980s. In the beginning of this movement, worksite health promotion programs were usually started and managed by trainers and trained program directors, some of whom were certified by one of several credentialing agencies that sought to professionalize the position. The role of the primary care physician in worksite health promotion programs was usually that of an adviser. In many cases, OEM physicians who served as corporate medical directors were reluctant to get their departments involved in worksite health promotion because they could not see the sustainable health benefit and feared that their energies would be detracted from more pressing issues of occupational hazard control. During the downsizing and delayering that followed, however, health promotion programs were often assigned to them anyway and in time became a part of the corporate medical department's structure. Many physicians enjoy the opportunity to encourage good health habits in an upbeat situation that these programs provide.

Worksite health promotion has been supported by a very large, enthusiastic commercial sector that advocates and markets powerfully for health promotion services that they would supply or manage. As is the case for health services generally, there is great interest in the private sector in franchising worksite health promotion services. This is particularly true because reimbursement for preventive medical services has been depressed but has the potential to rebound in mainstream medicine, as demonstrated by the public's huge out-of-pocket expenditures for prevention-oriented alternative care and nutrition. But in many companies, health promotion programs were seen as expensive nonproductive costs and were terminated during the 1990s.

Worksite health promotion programs may be based on company grounds or they may operate by encouraging or subsidizing employees to use a community facility. Some are directly run by the employer, but many of the most successful programs are sponsored through employee recreation associations. Management of such programs has become highly specialized and professional, but small-scale programs can begin on an inexpensive basis. Worksite or employer-sponsored health promotion programs offer an opportunity to link health promotion, cost containment, and self-management of health-care. Self-management will require a considerable educational effort to change people's perceptions of what they should do for themselves, when they should seek medical care, and whom they should go to when they need care. The worker's personal physician will be in a key position to support these changes and to reinforce that education.

Worksite health promotion programs target those health-related behaviors that are most appropriate to employed persons, who are generally between twenty and sixty-five years old and in good health. They tend to attract more youthful, physically fit, and middle-class workers who are already aware of health risk factors. Blue-collar workers, linguistically or ethnically isolated workers, workers in rural areas, or workers whose worksite is remote from headquarters tend not to participate, although there is evidence that they stand to benefit as much or more than white-collar, urban workers. Executives tend to prefer separate programs, but for ensuring motivation and credibility among employees it is also important that the executives be seen to participate in worksite programs themselves.

Worksite health promotion programs may play an extremely important and constructive part in an individual worker's healthcare if the worker is motivated to participate. It is a solid adjunct to personal prevention at home and a healthy lifestyle. The worksite program offers an opportunity to target individual risk factors. For example, a worksite health promotion program may be the most appropriate means for prescribed exercise programs, for nutritional counseling, or for support in lifestyle changes such as smoking cessation or weight reduction. In order for the physician to take advantage of this opportunity, the worker-patient and his or her personal physician should discuss the program and what opportunities are available.

Most worksite health promotion programs are not supervised directly by a physician on site, although many have physicians as consultants or advisors. When there is a special need or opportunity, the worker's physician should not hesitate to contact the physician associated with the program in order to maximize the benefit and to minimize the risk of that worker participating in the program.

Evaluation of the impact of worksite health promotion programs suggests that well-managed worksite health promotion programs succeed in reducing illness and healthcare utilization, improving employee morale, and encouraging lifelong good health habits. Self-selection and attrition remain major limitations to the evaluation of worksite health promotion programs. However, effectiveness is not the only reason for their popularity, and evaluation of effectiveness is not the only criteria used by management in deciding to support such programs. The programs are very popular among employees, so most organizations wish to retain them. Thus, like health insurance after World War II, it has been difficult for many employers to phase out worksite health promotion programs once they started, regardless of whether they are deemed to be successful. Some employers saw no reason to evaluate them, since their continued presence served a business need in retaining employees.

Companies that are more committed to health promotion tend to be larger and involved in high technology, in which case they are usually in competition for desirable employees, who tend to be younger, well-educated, and health conscious. The employees drawn to worksite health promotion programs therefore tend to be concerned with their health and already motivated. More women than men participate, and women tend to participate in more activities, particularly those that involve interpersonal skills, stress reduction, and weight control. Sociological theory and hard-nosed management experience both confirm that the motivating force behind the introduction of worksite health promotion programs is not cost effectiveness or the control of healthcare costs. In the view of many, it is the social importance of health promotion as a means for organizations to attract and hold desirable employees, to express their concern for employee's well-being, and to offset problematical cutbacks in benefits while maintaining the morale of the workforce.

Health promotion programs continue to have less visible influence among rural, working-class, and socially isolated subgroups than with urban, better educated, and more affluent North Americans. This class distinction may ultimately disappear due to social mobility and marketing.

Elements of Worksite Health Promotion Programs

Certain services and interventions are common and important as a part of worksite programs, as listed in Table 19.2.

Fitness programs are by far the most popular program elements and are seen by a substantial fraction of employees—usually younger and

Table 19.2. Typical Components of Worksite Health Promotion Programs

Health Education

Cancer prevention	Common minor illnesses
Heart disease	Child health
Mental health	Care of the elderly
Nutrition	Diabetes
Substance abuse	Allergies
Smoking	Automotive safety
Injury prevention	Families relations
Breast self-examination	Travel medicine
Back school (prophylactic)	Sports
Care of dependents	Aging
Hair loss	Cosmetic surgery

Preventive Medicine

Screening activities	*Intervention activities*
Hypertension screening	Smoking cessation
Diabetes screening	Dietary interventions
Glaucoma screening	Back school (rehabilitation)
Cardiovascular risk factors	Weight control
Pulmonary function testing	Stress reduction
Weight monitoring	Prescriptive exercise regimes
Breast examination	Unsupervised exercise
Stool occult blood	Hypertension control, monitoring

Personal Wellness and Self-Care

Anxiety disorders
Arthritis
Asthma
Chronic pain
Diabetes
Gastroesophageal reflux disorder
Headache
Hypertension
Osteoporosis
Pregnancy
Urinary tract infections

already fit—as a major employment benefit. Access to fitness facilities onsite or nearby in the workers' own home community is highly attractive to workers who are already persuaded of the benefits of fitness. It is also common for employees to organize their own informal fitness programs, such as lunchtime aerobics, with management cooperation. In the past two decades most large companies have enthusiastically joined this trend, often installing well-equipped fitness facilities at their headquarters and major locations and hiring trainers and coordinators to staff them. These facilities are very expensive and are cost-effective only when large numbers of employees are concentrated in one place. An alternative is for the employer to pay for memberships in local fitness clubs or gyms, although the identification with the employer tends to be less strong in this case. A key to the success of fitness programs beyond lunchtime aerobics is to make available a variety of levels of involvement so that workers can individualize their regimens according to need, preference, and personal schedules. Another key to the success of fitness programs is the availability of a sufficient number of showers. Fitness programs can be started on a shoestring as lunchtime aerobics and stepped up from there. Men, particularly, often see the facilities as an opportunity to regain or maintain athletic levels of fitness, but an emphasis on this level of commitment , and the monopoly of fitness facilities by hard-bodied regulars, may discourage participation by out-of-shape workers, who need the facilities the most. It is important that fitness programs encourage participation at all levels and discourage attitudes that promote a "jock" or "gym" mentality of personal competition, cliquishness, and singles cruising. Properly supervised, fitness-activity related injuries are much less common than unsupervised sports-related injuries and on balance appear to reduce the risk of workplace injuries among participating workers, although this has been difficult to document. Since workplace fitness programs are not oriented to athletes, persons of normal strength and coordination can set reasonable goals and attain them; the emphasis should not be on high performance. Fitness programs are fun and build morale among employees. From the point of view of management, fitness programs are excellent opportunities to build morale and team spirit among employees.

Nutrition and weight control are very popular program elements that tap into the concern of North Americans about their weight and eating habits. Because weight reduction is best achieved through reinforcement of diet and exercise behavior, it makes sense that group programs would be effective, although this remains unproven for the long term. Further, because objective nutritional education is hard to come by in daily life in a society devoted to product marketing, the nutritional counseling component of such programs is very popular. Weight control programs dovetail well with other health promotion activities, particularly fitness and cardiovascular risk factor modification, and lend themselves well to campaigns and institutional changes (particularly light cafeteria menus). They are good ways to start or to introduce a more comprehensive health promotion program in the workplace. One approach has been an incentive in which the employer makes a contribution to an employee's individual "cafeteria fund" (i.e., the company helps to buy lunch, but it has to be healthy), which demonstrates that simple measures to achieve gains are possible within the health promotion paradigm.

Smoking cessation programs are common, popular, and often effective, especially when combined with a change in corporate smoking policies that reduce opportunities to smoke. Help to stop smoking is very nearly an ethical necessity when smoking is abruptly prohibited in a facility or workplace. Because approximately one-third of smokers are thought to be sufficiently addicted to cigarettes to be unable or unwilling to quit on their own, corporate smoking cessation programs can provide a real community service.

Cardiovascular risk factor modification programs include all of the elements previously mentioned as well as regular cholesterol and blood pressure determinations. Managing individuals with clinical hypertension or major elevations in blood cholesterol is primarily a medical responsibility and is beyond the scope of worksite health promotion programs. However, such programs may be an opportunity for on-site medical facilities to monitor health at work for employees at risk. Cardiovascular risk factor modification in worksite health promotion programs plays a supporting role in modifying the health risk of the great majority of persons with normal blood lipid phenotypes who can control their level of risk within the "non-high-risk" group by simple dietary adjustments and exercise.

Stress management is a popular theme in health promotion programs and is sometimes introduced during critical transitions in the company, especially during times of layoffs. The topic is discussed in Chapter 13.

EMPLOYEE ASSISTANCE

"Employee assistance" is a term, adopted in 1974 by the National Institute on Alcoholism and Alcohol Abuse, that refers to an organized system to provide assistance to employees with personal problems, mostly related to substance abuse. Employee assistance is by definition a form of secondary and sometimes tertiary prevention, because it is designed to identify and stop the progression of an existing health problem and to assist the worker in obtaining skills and building the motivation to overcome it. The guiding philosophy of employee assistance is that the worker is more likely to recover and manage an addictive behavior or to break other health-adverse habits with the support of a community and when something the person values is at stake, like a job. Employee assistance is a way of helping troubled employees for their own sake, giving workers with problems a second chance, and saving value for the employer by retaining skilled and loyal employees.

Employee assistance programs (EAPs) identify workers with personal problems, refer them for treatment, support and motivate them to complete treatment, and assist in their rehabilitation. The majority of "broad brush" EAPs are really substance abuse and financial counseling programs with a relatively small primary preventive aspect, usually in the form of low-key health education. Participants in EAPs either self-refer or are referred to the EAP by management because of performance problems or positive drug screening tests.

(Drug screening is discussed in Chapter 18 because it pertains primarily to fitness for duty.) Most EAPs are focused on alcohol and drug abuse and mental illness, but many concern themselves with family and adjustment problems, financial mismanagement (particularly credit card overruns), grief management, adjustment crises (such as helping victims of crime or loss due to a disaster such as a fire), job burnout, stress in and outside the workplace, domestic violence, and mental illness. EAPs can be pivotal in the management of mental disorders, which is the second major category of disability in the United States and among the most costly diagnostic category for employer-sponsored health insurance, primarily because of long-term disability and duration of treatment and absence incidents. An important role of EAPs is helping the employee to reestablish balance in work and life.

EAPs usually do not provide on-site counseling and therapy beyond an initial session or crisis intervention. They identify workers with personal problems, refer them for treatment, monitor their progress, support and motivate them to complete treatment, and assist in their rehabilitation. The EAP also helps to determine fitness to return to work (see Chapter 18) and assists in the reintegration of workers.

EAPs are a very mature intervention strategy, with precedents going back decades, established protocols, and a wealth of empirical experience. The literature is summarized in one authoritative source, making this one of the few fields of public health that, uniquely, can be encapsulated in a single handbook, a work by Oher that has been through many editions and is considered the standard reference in the field.

An EAP operates primarily by self-referral of patients, who are then referred to local healthcare or counseling facilities. Some workers are sent to EAP programs by their supervisors as a condition of retaining employment when their job performance has suffered or they have appeared to be impaired. The employer is informed of the progress of the employee's rehabilitation and guarantees return to the same or similar work when recovery is sufficient. Confidential information, such as diagnosis, treatment, and the content of interviews, is not shared with management. EAPs usually do not provide direct treatment except for initial counseling. Instead, EAPs usually rely on existing community services.

If a worker presents signs of personal problems, anxiety, or substance abuse, that worker may be helped by self-referral to an employer's EAP, if one is available. In the absence of an EAP, the physician can perform the initial evaluation, triage, and, in some cases, begin treatment on an individual basis. Many employers will be cooperative and may assume costs for key or long-term employees if reimbursement under the health plan is not complete. It is not unusual for the cost of treatment to be shared between the employer and the health plan or a private insurer, depending on local arrangements. Maintaining patient confidentiality is essential at every step.

The ideal is of course voluntary referral by individuals who recognize that they may have a problem affecting their life and work. Obviously, some insight and honesty are required to recognize the symptoms, and people in denial may be incapable of recognizing the cardinal symptoms of alcohol abuse.

The emphasis should always be on voluntary referrals, but acceptance of mandatory referral may be necessary if the alternative is for the individual to be fired after a certain number of warnings. One cannot count on such people having the insight to refer themselves, however, and for that reason mandatory referrals are almost inevitable if a program is to be truly effective as an alternative to firing the impaired worker. Mandatory referral should only be used as a last resort, however, and every effort should be made to encourage voluntary referral, at least in part because the programs work better for those who have taken the initiative to refer themselves. This means promoting the program heavily and insuring that confidentiality is kept strictly. Privacy measures should be highly visible; for example, the EAP office should be off site and away from view of other employees. (Two hospitals on opposite sides of the island of Oahu, Hawaii, for example, each with EAP programs, had an agreement to take one another's employees.)

As a general rule, if an EAP program is operating primarily with voluntary referrals, it is doing well. If most of the participants are there because of mandatory referrals due to poor work performance, this suggests a problem with how the EAP is perceived. The program may not be trusted by employees, it may be overused by supervisors, it may not be sufficiently promoted, or the workers for whom it is intended may not view it as a viable resource for their problems.

The supervisor's role in an EAP should be kept limited but is essential to the process. The supervisor may play a very constructive role in identifying the problem since supervisors are often the first to see a decline in work performance or other indications that a worker is in trouble. The supervisor may also be able to arrange the worker's schedule and duties to accommodate participation in the program and to ensure easy return on completion. The supervisor, in short, cannot be kept out of the process but should be involved only to a limited extent in keeping with the confidentiality of medical information. The supervisor has no business receiving any sort of medical or personal information on the worker, although it is impossible to stop rumors and information through the shop grapevine reaching him or her. The supervisor is entitled to receive regular reports on the worker's fitness to return to work and to assume the duties required by the job. The supervisor does not need to receive any specific diagnosis or sensitive information, only whether or not the individual can do the job and if the individual cannot what the individual is capable of doing if there is evidence of impairment. The supervisor should also be told if there is any possibility that the individual could be a risk to others. In a humane and supportive working environment, the supervisor can be a big help in facilitating the return to normal working life of the recovering worker. It is important, however, for the worker, the supervisor, the company, and the union to be entirely clear on the ground rules ahead of time to prevent problems. There is obviously a fine line between a supervisor's human concern on the one side and meddling and paternalism on the other.

EAPs appear to be cost-effective for the employer, particularly in large organizations, depending on its structure and level of activity. It is not unusual for the cost of treatment to be shared between the employer and the health plan or a private insurer, depending on local arrangements.

There is a sharp distinction to be made between employee assistance programs and health promotion programs. The two types of programs should be kept distinct and under separate organizations. Employee assistance programs are very sensitive and should be tightly controlled, while health promotion programs should be more relaxed and activities are usually best done in groups.

Referral to an outside counselor or health professional for evaluation and treatment, rather than treatment by an internal unit within the organization, is generally preferable. Unless an employer is very large, it is difficult to preserve the confidentiality required when workers receive their care at the worksite. The employee assistance counselor should be isolated from the pressures of management (as, ideally, should the occupational physician), but in practice it is very difficult to stand alone in the organization against requests for information and certification to return an employee to work. Many effective programs rely on external agencies to provide treatment and medical or psychological evaluations and use their in-house counselor to monitor progress through regular reporting and discussions with the treating health professionals or for crisis interventions when necessary. This approach is also more cost effective, in general, than establishing an elaborate treatment program onsite. Having the evaluation and treatment at arm's length from the employer keeps a degree of objectivity, removes the suspicion that management might interfere, and reduces mistrust over the quality of care being given.

DISEASE/CASE MANAGEMENT

Employers have become increasingly interested in managing high-cost cases through assistance in scheduling, monitoring compliance, referrals to specialized care, convenient workplace health monitoring (through their occupational health services), education and behavioral medicine, pharmacy-care programs and tertiary prevention (interventions to prevent disabilities and disease progression). This trend, which is growing in strength in the business community, follows the observation that individualized risk factor intervention for high-risk employees results in more favorable outcomes that broad employee health promotion programs alone.

An example of the disease management approach is a program introduced by Lucent Technologies. Employees were screened for cardiovascular risk factors, and qualified high-risk employees were then supported through exercise/fitness programs, educational programs, dietary change, and individualized on-site counseling in the workplace. The program achieved a high level of employee satisfaction, identified 2.4 percent of the employees as having diabetes, and resulted in 17 percent of the employees beginning cardiovascular medication. On the other hand, in one employer-sponsored cardiovascular risk reduction program, employees who were followed up with structured programs after screening did not do as well as those who chose informal means of health risk management. Thus, there is much that remains to be defined and clarified in the disease/case management approach.

The principal conditions that major employers considered to be priorities (over 40 percent deemed highly important) are those that incur the greatest costs in productivity and health-related expenses: back pain, musculoskeletal disorders, depression and other mental disorders, repetitive strain injury, cardiovascular risk factors (hypertension, obesity and diabetes), substance abuse, smoking-related problems, and influenza. Arthritis and headache/migraine are also known to be associated with a disproportionate loss of productivity. However, employers rated their performance in managing most of these priority conditions as deficient. The conclusion to be drawn from these and other data is that there is a large performance gap in management of disorders connected with the greatest loss of productivity and that current models of intervention and behavior change are not meeting the need.

The movement for intensive case management is not well documented in the literature, unlike the abundant literature on the health promotion movement. Employers are engaging in this approach reluctantly, aware that it may be considered intrusive by employees and unions, and many employers believe that they are being forced, in effect, to assume responsibility for direct delivery of care, which is outside their core business and comfort zone.

Not as developed but equally important with respect to social benefit is the measure of the advantages of workplace-centered wellness programs to workers and their families: improved general health and vitality, reduced risk of catastrophic illness, enhanced employment security, enhanced productivity in non-employment-related activities, and protected social capacity, by which is meant the ability to play social roles as, for example, a parent, friend, community leader or civic participant.

WELLNESS AND PRODUCTIVITY MANAGEMENT

Employers today are confronted by severely rising costs and declining economic prospects, especially during the current recession, which have led employer-payers to consider new healthcare reform strategies. The strategy of wellness and productivity management emphasizes prevention, managed care, and marketplace mechanisms and has increasingly considered previously unacceptable measures that involve intensive case management, individual intervention, and personal tracking that would previously have been considered overly intrusive on the part of an employer. However, faced with the burden of paying for healthcare coverage, employers are increasingly assertive in their role as healthcare managers and see no alternative to managing their employees' health. What is new about this approach (which is not well documented in the medical literature) is that efforts are being more tightly targeted and the interventions are specifically designed to reduce high-cost outcomes such as chronic disability.

This framework emphasizes science-based health and human performance interventions intended to target opportunities for controlling costs and enhancing productivity. This would be achieved through reduced sickness incidents, improved case outcomes, decreased "presenteeism" (the presence of a worker on the job but not working at full capacity, due to low-grade illness or incapacity), and enhanced physical capacity to do the job. Most cardiovascular and mental disorders are the leading targets, and the intervention may take the form of health promotion programs or intensive case management for chronic disorders associated with high cost and the risk of disability, such as diabetes.

The prevailing philosophy of this strategy has been that health-care costs could be brought under control, or at least reduced into more manageable proportions, by reducing both the actual need and the demand for market-driven health services. This strategy encourages interventions targeted to prevent loss of productive years of life and to prevent disability, rather than the more traditional goals of extending life and preventing disease. For example, one major initiative undertaken by Thomas Jefferson University was to quantify lost productivity due to migraine headaches, on the theory that intensive management could result in considerable cost savings that would recover the cost of introducing and maintaining the program. This policy approach may require substantial cultural change to discourage risk-taking behavior, to devolve responsibility for personal health management (and triage) on the individual from a practitioner or system, and to manage individual cases through intensive case management, facilitated scheduling, or services and provider discounts (such as drug plans). The goals would be achieved by, respectively, health promotion (and self-care), managed care, and intensive case management.

As the attention of industry has shifted from cost control and loss reduction to productivity, the tools for measuring performance and assessing efficacy have also changed and have become much more sophisticated. Disease outcomes and the cost of disability are relatively crude measures. More sensitive financial and behavioral indicators have been developed to assess productivity on a micro level, for evaluation purposes, and to identify opportunities for intervention. These include the Health and Labor Questionnaire, the Work

Productivity and Activity Impairment Questionnaire, the Osterhaus productivity technique (based on frequency of presence and absence and developed for migraine studies), the MacArthur Health and Performance Questionnaire, the Work Limitation Questionnaire, and the Stanford Presenteeism Scale, among many others. The measures used to do this include time on task in the workplace, work quality, work quantity (productivity), interpersonal functioning in the workplace, and work culture. A comprehensive toolkit is now available from the American College of Occupational and Environmental Medicine.

An important aspect of productivity research is the financial gain to the employer of promoting health among employees. Current methodology stresses identifying the "break-even" point at which an investment in wellness covers the cost of operating a program. However, senior managers in industry are oriented more toward comparing alternative rates of return than either to loss reduction or covering costs alone. This strategy may backfire if unscrupulous managers use tactics to exclude high-risk individuals from the workforce or to make jobs more difficult for the disabled (fortunately, such tactics have been made more difficult with the requirements of the Americans with Disabilities Act) rather than modifying the work or introducing wellness programs. The OEM physician often faces a challenge in influencing senior management to do the right thing, but a good business case combined with ethics and a corporate policy spelling out commitment can be very persuasive.

RESOURCES

Boulware LE, Marinopoulos S, Phillips KA, Hwang CW, Maynor K, Merenstein D, Wilson RF, Barnes GJ, Bass EB, Powe NR, Daumit GL. The value of the periodic health evaluation (systematic review). *Ann Inten Med.* 2007;146(4): 289–300.

Swotinsky RB, Smith DR. *The Medical Review Officer's Manual: MROCC's Guide to Drug Testing.* Beverley Farms, MA: OEM Press; 2006.

U.S. Preventive Services Task Force. *The Guide to Clinical Preventive Services.* Washington DC, Agency for Healthcare Research and Management, updated annually. Available at www.ahrq.gov/clinic/uspstf/uspstopics.htm.

NOTEWORTHY READINGS

American College of Occupational and Environmental Medicine, ACOEM Health-Related Productivity Roundtable. *The Health of the Workforce and its Impact on Business.* Arlington Heights, IL: ACOEM; 2003.

American College of Occupational and Environmental Medicine, and The Benfield Group. *Strategic Management Needs in Health and Productivity.* Arlington Heights, IL: ACOEM; 2003.

American College of Occupational and Environmental Medicine, and the Office of Health Policy and Clinical Outcomes, Thomas Jefferson University. *Health-Related Work Loss and Productivity.* Arlington Heights, IL: ACOEM; 2002.

American College of Physicians, Medical Practice Committee. Periodic health examination: a guide for designing individualized preventive health care in the asymptomatic employee. *Ann Intern Med.* 1981;95:729–732.

Battista RN, Lawrence RS. Implementing Preventive Services. *Am J Prev Med.* 1988 (suppl);4(4).

Bertera RL. Planning and implementing health promotion in the workplace: a case study of the Du Pont company experience. *Health Educ Q.* 1990;17:307–317.

Bertera RL. The effects of workplace health promotion on absenteeism and employment costs in a large industrial population. *Am J Pub Health.* 1990;80:1101–1105.

Borland R, et al. Changes in acceptance of workplace smoking bans following their implementation: a prospective study. *Prev Med.* 1990;19:314–322.

Brady W, Bass J, Moser R, Anstadt G, Loeppke R, Leopold R. Total corporate health care costs. *J Occup Environ Med.* 1997;39:224–231.

Breslow L, Somers AR. The lifetime health monitoring program—a practical approach to preventive medicine. *N Engl J Med.* 1977;22:588–592.

Canadian Task Force on the Periodic Health Examination. The periodic health examination. *Can Med Assoc J.* 1979;12:1194–1254.

Canadian Task Force on the Periodic Health Examination. The periodic health examination: 1. 1984 update. *Can Med Assoc J.* 1984;130:1278–1292.

Charap MH. The periodic health examination: genesis of a myth. *Ann Intern Med.* 1981;95:733–735.

Conrad P. Worksite health promotion (special issue). *Social Sci Med.* 1988;26(5):485–575.

Goldbloom R, Battista RN, Haggerty J. The periodic health examination: 1. Introduction, 2. 1989 update. *Can Med Assoc J.* 1989;141:205-207, 209–216.

Green H. *Fit for America: Health, Fitness, Sport and American Society.* New York: Pantheon Books; 1986.

Gross PA, Cataruozolo P, Mitofsky W, Furnari M, Crupi T, Skurnick JH, DeMauro P, Statmore G, Moogan M, Berdy J, Sokol C. Implementing preventive health measures: a pilot study. *Clin Perform Qual Health Care.* 1999;7(2):52–55.

Guico-Pabio CJ, Cioffi L, Shoner LG. The Lucent-takes-heart cardiovascular health management program: successful workplace screening. *AAOHN J.* 2002;50:365–372

Guidotti TL. Adaptation of the lifetime health monitoring concept to defined employee groups not at exceptional risk. *J Occup Med.* 1983;25:731–736.

Guidotti TL. Comparative models for workplace-centered wellness. *J Health Productivity.* 2008;3(1):15–21.

Han PKJ. Historical changes in the objectives of the periodic health examination. *Ann Intern Med.* 1997;127:910–917.

Health Promotion Research Methods: Expanding the Repertoire. Conference overview and selected papers. *Can J Public Health.* 1992 (suppl 1); 83.

Health Promotion: A Discussion Document on the Concept and Principles. Copenhagen: World Health Organization Regional Office for Europe, ICP/HSR 602, 1984.

Hopkins WG, Walker NP. The meaning of "physical fitness". *Prev Med.* 1988;17:764–773.

Keating DP, Hertzman C, eds. *Developmental Health and the Wealth of Nations: Social, Biological and Educational Dynamics.* London: Guildford; 1999.

Labonté R. Population health and health promotion: what do they have to say to each other? *Can J Pub Health.* 1995;86:165–168.

Lalonde M, Health and Welfare Canada. *A New Perspective on the Health of Canadians.* Ottawa: Health and Welfare Canada; 1975. [The Lalonde Report]

Mullan P. *The Imaginary Time Bomb.* London: I. B. Tauris; 2000.

Ockene JK, Edgerton EA, Teutsch SM, et al. Integrating evidence-based clinical and community strategies to improve health. *Am J Prev Med.* 2007;32:244–252.

Oher JM. *The Employee Assistance Handbook.* New York: Wiley; 1999.

Ozminkowski RJ, Goetzel RZ, Santoro J, Saenz B, Eley C, Gorsley B. Estimating risk reduction required to break even in a health promotion program. *Am J Health Promo.* 2004;18:316–325.

Pelletier KR. A review and analysis of the clinical- and cost-effectiveness studies of comprehensive health promotion and disease management programs at the worksite: 1998–2000 update. *Am J Health Promo.* 2001;16:107–116.

Pescatello LS, Murphy D, Vollono J, Lynch E, Bernene J, Costanzo D. The cardiovascular health impact of an incentive worksite health promotion program. *Am J Health Promo.* 2001;16:16–20.

Pollmar TC, Brandt ENJ, Baird MA. Health and behavior: the interplay of biological, behavioral, and social influences. Summary of an institute of medicine report. *Am J Health Promo.* 2002;16:206–219.

Russell LB. The role of prevention in health reform. *N Engl J Med*. 1993;329: 352–354.

Sagan LA. *The Health of Nations: True Causes of Sickness and Well-Being*. New York: Basic Books; 1987.

Schneider WJ, Stewart SC, Haughey M. Health promotion in a scheduled cyclical format. *J Occup Med*. 1989;31:443–446.

Sciacca J, Seehafer R, Reed R, Mulvaney D. The impact of participation in health promotion on medical costs: a reconsideration of the Blue Cross Blue Shield of Indiana study. *Am J Health Promo*. 1993;7:374–383.

Scofield ME, ed. Worksite health promotion. *Occup Med*. 1990;5(4):653–876.

Self-Care Institute. *Demand Management Handbook*. Washington, DC: Partnership for Prevention; 1996.

Stein AD, Shakour SK, Zuidema RA. Financial incentives, participation in employer-sponsored health promotion and changes in employee health and productivity: HealthPlus health quotient program. *J Occup Environ Med*. 2000;42:1148–1155.

Terris M. The distinction between public health and community/social/ preventive medicine. *J Pub Health Pol*. 1985;435–439.

World Health Organization. *The Ottawa Charter for Health Promotion*. Ottawa: World Health Organization, Health and Welfare Canada, and Canadian Public Health Association; 1986.

20 OCCUPATIONAL HEALTH SERVICES

An occupational health service (OHS) is a facility or unit that provides healthcare and prevention services to workers. In this chapter, the term is used to refer to staff and facilities providing medical care, with or without support services. An OHS in this sense is analogous to a "service" in a hospital. (For some reason, OHSs are rarely called "occupational medicine services.") OHSs normally consist of an occupational medicine clinic and supporting services for hazard control, wellness, and evaluation. They may be inside the organization or outside, providing services on contract or case by case.

OHSs have a medical orientation and provide healthcare services. The units called "occupational health and safety departments," on the other hand, manage workplace health protection but do not provide healthcare. Occupational health and safety departments are within the organization but are not necessarily comprehensive; they may contract out for services such as occupational (industrial) hygiene.

Every OHS has its own mission and reporting relationships. In general, the purposes of an OHS are to:

- Manage injuries, illness, and disability resulting from work
- Protect employees from occupational risks where they work

- Prevent disability by providing or managing the highest level of care followed by support during recovery and rehabilitation as needed
- Achieve the highest practicable level of health and productivity among all employees of the enterprise for which it is responsible
- Ensure that work capacity, production requirements, and job requirements match
- Support the business, that is, assist in the management of workers' compensation, insurance, administration, monitoring, and productivity

This chapter will discuss the role of various types of OHSs, their organization, their operation, and their limitations.

THE OCCUPATIONAL HEALTHCARE SYSTEM

The occupational healthcare system exists in parallel with the larger general healthcare system in North America. The general healthcare system is undergoing rapid and fundamental change in the United States, as is well known. By comparison, the occupational healthcare system is less well known and much less well understood in its complexity. The occupational healthcare system is separately financed and is organized around different principles than the general healthcare system. The two systems share practitioners and facilities, but they function very differently in the service of each system and often interact poorly.

The currently decentralized and individualized approach to providing medical care has fragmented care and resulted in a diffuse and sometimes incomplete network of practitioners providing OHSs. These practitioners primarily serve a centralized workers' compensation system and coexist with medical services sponsored by larger employers. Large parts of the system, such as the appeals process in workers' compensation and the in-plant occupational health and safety activities, have become invisible to the average practitioner in the community.

OHSs are often the historical basis for general systems of health-care. In many countries, and in North America in times past, OHSs have been the basis for providing general healthcare in newly urbanized or settled areas of industrial development. The railroads played a major role in establishing hospitals and supporting physicians outside the major cities in both the United States and Canada in the eighteenth century, for example. In Venezuela, health services for the general population in the western part of the country developed from medical services provided for the employees of oil companies. In Mexico, the financing of individual health services started through the employment-based social security (*seguridad social*) systems. In the United States, innovations in healthcare financing for employees and their dependents laid the foundation for health maintenance organizations, capitated reimbursement, and integrated hospital systems.

Characteristics of the System

Occupational healthcare as provided by the physician is part of a much larger, complex system. The system is built on different assumptions than the general or personal healthcare system. In a traditional fee-for-service setting, the primary relationship is that between physician and patient, with the insurance carrier or other third-party payers now playing an increasingly active role, as illustrated in Figure 20.1. OHSs, on the other hand, are often five-sided relationships involving the physician, the patient, the employer, a government regulatory agency, the workers' compensation board and

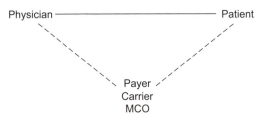

Figure 20.1. Relationship of the physician, patient, and other stakeholders in general medical care.

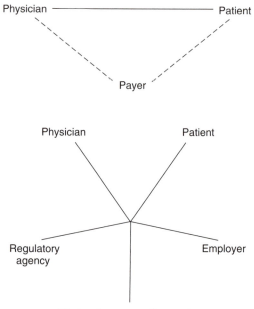

Figure 20.2. Relationship of the physician, injured worker and other stakeholders in occupational medical care.

carrier, and often a union as well, as illustrated in Figure 20.2. Among these stakeholders, information circulates subject to legal requirements and accepted rules of confidentiality. Authority for decisions and responsibility for compensation do not rest mostly or even primarily with the physician but are shared according to the roles of each player. The physician often acts as an agent reporting to the employer or to the carrier rather than on behalf of the individual patient, as in the case of independent medical evaluations. Figure 20.2 illustrates these differences. Ethical dilemmas predictably arise when these responsibilities conflict, but the legal relationships are fairly well defined.

Occupational medicine services may be divided into two categories: (1) curative and ameliorative and (2) preventive (Table 20.1). Curative and ameliorative services are intended to cure or to limit disease or to manage an existing problem. Preventive services seek to

Table 20.1. Occupational Medicine Services

Subsets of Services	Curative/Ameliorative	Preventive
"Industrial medicine" (traditional name, not a recognized specialty)	Acute and chronic care Disability evaluation	Pre-placement and periodic screening
Occupational hygiene (teamwork required)	Health hazard evaluation Compliance with government regulations	Consultation Worker education Surveillance Monitoring
Personal health (individual health)	Employee assistance programs	Health promotion (enhancement)

avoid exposure of the worker to hazards, to detect disorders at an early and potentially curable stage, and to limit disability. The physician's responsibility is first to the patient whether in treating occupational disorders or intervening and educating to avoid the development of preventable illness. It is the employer's role to deal with the economic and public relations aspects of a problem, not the physician's role. Table 20.2 provides a breakdown of the tasks performed by a physician-led regional medical office of one large utility in the

Table 20.2. Distribution of Services Provided by or Under the Supervision of a Physician for a Large Utility in a Representative Year

Management of work-related injury or illness, clinical	30 percent
Fitness-to-work evaluations, other than pre-placement	25 percent
Absence review, certifying return to work after illness, and reviewing personal healthcare issues	20 percent
Counseling and arranging referral for employee assistance	8 percent
Periodic health evaluations, either surveillance mandated by regulation, or voluntarily for employees at elevated risk	8 percent
Management of minor personal health problems, clinical	6 percent
Pre-placement evaluations	3 percent

United States. It illustrates the distribution of work in an industry without unusual hazards.

In occupational medicine, the diagnosis is often the beginning rather than the end of the evaluative process. This is particularly true for occupational illnesses due to workplace exposures and for repetitive motion injuries. The related but distinct questions of the exposure responsible, the work-relatedness of the condition, and the expected degree of disability are sometimes more important than a precise diagnosis because on such questions hinges eligibility for compensation, prognosis for rehabilitation, fitness for future work, and prevention for the protection of other workers.

Prompt and effective treatment of the injured worker can save that individual from unnecessary disability. An early return to work, when medically indicated, can also assist in rehabilitation. Acute care in an occupational healthcare setting, however, is more than a simple service function as it might be in a hospital emergency room. Opportunities exist within a well-organized occupational healthcare system to use the lessons learned from each injury, either singly or as aggregate statistical data, to prevent future injuries. The ultimate goal of an occupational health intervention, of course, is to control the hazard that led to the problem in the first place.

The physician never acts alone in an occupation-related case. Each action is reviewed and closely monitored behind the scenes, whether the physician is aware of it or not. Workers' compensation carriers require telephone authorizations after the initial visit, copies of the medical record, and supplemental reports before payment is authorized.

Another aspect of delivering occupational healthcare is the importance of accurate and segregated medical records. These records are subject to review not only by the patient, but also by the insurance carrier, the employer, or outside consultants when a claim is appealed. In disputed cases, medical records are subpoenaed. Occupational health records must be maintained separately from the patient's personal medical records to prevent inadvertently breaking confidentiality. The occupational health record should not include personal or medical information that is not directly pertinent to the workers' occupational health, such as incidental past medical history (which may include much confidential material of no concern to other parties), detailed family history, correspondence about billing, or any remarks on the patient's character or that of the employer. The rules for disclosure and for authorizing release of information by the patient are spelled out in occupational health and safety regulations. Occupational health records should be maintained for at least thirty years (in keeping with the OSHA standard for retention of medical records) and preferably indefinitely.

A clear understanding of the occupational health and safety and the workers' compensation system will prevent unnecessary problems and administrative burdens. Information on how each system operates is available on request from the appropriate federal, state, or provincial agency, workers' compensation board, or from workers' compensation insurance carriers. Information on maintaining occupational medicine records is available from the government agencies responsible for occupational health and safety.

OCCUPATIONAL HEALTH PROFESSIONALS

Teamwork, administrative ability, and versatility play a greater role than in other specialties. The new occupational and environmental medicine (OEM) physician soon finds that he or she depends on other skilled health professionals, such as occupational health nurses, safety engineers, and industrial hygienists (engineers trained in the recognition and control of health hazards in the workplace). Each of these professional groups has its own training, certification, and licensing arrangements; the OEM physician relies as heavily on these skilled professionals as a surgeon relies on the operating room team. Some of the professions are listed in Table 20.3. For ease of communication, it is useful to know about the background and role of the principal occupational health professions.

There are two types of OEM physicians traditionally found in employer-based facilities: the "plant physician" and the "corporate medical director." Since the mid-1980s, most OEM physicians are

Table 20.3. Occupational Health Professions

Occupational Medicine
Occupational Health Nursing
Industrial Hygiene
Ergonomics
Safety Engineering
Radiation Health
Occupational Audiology
Toxicology
Epidemiology
Risk and Liability Control
Employee Assistance Management
Vocational Rehabilitation
Fitness and Health Promotion Program Management

based in the community and practice out of their own medical offices or other OHSs; they are formally called "community-based occupational medicine practitioners" (and often informally call themselves "occ docs," pronounced "ock-dox"). "On-site medical practitioners" may be as good a name as any for the increasing number of medical practitioners who practice in "on-site clinics," general medical clinics in stores and factories. This trend only began in 2006 but has grown rapidly. On-site practitioners are not OEM physicians, but they are sometimes called upon to provide basic services, such as pre-placement evaluations.

"In-plant services" are provided inside the employer's facilities, usually by a practitioner hired part-time by the employer. A "plant dispensary" or infirmary may employ a plant physician and an occupational health nurse whose responsibility may range from simple triage and first aid to fairly comprehensive primary care. Plant physicians have no direct authority in setting corporate policy. The corporate medical director, on the other hand, is usually based at the headquarters of the organization.

Corporate medical directors usually see only a few selected patients with special problems and spend most of their time managing and contributing to policy on health-related matters within the company.

Community-based occupational medicine practitioners became a majority in the 1990s, reflecting outsourcing and downsizing in corporate medical departments. Increasing numbers of trained OEM physicians started practicing outside industry in clinics, group practices, and other community-based medical facilities. Paradoxically, the total volume of occupational medical services seems to have dramatically increased at the time, probably because the new availability of such services in the community attracted midsize and smaller employers that previously did not access OHSs. By 2000, the total number of practitioners had increased disproportionately to the number of physicians leaving industry and the number of specialists finishing training programs, indicating that more practitioners were recruited into the field in midcareer. A small number of physicians, mostly specialists in occupational medicine, maintain full-time private practices exclusively directed to disability evaluations, assessing causation and work-relationship, and reviewing cases under appeal or litigation.

On-site medical practitioners are mostly family physicians, who practice primary care rather than the full range of OHSs. To date, these clinics have not employed OEM physicians. However, the convenience and low cost of the model means that inevitably the practitioner will be asked to perform many services in OEM.

An "occupational health nurse" specializes in OHSs, almost always in an in-plant setting. Occupational health nurses are trained in health education, occupational health, disease recognition, rehabilitation, and administration. The specialty is highly regarded within nursing for its relative autonomy and level of responsibility. "Occupational health nurse practitioners" perform midlevel practitioner duties in the workplace, much like plant physicians. The principal organization for nurses in the field is the American Association of Occupational Health Nurses. Since 1972, there has been a specialty board certification in North America for nurses in the field.

An "occupational hygienist" or "industrial hygienist" is a professional specialized in the recognition, evaluation, and control of occupational health hazards. The training includes engineering solutions, ventilation, analytical chemistry, mathematics, and toxicology, usually at the master's degree level. Board certification is provided by the American Board of Industrial Hygiene and is quite rigorous. The principal organization for industrial hygienists in both the United States and Canada is the American Industrial Hygiene Association, which has many local chapters.

A "safety engineer" is responsible for the recognition and control of safety hazards. Their preparation is usually not at the graduate university level. Many safety professionals have obtained their training in short-term, intensive institutes or seminars. Often, safety professionals have worked their way up through experience and continuing education from positions as foremen or supervisors. Their training usually emphasizes physical hazards, fire protection, and safety education. In the United States, the American Society of Safety Engineers and the National Safety Council are the leading professional and general membership organizations concerned with safety. The Canadian Society of Safety Engineers and the Canada Safety Council are the major general safety organizations in Canada. There are many associations concerned with safety in particular industries and many more committees and working groups within trade association and industry groups.

A "work evaluation" or "rehabilitation counselor" is a consultant called into a case by the workers' compensation or other insurance carrier to assess the work skills, physical tolerances, specialized training, and motivation of the worker. The assessment is used in judging disability in workers' compensation cases. Work evaluation counselors are usually trained at a bachelor's or master's level and often have backgrounds in rehabilitation and physical therapy as well.

An "audiologist" is a health professional specializing in the evaluation of hearing disorders. Audiologists are usually trained at the master's or doctoral level in behavioral audiometry, the physiology of hearing, speech pathology, acoustics, and psychological aspects of hearing impairment. Audiologists usually work closely with physicians in the diagnosis and evaluation of hearing impairment. Audiologists are not to be confused with occupational hearing conservationists, who are technicians with a certification from the Council of Accreditation in Occupational Hearing Conservation, which attests to their skill in performing audiometric evaluations of workers exposed to noise. Occupational hearing conservationists are technicians trained in the proper procedures for conducting screening, but not necessarily diagnostic, audiograms in working populations.

OCCUPATIONAL HEALTH SERVICE FACILITIES

The role of the OHS is to provide assistance both to management and the employee/worker so that the worker is not harmed in the course of work. To fulfill this role, the OHS facility must be and also must be perceived to be objective and impartial, whether it is part of the management structure or an external healthcare provider. The operational responsibility for sound occupational health and safety practice lies with the people who do and supervise the work: the employee, operating personnel, and managers. The OHS exists to serve them; it can assist, but it cannot be in all places at all times. Its role is that of consultant, troubleshooter, teacher, auditor, and advocate. It cannot function as a policeman, personnel officer, or scapegoat and remain effective.

Most routine occupational health services are simple in their execution. Employers are not always aware of differences in quality among potential providers of occupational health services and may not see any reason to pay a premium for quality when "adequate" will do, insofar as acute care for simple injuries is concerned. Perceived quality of care, beyond adequate, is not usually a consideration. Although the worker receives occupational healthcare in the role of "patient," it is usually the employer (sometimes the carrier) who selects the provider of care and plays the role of "consumer." In this situation, the major incentive governing the behavior of the "consumer" is to control costs, not to maximize benefit.

The decision by the management of an employer to develop an in-house capability to provide or to contract with an outside medical provider for an OHS and how the arrangement shall be structured must reflect the realities within both the organization and the community of which the organization is a part. Among the considerations that managers should take into consideration are the following:

1. Is qualified medical care (i.e., from physicians knowledgeable about occupational disorders) available in the community and easily accessible?
2. Do operations within the organization require special insight or expertise because of particular hazards, unusual technology, or the potential for injuries?
3. What are the pertinent regulations regarding occupational safety and health?
4. What has been the past experience of the organization and what is its expected future growth?
5. Who are the employees, what is their social, ethnic, and economic background, will they use the facility, and can the facility effectively meet their needs in communication and for prevention and health promotion?
6. How much of an investment is the organization prepared to make?

Types of Occupational Health Facilities

Occupational health facilities can be divided into "in-plant" and "external" facilities. Until recently, in-plant services dominated the delivery of occupational healthcare.

In-plant services are provided within the employer's facilities and almost always by a practitioner employed by the employer. In-plant services are practical only for larger firms. Within the last two decades, "off-site" or community-based healthcare facilities have displaced in-plant services as the principal form of organization for providing healthcare. Many practitioners, especially family physicians, provide such services in the course of their practice out of their own office. The major facility of this type at present, however, is the free-standing "occupational medical clinic," a medical group or practice more or less devoted to providing healthcare on a contract or fee-for-service basis with local industry. (In past years, the term "industrial medicine clinic" was often used, implying an inferior level of care.) Large multispecialty group practices, particularly in the east and southwest, have been developing occupational medicine services as a major new thrust. Hospital-based OHSs are becoming more prominent. At one time, there were many union-sponsored occupational health centers, but now only a handful of labor-oriented occupational health clinics exist, principally in New York and Canada, most notably the provincially funded Occupational Health Clinics for Ontario Workers (OHCAW). Government agencies may have medical clinics for their own employees. The military maintains occupational health clinics for both active duty and civilian personnel and in the aggregate constitutes a major subset of the occupational healthcare system.

OHSs in industry can be divided into "in-plant" or internal and "off-site" or external facilities and services. Internal services are overseen by a plant physician or occupational health nurse. On the corporate level, discussed later, a corporate medical director may oversee the in-plant services or coordinate and supervise the delivery of care by off-site contract physicians, or a combination of both.

Occupational medical services may take one of four basic forms:

- Internal, serving one employer
- External or "community-based," serving one employer or, more often, one industry
- Internal, serving multiple employers
- External or "community-based," serving multiple employers

Internal, Single Employer

Internal OHSs serving one employer are typical of large corporations, large single plants, and public agencies of cities and higher levels of government. They exist on two levels: the in-plant health service and the corporate medical department. In the past, the in-plant health service usually went by the name of infirmary, dispensary, or clinic; today it is usually called the occupational health or employee service. It is a facility where medical care above basic first aid can be rendered to ill or injured employees and where programs of a medical nature for prevention and health promotion are organized and implemented. It may be supervised by a suitably trained nurse or by a physician and is often staffed by both with the physician available by contract at designated times during the week. The in-plant health service is the first level of care, providing initial treatment and evaluation for fitness to work but rarely managing complex or difficult cases, which are usually sent outside to local practitioners. Unless a plant presents an unusual or particularly serious hazard, such as a shipyard, or it is in an unusually isolated location, it is generally unwise for the in-plant health service to provide specialized or major surgical care because of legal liability and the cost of maintaining adequately equipped facilities.

On-site general medical clinics represent a rapidly emerging model, newly introduced in 2006, although similar arrangements existed in the early twentieth century. Some companies, led by Wal-Mart, have opened general medical clinics in their stores and factories. The objective is to provide additional services to customers that add to convenience, increase sales, and make the store indispensible to the community. Wal-Mart began with plans for 400 such clinics and contracted with providers to staff them. At least one, Checkups, subsequently closed twenty-three facilities in 2008, but this contraction appears to have been due to inadequate financing rather than because business model was unsuccessful. Major drug store chains have opened similar clinics in their stores, including CVS and Walgreen's, with 200 clinics. Major employers such as Disney,

Toyota, and Harrah's Entertainment have opened clinics in their plants and office facilities as well but not to attract customers or visitors. These clinics operate with the objective of reducing health-care costs, time lost due to scheduled and emergency medical care, sickness absence, and presenteeism (when an employee is at work but not functioning due to a health problem). The on-site medical practitioner is not an OEM physician but is often called upon to perform basic procedures such as injury care and pre-placement evaluations. At least one contractor, CHD Meridian, offers a range of services including fitness-for-duty evaluations, pre-placement evaluations, employee assistance, acute injury care, impairment evaluation, and some health education programs; and markets its ability to handle workers' compensation cases. This model represents a potential opportunity for OEM physicians who wish to provide primary care as well and will probably do well in the current recession because of low cost and convenience.

Community-Based, Single Employer

External services serving a single employer or a single industry are common in the form of individual physicians or consultants who do part-time work, usually on an as-needed basis, for a particular company or public agency or a narrow range of companies in the same economic sector. Usually, this activity supplements a private practice, but it can be part of a physician's retirement activities or the result of a special relationship or prior experience with the agency or company or a specialized industry, such as aviation, with particular needs.

Internal, Multiple Employers

Internal programs providing services to multiple employers are of three general types: (1) in-plant services open to subsidiaries and affiliates of a larger company (essentially an extended form of the internal-single employer approach), (2) in-plant services open on a contract or fee-for-service basis to other small local companies (a variant of the external, multiple-employer approach), and (3) contractual arrangements by which an OHS provides limited in-plant services for several employers at the same time. The first two are more common in other countries where the healthcare system is not well developed or where "polyclinics" (healthcare centers serving the needs of a particular population) were once organized by industry or employment, as in Eastern Europe. The most common situation of contractual arrangement serving multiple employers with in-plant services is when a physician or occupational health nurse works part-time in more than one plant, practicing in the plant facilities.

Community-Based, Multiple Employer

External services serving multiple employers predominate in the occupational healthcare system. They include individual physicians, group practices, hospitals, and clinics that accept patients from several local employers on a contract or fee-for-service basis. OHSs serving many employers are in a relatively poor position to influence management and are at a disadvantage (and are not always motivated) in providing services in prevention or control of hazards. This is probably the only practical model for providing services to small enterprises, however, given the high overhead costs of maintaining internal services for small numbers of employees.

Several models exist for the provision of occupational healthcare to many employers. The most common are:

- Occupational medicine in primary care practice
- Consultation practice in occupational medicine
- Multispecialty group practice
- Hospital-based clinic
- The occupational health center (successor to the "industrial medicine" clinic)

The delivery of occupational health services at a high standard requires administrative skills beyond office management. To communicate successfully with all parties, including workers' compensation boards, employers, workers, regulatory agencies, and insurance carriers, requires special skills and the ability to appreciate a problem from many points of view. Clinical occupational medicine practice often requires the screening of large groups of well persons, in situations in which price is a factor. The various models of occupational healthcare facilities do not do equally well on these requirements.

Independent OHSs, as combined with primary care, as a consultation practice, or freestanding occupational health center, are entrepreneurial activities in which the business plan centers on the success of the OEM practice, which depends on the practitioner for quality of care and delivery of service. Sponsored OHSs, which are part of a hospital or group practice, are business-driven entrepreneurial activities in which the service is expected to fit in with a broader business plan and depends on the practitioner for quality of medical care but on the institution for delivery of service and support.

OHSs that are owned, operated, or embedded in healthcare institutions, such as multispecialty group practices and hospitals, face a common set of problems that is discussed in the subsection on operations.

Occupational Medicine in Primary Care Practice

Individual practitioners and hospital emergency rooms deal with innumerable occupation-related cases as a matter of routine, usually providing only acute or episodic care. This diffuse network of practitioners is the most widespread network of providers, but its capabilities are limited by the lack of available technical expertise; the absence of well-exercised skills in aspects of care management unusual or unique to occupational medicine practice; and the constraints on time, energy, and resources that can be invested in a narrow aspect of private practice. Most primary care physicians who do occupational medicine "on the side" are family physicians or emergency medicine specialists, although some are internists.

Primary care physicians have a decisive role to play in the private practice of occupational medicine. There are nowhere near enough OEM physicians to see all occupational injuries and illnesses. Primary care physicians will provide the major share of OHSs for the foreseeable future—and probably well beyond. Physicians may choose to emphasize occupational medicine in their practice for a number of reasons:

- To gain an additional source of revenue
- To obtain an additional source of patients for general care
- To meet the need for services in the community
- To conduct clinical research or to provide education and training
- To pursue a personal interest

There are inevitably practical problems for the primary care physician working in OHSs. These include the large administrative burden that falls on the physician because of the need to prepare claims and numerous reports, frequent legal actions involving the physician as a witness, and the need for frequent reporting to employers. On the other hand, the concept of prevention is directly compatible with the missions of family practice and internal medicine, in particular.

The greatest drawback to the incorporation of occupational medicine practice into primary care is the patient-centered role one plays in primary care versus the client-enterprise-provider relationship of occupational medicine. There is also a distinct difference in culture among different specialties. The cultural dimension goes deeper than a lack of understanding among primary care physicians about occupational health services, although that can be an obstacle. The world of occupational medicine is quite different from that of most other specialties and requires a detached view of the injured worker's problems that differs from the patient advocacy role in primary care. The practice of occupational medicine can be very disconcerting to physicians oriented to traditional primary care.

Family practitioners are in an excellent position to provide the wide range of clinical services, including minor injury care, that may be needed. The family physician is trained and acculturated to be the advocate of the patient, to provide a high level of basic care, to establish long-term relationships and continuity of care, and to know when to refer patients to a specialist for clinical care. This role may conflict with the need in occupational medicine to report findings that may not appear to be in the patient's immediate interest (such as a lower rather than a higher level of impairment), with the extensive documentation needs that are essential to occupational medicine (especially in workers' compensation), to separate the patient's satisfaction with objective criteria in making decisions about fitness to return to work, and to know when a work-related problem requires investigation and consultation with professionals outside the world of medical specialties, such as occupational hygienists.

The internist brings strength in analysis and deductive reasoning that is particularly important in occupational disease cases. Internists are trained and acculturated to be master diagnosticians, but the diagnosis itself is often less important in occupational medicine than causation and impairment. Internal medicine training is often weak on musculoskeletal disorders and toxicology and may not provide some of the relevant clinical skills.

Emergency physicians are trained and acculturated to provide excellent care in urgent situations and have diverse clinical skills, but the care they give is episodic. Physicians with such training need to be prepared for the other side of occupational medicine practice, the preventive services, and the need for tracking recovery over weeks and months, in addition to monitoring people who have nothing much wrong with them. The few emergency physicians with training in toxicology are particularly well equipped to deal with occupational diseases.

The occupational healthcare system is an often complex network functioning somewhat isolated from the mainstream personal healthcare system and subject to its own internal tensions and forces.

One of the issues OEM physicians continually face is the assumption that they perform mainly acute injury care that can be handled equally well by primary care practitioners. Occupational medicine practice, particularly at the higher levels, tends to be less clinical and more administrative and cognitive in the skills it demands, requiring a deeper knowledge of population health, toxicology, fitness for duty, occupational hazards, functional assessment and the workers' compensation system. The OEM physician must deal continually with strong economic, political, and social pressures even above the present complexities of medical practice. These include workers' compensation, disability claims, lawsuits, government regulations, labor-management relations, budgeting, and other issues far from usual office practice.

Any physician moving into OEM practice from a primary care specialty is welcome but is well advised to take the time to prepare by mastering essential skills in OEM. Some physicians simply choose not to make the investment and therefore do not practice at a high level.

Consultation Practice in Occupational Medicine

A small number of full-time private practitioners in OEM, who are usually located in major cities, practice primarily as consultants. Their practice may be associated with academic institutions or independent, whether or not they hold an academic appointment.

In the setting of academic institutions and teaching hospitals, occupational health consultation clinics combine clinical practice with teaching and research. Most patients to such clinics come by referral from other physicians. They mostly serve as independent medical examiners in workers' compensation cases, as expert witnesses in disputed cases, and as consultants in toxicology, epidemiology, and often aerospace medicine. (Many aerospace medicine specialists also practice general occupational medicine.) The organization representing such clinics is the Association of Occupational and Environmental Clinics.

Consultation practice in occupational medicine today increasingly requires meaningful credentials and several assured sources of referrals. A referral network normally comes from visibility, reputation, success in managing certain types of cases, and extensive contacts with employers. If one wishes to develop a referral practice, one must ask where these cases are to come from, who will see them first, and why they should be referred to a particular consultant over another.

Occupational medicine is practiced in a fishbowl. Opinions and findings are under review by workers' compensation boards, employers, insurance carriers, and frequently unions. Each is a potential source of or a potential obstacle to referrals. They are very sensitive to inadequate documentation, incomplete records, and delayed reports and react silently by steering referrals elsewhere.

Complex cases, those which are most likely to be referred to a consultant, often go to court or to arbitration, and the physician must be prepared and be seen to be prepared to stand behind opinions and reports. The suitability of a physician as a possible expert witness when the possibility of litigation exists is often a factor in the selection of a consultant in a given case. The physicians' formal credentials in occupational medicine become important in such situations. (See Chapter 23.)

Occupational medicine consultation clinics, unlike primary care clinics for occupationally related injuries, are seldom profitable in the private sector unless overhead is kept to a minimum and referrals include many "high-value" cases (high value in this sense only in terms of financial worth, of course), which may involve medicolegal support, independent medical evaluation, or high-value services such as exercise testing and cardiopulmonary evaluation. One way to keep costs low is to rely instead on tests performed by lower-paid staff and limit the patient-physician interaction to situations where the physician is most needed: a highly focused interview and examination. One way to encourage a steady flow of high-value cases is to associate with one or more OHSs that provide acute injury care and a primary care level of healthcare to injured workers. Acute-care facilities generally prefer not to deal with complicated cases or cases of occupational disease and are happy to refer them in order to get them out of their system, which is geared to high-volume care.

Multispecialty Group Practices

Multispecialty group practices are partnership organizations in which specialists in compatible areas of medical practice engage in a relationship in which common expenses and resources are shared, whether in a single large clinic or a network including satellite clinics. Group practices are often faced with intense competition and feel the need to capture groups of patients, as in health maintenance organizations and similar prepaid plans. Group practices in the United States have often entered OHSs to "lock-in" large groups of employees that are then expected to use the OHS services for their personal health needs and those of their families. Historically, multi-specialty group practices have done well in providing occupational health services, and most of the larger practices have at least some physicians involved on a routine basis.

Multispecialty group practices do have certain disadvantages. They have usually developed as providers of personal healthcare and often developed occupational healthcare services without appropriate preparation. Group practices tend to enter the field by either creating within themselves new services staffed by physicians recruited for the purpose or by using the personnel they have on staff already, qualified or not. As the OHS develops, it frequently finds itself subordinated to personal health services whenever decisions are made regarding allocating resources, recruiting staff, marketing, and opening satellites. For this reason it is advisable to keep the administrative structure of the OHS as autonomous as possible within the group, even at the expense of some duplication. Administrators who are not sensitive to employer's concern over lost time may see no need to expedite registration and waiting periods. One of the major criticisms of group medical facilities by employers is that because occupational injuries are no more important to the group than nonoccupational injuries, an injured employee may have to wait longer to be treated because the injured employee will be competing with nonoccupational injuries for available physician time. Groups suffering financial problems or poor cash flow may also be tempted to shift overhead expenses onto the apparently lucrative occupational services contracts, raising costs to employers and destroying the attractiveness of the group-based option.

Hospital-Based Occupational Health Clinics

Hospital-based OHSs have been introduced in many large institutions in the United States. More recently, community hospitals have entered the field in large numbers. Most hospitals have promoted their services through selective business contacts rather than media advertising. Like group practices, the incentive for hospitals is to cultivate a patient base likely to enroll in their health maintenance organizations and to use the hospital and its outpatient clinics for their personnel healthcare. Some hospitals do a very credible job providing specific occupational health services, but others develop their programs as a marketing device, with little real commitment of resources or quality assurance.

Most of the services are relatively rudimentary, operating either as an extension of emergency room care or an isolated community outreach program. A few, however, are well developed and comprehensive in their provision of services. Pacific Presbyterian Medical Center in San Francisco has provided an extensive service for many years. Many academically oriented medical centers that have offered such services in the past did so as part of training programs in occupational medicine. Many hospitals are using occupational health services to build up "wellness," or health promotion, programs, and virtually all expect the services to increase utilization of other hospital departments such as radiology, clinical specialties, and laboratories. Unfortunately, the fees charged by hospitals for routine services such as chest films are often noncompetitive in the marketplace.

Occupational Health Centers or Clinics

"Occupational health centers" or clinics are free-standing facilities, serving many employers in a well-defined geographical area such as a town or an industrial park. Although not a new phenomenon, these clinics have become attractive models for entrepreneurs interested in providing direct healthcare services in settings with low overhead. Their patients are generally drawn from local employers, with whom they have contracts or informal arrangements to provide services, emphasizing episodic care of injuries or illnesses on an acute basis and periodic health evaluations as mandated by law or by company policy. The occupational health center is characterized by certain basic features: a central facility serving multiple client employers, expansion of medical staff with primary care providers, an emphasis on medical care with less involvement in prevention, close attention to market trends, and a relatively small nursing and support staff. Their revenues are generated primarily from workers' compensation fees for the former and third-party payments from the employer for the latter. In a few cases, they have grown quite large and diverse. In general, however, they grow by establishing satellites or spin-off clinics and by creating larger healthcare systems composed of several clinics.

Occupational health centers focus on cost-effective management of minor trauma and pre-placement evaluations. The business model emphasizes high-volume care, triage for cases that are complicated, and high efficiency of operations to keep overhead under control. The primary advantage to injured workers and employers is rapid access to care, early return to work, one-stop provision of all essential services, and correct and timely reporting and filing of paperwork, especially that required by workers' compensation and the U.S. Department of Transportation for commercial drivers (which is very time sensitive).

Occupational health centers are a new generation of service that grew out of the "industrial medicine clinics" of an earlier era, peaking in the 1970s and early 1980s. At that time, industrial medical clinics generally had a reputation for marginal quality of care and isolation from the mainstream of occupational medicine. One exception was the Detroit Industrial Clinic, which was a model of its type. During the outsourcing of the 1980s, many well-qualified OEM physicians left corporate medical departments and entered practice in the community, and other physicians entered occupational medicine practice because of the new opportunities. Employers that had previously been served by in-house health services were more demanding in their expectations. The result was a substantial upgrading in that sector of healthcare.

The proliferation of occupational health centers and the emergence of these facilities out of the old industrial medicine clinics have led to many favorable changes in OHSs. It has made services that were previously available only to major employers easily accessible to small enterprises. The sector has consolidated in recent years and is now heavily dominated by a few providers, the largest of which is Concentra.

CORPORATE OCCUPATIONAL HEALTH SERVICES

Large employers, by definition, have more than 1,000 employees and often need a full-time, in-house corporate medical department. Sometimes this corporate service acts primarily to coordinate a network of individual healthcare providers at scattered workplaces, either plant physicians or community physicians receiving employees at their own facilities. In other organizations, the corporate medical department primarily manages contract services and personnel that perform OHSs as needed. After the downsizing and delayering of the 1980s, many large corporations outsourced most of their occupational health and safety services, including medicine, to external providers. Often, these providers were their previous employees. The result was that there are many fewer corporate medical departments today than twenty or thirty years ago, but the total number of providers is greater. The corporate medical departments that have survived often assumed a broader span of responsibility, including occupational health, health affairs management (such as insurance and managed care issues), safety, and the environment. Recently, many corporate medical departments were beginning to hire again, in small numbers, to bring OEM physicians back into the organization to assume responsibility for this expanded portfolio and to manage the fragmented contractor relationships that developed after their OHSs were outsourced.

Corporate Medical Department

The corporate medical department is a unit within the management structure that reports at a high level and participates in policy formation and decision making. The corporate medical department is headed by a physician, usually with an executive title and position, who directs and reviews the provision of healthcare within the organization, including its plants and other worksites, the headquarters staff, and the medical aspects of the benefits packaged for employees. At the corporate level, direct medical services may be provided to local or headquarters staff or in the evaluation of individual problem cases, but this function is secondary to that of coordinating and advising on health-related matters within the organization.

The single most important determinant of cooperation in matters regarding occupational health and safety is a clear and explicit corporate policy statement, widely distributed, reinforced with regular application, and referred to often in business communications. This clear commitment should be reflected in personnel policies and budgeting and cited throughout the corporate policy manual. Among its other elements, the policy should hold all personnel accountable (including top managers, supervisors, and workers on the shop floor), commit the employer to meet or exceed applicable government regulatory requirements, hold contractors on-site equally accountable for unsafe practices by their own employees, and commit management to regular review and reporting of their performance in health and safety.

The physician should report at the highest levels of management, preferably to the chief executive officer or at the vice-presidential level, to be maximally effective. This ensures that issues in occupational health and safety are reported without distortion or censorship and permits the corporate medical director to convey a set of priorities that may not be shared by midlevel managers. It sends a signal throughout the rest of the organization that occupational health will not be subordinated to other priorities.

Occupational health and safety deals with working conditions and hazards and other issues of the quality of life for workers. Ill or injured workers contribute to absence from the job, and their paperwork is usually handled by the personnel office. Many employers have therefore placed their occupational health and safety units within the personnel or "human resources" department. The advantage of this system is that it appears to be tidy administratively and facilitates the handling of absence data and claims for workers' compensation. The disadvantage is that it undermines the integrity of the occupational health and safety unit. Placing it so close to the human resources offices and functions compromises the perceived and, usually, actual independence of the occupational health and safety unit. It also tends to push issues involving absence onto the OHS, when this is properly a human resources function, not a medical function. It becomes too easy for HR managers to request (and insist upon) access to information to which they are not entitled. Workers seeking help or involved in exposure-related issues draw the conclusion that the HR manager is watching their actions and that they will be laid off for complaining or for becoming injured or ill. Often, this concern is justified because the personnel officer does not understand the proper limits of his or her authority. Physicians practicing in such an arrangement are severely compromised, appearing to be too close to management to be trusted. The inevitable result is withholding of information, refusal to cooperate, reluctance to accept medical judgments as authoritative, and suspicion of any new health-related projects.

Even worse is placement of the occupational health and safety unit in a department of labor relations. Preoccupied with issues of union negotiation, managers in these departments often tend to withhold or censure information that should be shared freely with workers. The occupational health and safety unit is often dragged into the middle of labor-management disputes and forced to declare itself on the side of management. This forced display of organizational solidarity may please management, but it inevitably destroys the credibility of the occupational health and safety unit and turns the service and all associated healthcare professionals into adversaries of the worker. Without confidence in the unit, workers will not only withhold information and fail to cooperate, but many actively resist programs that might benefit them because they are seen as being imposed by management and subject to a hidden agenda.

Although managers understandably wish for all senior employees in their organization to be on the same team, close identification of occupational health and safety personnel with line management is the kiss of death for their ability to work closely with workers. Since this ability is key to their effectiveness, the employer is much better off accepting that the OEM physician, nurse, or hygienist is a professional within the organization who must function somewhat independently and must avoid an adversarial role with workers. At the same time, the OEM physician, nurse, or hygienist must be capable of understanding management systems and objectives and communicating with management in language that can be understood.

A successful corporate OHS is one that is appropriate to the needs of the organization it serves, efficiently managed, ethical and respectful in treatment of the worker, and effective in relation to cost. However, in order to survive and be successful, the corporate department must constantly justify its existence to senior management, especially financial officers of the company. Corporate OHSs are very vulnerable as business units because they do not directly produce goods and services, they are perceived as "consumptive" cost centers (units that cost money but add little value), and are hard to evaluate, especially if they are successful.

All large organizations have a common basic structure. The "line of authority" extends from the top leader to the employee at the lowest level. Along this line all management decisions and orders are conveyed relating to the goods or services that are the business of the organization. The staff line, perpendicular to the line of authority, supports it by providing necessary services such as financial, legal, human resources, and occupational health and safety. Occupational health and safety is intrinsically a staff rather than a line management function, but it must necessarily be a line responsibility if safe work practices are to be followed consistently. The occupational health and safety staff cannot be all places at all times and cannot know the workplace as well as the workers who are assigned there regularly. If staff bear the primary corporate responsibility for occupational safety and health, the line managers may not be as responsive or interested and hazards will not be corrected. Individual managers and supervisors must be individually responsible for the safety performance or injury experience in their areas or responsibility and should be individually evaluated for performance in this area just as they are on productivity.

On the organization chart, the corporate medical director is in a "staff" position, providing support services and assistance to top management, rather than in a "line" position of direct authority over production and services. Those occupational health personnel under the direction of the corporate medical director should cultivate close relationships with line personnel, however, in order to ensure cooperation and full understanding of the production process and options for control of potential hazards.

An important role of the OEM physician in a corporate medical department is to manage contract services, such as audiology and hearing conservation. A successful service is rarely found "off the shelf." Obtaining the right system to meet the needs of the employer requires careful analysis and good planning. The variety of "packaged" occupational health programs for sale in the marketplace does not obviate the need for planning and evaluation because many of these package deals may be of little or no value to the employer and may not provide a service of acceptable quality for the worker. They may be poorly conceived, badly implemented, inflexible, or unsuitable to the employer's particular situation. Lacking a plan and carefully considered expectations, an employer can easily fall into the trap of paying for a system or program that fails to meet the real need.

The department should have a close working relationship with the safety and occupational hygiene functions. Safety and hygiene usually report to an operating manager, possibly with other responsibilities for risk and loss control. Once a company has grown to around 3,000 employees, a single administrative grouping of health, safety, and hygiene should usually be formed under a senior manager, preferably the medical director if the medical director has management skills for the responsibility.

The current trend is to consolidate health, safety, and environmental affairs into an overall "HSE" department. HSE departments combine health, safety, and environmental management, often under the leadership of a manager specializing in the field. In such arrangements, the OHS may be a unit within the HSE department, the non-medical OHS and environmental functions may be integrated into the management structure of the OHS, or the physicians in the organization may be part of a team addressing HSE issues with additional clinical responsibilities. A few organizations, most notably International, a large truck manufacturer, have incorporated security into the HSE department, giving it a broad mandate for business continuity and protection of the enterprise. (See Chapter 22.) Very recently, this trend has included environmental sustainability in the portfolio of the HSE department. Such departments, which are becoming increasingly common, combine environmental health concerns of the type discussed in Chapter 12 with broader issues of sustainability outside health, such as energy conservation, recycling, reducing carbon emissions, and green technology.

All organizations benefit from an explicit occupational health and safety policy that specifies their responsibilities to their employees and their employees' responsibility for safe work practices. A model occupational and environmental health policy, one that could apply to any company large enough to have a corporate medical department, will confirm the company's commitment to protect the health and safety of its employees and of persons living or working near company operations and will assign responsibility for the actions and decisions required to maintain this commitment.

Labor–Management Relations

Each employer has its own pattern of labor-management relationships, unionized or not. Sometimes there is a mixture of both, as when a union represents some workers but others in another division or certain jobs are not organized. The responsibility for protecting worker health rests squarely with management. In the non-unionized setting, management must fulfill this obligation with no less diligence than is required when it has a union looking over its shoulder. In either case, effective policies and procedures to protect employee well-being should be in place. These should be based on a moral commitment that protecting employee well-being is a fundamental principle of doing business.

Whether a plant, company, or agency is unionized or not becomes important to the role of the OHS, but it is difficult to generalize how interaction with a union affects day-to-day operations. When employees are organized in a plant, the union may negotiate for improved working conditions as part of collective bargaining. In general, an OHS that is the direct product of collective bargaining is vulnerable to abrupt changes in policy, to financial cutbacks, and to being used as a pawn or distraction in contract negotiations. The OHS may be mistrusted by management as an unwarranted benefit for employees or may be seen as a beneficent gesture or concession, demonstrating the employer's good will and responsiveness; this is not necessarily desirable, as it can degenerate quickly into a patronizing and paternalistic attitude that turns into sour resentment at the slightest problem or conflict. It takes real effort to preserve the OHS as neutral ground in such circumstances and requires a commitment from both sides. This commitment can only come from a mutual understanding of the OHS and its actual role in the workplace, regardless of what either party would like it to be for their own purposes. In unionized plants, the local often intervenes in individual claims as well as advocating changes in the workplace and acting as a conduit for complaints regarding working conditions. The union representative may assist the employee in filing a claim, arguing an appeal, or researching the background to a complex problem. Unless allowed by a clause in the collective bargaining agreement, the union representative is not entitled to personal medical information (other than fitness to work) any more than the representative of the employer, but the employee is free to release medical information to whomever they wish and will do so if the union is taking up the case. A collective bargaining agreement, on the other hand, is a contract binding on all parties until it expires. If the contract stipulates that specific information is to be or can be released, that constitutes valid authority to do so.

The negotiated collective agreement between an employer and its union (or unions) sets the tone of the relationship and lists many of the rules of behavior for the workforce in a unionized plant. While the collective agreement in no way removes the employer's right to run its own affairs, it binds management and the workforce to a contract. These rules are in force for the life of the collective agreement, which includes an arbitration mechanism for settlement of disputes. Issues concerning the well-being of workers, individually and as a group, form an important and often controversial part of collective agreements. Sometimes the terms of the agreement contain only broad standards, but others set down very specific policies and procedures.

All such collective agreements insist upon some form of worker participation in programs that deal with worker health and safety. A common stipulation (especially in Canada) is the joint health and safety committee. The powers of these committees vary greatly, ranging from total control of health and safety matters to serving merely as discussion groups. They provide a valuable opportunity for management and workers to come together to solve problems in the workplace, if the participants can keep focused on occupational health and safety.

Occupational Health and Safety

Nonmedical functions, such as safety and occupational hygiene, may be organized as separate departments within an organization or incorporated into the management structure in an integrated occupational health unit. Sometimes specific nonmedical services are obtained by contractual agreement from an outside supplier and simply coordinated by an internal manager. Regardless of what form of organization is selected, it is essential that there be clear lines of communication and a close working relationship between the essential nonmedical functions and the medical department. Otherwise, efficient prevention and problem solving are impossible, and solutions to problems are often postponed or resisted because of personal or political agendas.

Among large employers in government and industry, a distinction is usually made between "occupational health" and "occupational safety." "Health" in this context is presumed to refer to occupational diseases and the control of chemical hazards in the workplace. Although it is recognized that there is substantial middle ground, the two are usually considered separate areas of authority and are usually under the responsibility of separate management units. Table 20.4 compares the general approaches of "health" and "safety" as they are divided in many organizations.

Health is the newer area conceptually, reflecting increasing awareness and regulation of chemical hazards and hazards intrinsic to industrial processes. Health functions are usually conducted by occupational (industrial) hygienists. The management unit may be headed by a hygienist or an OEM physician, although sometimes this area is combined with loss and liability control functions under the direction of a manager with an appropriate administrative background. Health is usually perceived as highly technical, somewhat arcane, and primarily an issue of minimizing the risk of an adverse effect or citation under government regulations by controlling levels of exposure in the workplace.

Safety is a more traditional concern of management and has arisen out of efforts to prevent accidents, respond to emergencies,

Table 20.4. Comparison between Health and Safety Approaches

Safety	Health
Numerous specific problems, "low tech"	Numerous specific problems, "high tech"
Macro-management cost-effective	Micro-management cost-effective
Workplace audits	Workplace environmental monitoring
Periodic health evaluation not effective	Periodic health evaluation has role
Diagnosis obvious	Diagnosis often subtle
Traditionally addressed physical and mechanical problems	More recently has addressed ergonomic problems

Middle Ground
Repetitive strain/cumulative injury
Chemical burns
Physical hazards of toxic chemicals
Disaster planning
Rehabilitation from injury
Drug abuse
Identifying risk factors underlying injuries

fight fires, and monitor the presence and handling of physically hazardous exposures in the workplace. These include flammable and explosive materials, high-voltage electricity, open flames, compressed gases, and mechanical hazards, such as unguarded equipment, motor vehicles, ladders, and scaffolding. Safety issues are usually dealt with by safety professionals trained in short courses after spending time as workers or foremen. The management unit is usually much larger than a health unit and is more closely tied to production units than health units. Safety personnel usually have greater visibility on the shop floor and are better known to rank-and-file workers. Of necessity, parallel safety units must exist in every plant the employer has.

Conflict between health and safety units, and between both and a separate medical unit, is common and typically reflects inadequate resources given to each or issues of authority over the large number of issues that fall into the "middle ground" between the two (or among the three). A more conceptually useful approach may be to consider health and safety as two ends of a spectrum of issues (Table 20.4). This model seems to work well, in general, but is difficult to put into place when the past model of organization has kept the functions separate and reporting lines have become rigid. A major concern in merging units is the allocation of limited resources to one or the other area: who will gain and who will lose.

FACILITIES AND OPERATIONS

OHSs operate on the level of acute and primary care or on the level of referral and specialty consultation, but usually not both. The reason is that the former requires a high-volume, clinical service–driven model that depends on efficient delivery of services and speed and accuracy in completing paperwork, especially for workers' compensation, and is generally reimbursed by billing systems based on service codes. The latter is a high-value-added, low-volume, cognitively driven model (meaning that the physician's expertise and knowledge are more important than clinical skills such as suturing) that requires a heavy investment of time in each injured worker and is generally reimbursed by invoice at an hourly rate. The two models are not compatible in a single business model and have very different implications for staffing, equipment, and spin-off of ancillary services. This section primarily addresses the high-volume, acute-care business model.

Location

Locations best suited for OHSs are areas of industrial growth. In particular, lower-technology industries, such as assembly line manufacturing or automotive repair, tend to produce more work-related injuries and illnesses than capital-intensive high-technology or automated industries. Labor-intensive industries, particularly those employing large numbers of untrained or partly trained workers with a high turnover, such as fast food operations, tend to produce more acute injuries. Older, lower-technology manufacturing industries are more likely to result in occupational injuries, while higher-technology injuries often present exotic problems in toxicology and ergonomics. Virtually all industries, including service industries with mostly desk jobs, generate large numbers of back complaints. Office operations and financial or information service industries require a larger proportion of preventive and educational services and may create a greater demand for health promotion activities. Particular locations will tend to attract one type of industry. Large employers will often be surrounded by many smaller ones providing support services and goods. In many cities, the downtown area is changing to a service core and manufacturing-related industry has moved to the periphery. Older health facilities serving the downtown area must consider whether the mix of services they have provided is now appropriate for their local industrial base.

Some healthcare organizations attempt to provide both personal and occupational healthcare in the same facility and locate in areas where there is growth in residential population. Residential population means little for OHSs because industry is seldom in the same neighborhood. Clinics or other facilities in a residential community are often in a poor position to provide occupational services to employers in the industrial parks or districts where those same potential clients and patients work. One clinic in San Diego, for example, was established in a commercial area on the periphery of a large suburb in a metropolitan area in a location selected to be convenient both for young families in a residential area of that same suburb and to industry in an adjoining city. The building was accessible only by car, separated by a hill from a local housing development and by enormous parking lots from a shopping center. Mothers with children and the elderly found the location highly inconvenient, even though on a map it appeared to be close to a concentration of homes. The major employer in the area never sent injured workers to the clinic because several physicians were within a shorter drive, even though this employer was on the same street. Professional marketing services costing thousands of dollars were engaged to promote utilization of the clinic but had little effect. After three years, this satellite had to be closed because it had served neither industry nor residents adequately. The location, having been compromised in order to satisfy both groups, satisfied neither since it was poorly located to serve the residential area and situated even worse to serve the occupational market. During its brief period of operation, several small industrial medicine clinics established themselves much closer to the primary market for OHSs.

Facilities

The siting and design of the clinical facility itself should be undertaken with care and preferably designed by reference to a successful model. It is impossible to describe a design that meets the needs of all organizations. Advice from consultants in both architecture and occupational health and visits to other facilities are always good ideas before one commits to construction and purchase of equipment. This section, therefore, will concentrate on general principles of space allocation, access, configuration, interior fixtures, and equipment.

Medications to be stocked are the minimum needed for the symptomatic relief of common occupational disorders or personal illnesses affecting employees on the job. Although occupational physicians cannot substitute for family physicians in providing comprehensive care, it is not unreasonable to treat common complaints in order to prevent unnecessary time off work. It is usually not cost-effective for occupational health clinics to maintain clinical laboratory apparatus beyond a bench centrifuge, microscope, and simple office testing supplies unless they are remote and must function as a self-contained infirmary. It is usually not cost-effective to acquire radiologic apparatus unless the industry is one at high risk for serious injuries and the site is a large one. Maintaining quality assurance for such services can be a serious challenge when the volume of cases is low and there is a temptation to raise revenue, which increases costs to the customer (the employer or insurance carrier) by unwarranted utilization in an effort to justify use of the equipment. Usually, a nearby clinic or hospital can provide the support services needed and indicated at a lower unit cost, with a better guarantee of quality assurance and without an incentive to over-order tests.

An OHS should be able to provide a realistic cost-benefit analysis for the organization of which it is a part or that uses it for healthcare services.

Staffing

The physician cannot be truly effective in managing an occupation-related case in isolation. Occupational health nurses are the essential occupational health professionals in most employer-based facilities and can deal independently with many cases. A complex case absolutely requires the participation of other professional experts. These may include occupational health nurses, occupational hygienists, audiologists, toxicologists, epidemiologists, engineers, radiation physicists, and many others.

As with all medical facilities, the staffing of an OHS depends on the mission of the organization and the health patterns in the industry and community. The number of patient encounters expected per year is a significant determinant of the size of the service overall and its projected capacity. The type of injuries or illnesses to be expected determines what special equipment should be readily available and what specialty coverage should be arranged. Close proximity to a hospital or large group practice, with the potential to receive referrals to specialists, makes a big difference in staffing; but if there is no such institutional support in the area, easy access on a timely basis to specialty services may require that the OHS have its own designated staff or working arrangements with local consultants. The administrative responsibilities of the service and budgetary constraints shape the nonmedical staffing of an OHS. The anticipated peak utilization of the service and variations through the year dictate short-term hiring and whether special services (such as audiometry) are contracted out rather than performed in-house.

As with all medical facilities, the staffing of an OHS depends on the mission of the organization, the health risks in the industry, and access to supplemental assistance in the community. Some factors to consider are:

- Number of patient encounters expected per year
- Type of injuries or illnesses to be expected
- Degree of organizational autonomy enjoyed by the service
- Administrative responsibilities of the service
- Budgetary constraints of the organization
- Anticipated peak utilization of the service and variations through the year

Peak needs should never be the basis for full-time staffing projections, as they burden the operation with redundant staff during most of the year. Peak load can be reflected in the budget for employing part-time personnel for assistance during these times. Seasonal industries usually schedule periodic health surveillance during their lightest months, to minimize disruptions to production.

Staffing formulas for OHSs without particular physical or chemical risks have followed a rough rule of thumb for many years, despite economic changes. A plant physician on at least a part-time basis becomes cost-effective for about 1,000 employees and on a full-time basis for more than 2,000. An occupational health nurse is usually needed for more than 300–500 employees and for every additional 750–1,000 employees. A safety officer and access to medical care nearby is generally adequate for an employee population of less than 200. A full-time occupational hygienist will usually be required at about 500 employees in manufacturing, but part-time consultants may be used for much routine work and for special problems. These crude guidelines do not take into consideration the increased risk and special hazards in some industries. An occupational health nurse may be quite sufficient for several hundred employees in an office building, but an occupational hygienist may be essential for a small company in a high-risk industry. There is no simple formula for staffing an OHS, but for medium-risk industries the above rule of thumb will not be far out of line.

Record Keeping

An OHS must maintain at least two types of records: personal health records and exposure records.

Medical records contain confidential information and should never be accessible to unauthorized personnel, including management. These records:

- Document significant exposures sustained by the worker
- Match the worker's health and fitness for duty and job requirements (see Chapter 18)
- Document the worker's health on entry for fitness to work determinations,
- Summarize the results of periodic health surveillance (see Chapter 5)
- Document compliance with regulatory requirements

Exposure records are the results of environmental monitoring or group data on personal exposure; they are not necessarily confidential unless they identify individuals. The U.S. Department of Labor issued a ruling in 1988 on access to medical records that requires that exposure records be kept for all workers, even those exposed to little or no hazard in the usual work environment. Workers have access to their own exposure and medical records, with copies to be provided free of charge.

Both types of records are normally the property of the employer or whoever caused the record to be created in the first place. However, workers must consent to the release of any information that identified them as individuals, even to their own union. Anonymous data (with all identifiers deleted) and group exposure data may be shared but not personal medical records, which cannot be individually reviewed by any party other than the worker or an authorized health professional; management representatives are not entitled to view the record, even if identifiers are removed. Only the worker can authorize release of health information from the medical record and sharing of the information with other parties. An exception to this general rule is when records are subpoenaed for litigation or become part of a disputed workers' compensation claim or are requested under the legal authority of OSHA or NIOSH.

Records must be retained at least thirty years after termination of employment to permit review in case chronic or latent health problems are identified. These records should always be transferred to a responsible recipient or government agency if the employer or clinic goes out of business. If there is none, the records are to be transferred to the Director of NIOSH in the United States. This is probably rarely done.

Certain exemptions to the record access regulation have been made. Research is permitted, but individual identification of workers is not allowed without explicit permission. Employee assistance records are considered separate from the medical record if they are maintained in a different file; they remain confidential but are not subject to the record retention requirement and do not have to be disclosed when the medical records are subpoenaed or requested by OSHA. Also, employees who leave the employer after less than one year employment may be given their medical record to take with them, and copies do not then have to be retained and stored by the employer.

It should be noted that chest films are considered integral parts of the medical record, subject to the rule of thirty-year retention after termination. Old films therefore cannot be processed to reclaim the silver until the retention period is over.

Employers are responsible for ensuring that the procedures are followed and requiring healthcare providers outside their organization to follow these same regulations. In the present climate of increasing litigation, it is wise to be prudent in obtaining written authorization for all transfers of confidential information.

Marketing

In the current competitive environment, marketing is necessary to preserve financial viability, but is also essential in order to respond in a timely manner to clients' needs. This second role of marketing is just as important as salesmanship. Marketing must be considered not only as a means of promoting a product or service but also as a means of determining what the consumers of that product or service require and adapting to the needs of the consumer. Applied to occupational medicine, marketing means listening carefully to understand the needs of the "consumer" of occupational health services, which is usually the employer, and providing services of high quality and convenience for benefit of the recipient of care, which is the worker.

Services should be designed to satisfy the needs of employers and the expectation of workers. Healthcare facilities and individual physicians providing occupational health services must accommodate the needs and preferences of injured workers in order to retain their share of the "market" of customers, the employers who send injured workers to them, and clients—the workers who choose them when seeking medical services. If employers perceive the waiting periods as excessive, and workers (clients or patients) come back dissatisfied, the facility will quickly lose customers (employers).

Occupational health services should not be used as a "loss leader" offered for the purpose of expanding the patient base for personal healthcare. The economic viability of OHSs should be the business reason for establishing a for-profit clinic or satellite. This economic viability can be guaranteed in part by establishing agreements, either by an informal letter of agreement or formal contract, with local employers to utilize the services of the new satellite on a trial basis.

Satellites that are not economically successful within a reasonable time period should be closed and the resources used elsewhere; attempts to repurpose them, such as converting family medicine offices to occupational health centers, usually do not work.

Marketing Principles

Employers entering into contracts with medical facilities for the provision of basic care select the provider on criteria quite different from what would be applied by a patient seeking a relationship with a personal physician. Six principles underlie the marketing of an OHS and distinguish it from marketing for general health services:

- The facility should be located where the workers work, not where their families live.
- The services provided by an OHS are sensitive to price; perceptions of quality differentiate providers within a price range.
- The facility should adapt to local needs and provide good service to local employers and their workers.
- A mix of large and small client employers is more stable than reliance on a single employer, however profitable.
- Occupational and personal health services should be kept strictly separate.
- The services provided by the OHS must be delivered in a timely fashion: waiting time must be minimal, turnaround time for reporting and paperwork must be quick, and reporting to the employer regarding fitness for duty should be timely.

The first rule is to locate where the workers work, not where their families live. To build up an OHS, medical care must be taken to the worker. The workers will not be sent long distances by the employer for care if alternatives are closer. Some studies suggest a limit of about three miles in urban areas. It is highly unusual for employers to send their workers with minor injuries across town just to be seen at a clinic with a good reputation. As well, any facility that intends to provide U.S. Department of Transportation (DOT) commercial driver evaluations on a large scale had better be located on a main highway with high visibility, good access, and nearby parking for trucks.

Employers considering referral to an OHS are sensitive to price more than to quality. Medical services are exceedingly difficult for the lay person to compare in terms of quality. Employers are more likely to select a provider of medical care on the basis of cost and convenience of location and hours rather than attempting the difficult task of comparing medical capability and credentials of the staff. Employers, especially small enterprises, are persuaded that most routine services, such as acute care for injuries and pre-placement evaluation, do not require extensive specialty care and are within the capability of any qualified physician. Rightly or wrongly, adequate is perceived as good enough and a reputation for excellence counts for little among managers if the injured worker is not seen as requiring fancy care. This attitude also holds true for periodic health evaluations (except for executives), workers' compensation management (until a company has a difficult case), and other forms of fitness-to-work evaluation and applies to rehabilitation services. It does not apply to specialized care for occupational disease, independent medical evaluations, or consultation for preventive services. Within a price range, however, employers will generally choose a provider with a superior reputation or higher visibility to start with but will experiment with new or unfamiliar providers if they can be convinced that time lost will be minimized, case management is more focused, and that the management of workers' compensation paperwork is expedited and taken seriously.

The third general principle is that the OHS must adapt to local needs. As downtown industry is replaced by a clean, white-collar office and service workforce, the demand for specific occupational healthcare services will be far different. Expansion of an existing clinic in the downtown area may be less advisable than, for example, the development of a satellite in a rapidly growing suburb from the standpoint of caring for injuries. A downtown location may make sense if prevention-oriented and health promotion programs are added to the range of services. The type of industry in the area will matter a great deal in generating demand for services, but some problems, such as back pain, are important in virtually every industry and office. Nothing creates dissatisfaction faster than services not being available as described. Services that are being marketed must be in place before they are heavily promoted or the facility will rapidly lose credibility among local employers.

The fourth general principle is to seek a mix of contracts or client employers. Although it is desirable to have big clients to ensure a high volume of services, it is dangerous to depend on a few big contracts that could disappear overnight, particularly those representing employers in the same industry subject to the same market trends. Successful OHSs usually develop a mix of large and small businesses in a variety of industries. Small business, of course, is "big" business in the aggregate and is just as important as big business itself in supporting a stable and profitable OHS.

The fifth principle is that the OHS must be separated from facilities providing personal healthcare services. The flow of occupational patients should not be mixed with family or primary patients. The expedited, time-sensitive flow of an OHS meshes poorly with primary care for the family. When occupational medicine is mixed with primary care, injured workers wait their turn behind patients awaiting general medical care, crying infants, and elderly and pediatric patients, who are often taken before them out of courtesy because most workers are or look healthy. This causes unavoidable delays and long waiting lines (which both workers and employers dislike), results in what employers perceive as lost productivity, and often promotes an unfortunate attitude on the part of the staff that the patient is "just workers' comp" (in years past the phrasing would be "just an industrial") and can wait. There is no equitable way to get around this problem in a shared facility. Giving priority to workers simply does not work in a clinic situation. Patients who are waiting to be seen, especially with children, feel slighted when workers with minor injuries or a seemingly administrative reason for the visit, such as a pre-placement evaluation, bypass the line. Except for small, individual, private practices, therefore, it is best to insist on a strict separation whenever possible between OHSs and general medical services, preferably by putting the two in separate facilities altogether. There are really no effective halfway measures. At a minimum, waiting rooms should never be shared.

Occupational medicine practice is fundamentally about timely care within a system that requires timely reporting. Employers need and expect fast service, rapid reporting, and adequate quality of care, which, as they see it, is reflected in accurate and complete paperwork that is filed without delay. Time off the job because of injuries or routine evaluations costs the employer money that the smaller business in particular can ill afford to lose. Uncertainty over how long the employee will be away from work compounds the loss by causing confusion, inefficiency, and difficulty meeting schedules.

Representation and Communication

Direct face-to-face contact between marketing representatives and the employer's representatives is absolutely required for effective marketing. Most physicians are not good at this, and their time is much too expensive to take on this function, beyond initial visits to a new client. Physicians are often too threatening and imposing to nonphysicians to be effective marketing agents. They will usually be treated with less candor compared with a nonphysician. A good marketing representative, on the other hand, can visit at regular intervals to trouble shoot problems and will get a more candid view of problems or complaints. Properly trained and instructed, a marketing representative can serve as the eyes and ears as well as the human face of the healthcare facility, but caution must be exercised to keep the overenthusiastic types in line. It can be very dangerous—and expensive—to turn marketing responsibilities over to a contractor or independent representative who stays away for long periods without supervision.

Marketing representatives must be careful not to oversell the capabilities of the clinic and must not be too quick to agree to employer's requests for specific services since some of them may be ill-advised. For example, one marketing representative committed a clinic to perform routine back x-rays for screening purposes on new employees, a procedure that is not acceptable practice. The representative had spent considerable effort selling local industry on the need for this unnecessary service, and the clinic was put in an extremely embarrassing position. Experience has shown that the best marketing representatives for occupational health facilities are relatively conservative in appearance, appear professional in manner, have some health-related experience themselves, and are willing to work closely with the professional staff of the facility. Former pharmaceutical representatives are often excellent candidates.

Clear lines of communication with both employers and also with workers using the facilities ensure that needs are met in a satisfactory manner. Web sites are, of course, essential for marketing and communication and absolutely necessary if an employer seeking a service is to find the facility. However, they are not enough. Web sites are passive media, accessed only if the employer is looking for them. Other media are required to bring the facility to the attention of local employers and to establish its niche in the community.

One way to promote such communication is by circulating to the persons responsible for workers' compensation and occupational health matters in each employer's organization a newsletter giving tips on health that can be reproduced for employees, news of the healthcare facility and its personnel, and items of significance to local industry in occupational health. This gives the healthcare facility visibility and promotes a more personalized relationship with the employer that makes it more difficult for the employer to break abruptly without explanation.

An OHS does not imply the same commitment to continuing care as a family practice or a health facility serving personal healthcare needs. The management of occupational injuries and illnesses is usually episodic, and only some cases require continuity of care.

Hence, there is a less personal commitment to healthcare than one expects in a primary care setting, such as family practice. If employers are not satisfied, they will often simply send injured workers elsewhere. Employers can and do shift their preferences for providers and feel no obligation to explain why. Following up with employers and obtaining feedback, while respecting the limits on their time and patience, are an important part of the art of marketing.

Marketing Strategy

A marketing effort dedicated to OHSs should have its own budget, a strategy to reach a broad range of local employers, and a sincere effort to provide empathic and satisfactory service to workers. It should be responsive to its clients in the form of facilities, staff skills and training, and quality assurance that is consistent with its claims. This cannot be achieved when the waiting room is shabby, parking is inaccessible and expensive, clinic hours are limited, and the staff does not behave in a professional manner. The facility has to "walk the talk" if marketing is to yield sustained results.

A sound marketing strategy requires knowledge of the range and levels of services that can be provided matched to the potential customers for these services, the employers. (The employees are the clients, if they are well, or the patients, if they are injured, but are not customers unless they choose the OHS themselves.) Table 20.5 lists various services that might be provided by a large OHS. The marketing strategy should be based on a realistic assessment of economic activity in the area, one that takes into account all industrial sectors and not just the most visible or prestigious ones, and it should utilize current profiles of employers across a wide range of sizes and sectors, not just the largest or most prominent employers.

Figure 20.3 is a diagram known as a "marketing cube" that allows a three-dimensional representation of the possible combinations of levels of service, range of services, and users or "consumers" of these services. A marketing cube presents three dimensions of OHSs: range of service, users of service, and level of service. Each subdivision of

Table 20.5. Core Functions of an OHS

1. Acute care for injured employees.
   1.1. Providing care on site
   1.2. Monitoring care given off site
2. Pre-placement evaluations
   2.1. Assessing functional capacity to do the job
   2.2. Assessing need for accommodation under the Americans with Disabilities Act
3. Functional evaluation of employees after hire
   3.1. Fitness-for-duty evaluations that assess the recovery and functional capacity of injured employees to return to work and what accommodations may be needed
   3.2. Impairment evaluation for injured workers with permanent impairment and workers' compensation claims
   3.3. Certification of time off work for workers with a nonoccupational illness or injury. (This is often performed by other physicians.)
4. Review of workers' compensation claims for causation.
5. Periodic health surveillance of employees exposed to a particular hazard such as noise, chemicals, dusts, or radiation (typically takes the form of a medical examination, often conducted annually)
6. Investigation of exceptional hazards, disease outbreaks, unusual injuries, fatalities, or other emerging issues
7. Prevention, health promotion and educational programs designed to enhance the health of employees and to increase productivity
8. Management of the health problems of employees on-site, to reduce absence and disability
9. Advice and consultation to management on issues of health, health and workers' compensation insurance, and regulatory issues in occupational health
10. Disaster planning and emergency management on or off site
11. External communications on health issues, as with local public health agencies and local physicians
12. Managing relations between the organization and local hospitals and the medical community
13. Employee assistance programs, for employees with problems involving alcohol and drug abuse or other addictive behaviors, such as gambling, that interfere with work

(*Continued*)

Table 20.5. (*Continued*)

14. Executive wellness programs, such as special medical evaluations or monitoring health problems among senior executives

Larger and more complex organizations may also involve the occupational physician in managing environmental risks, product safety, contracting for health services, representing the organization in industry-wide health activities and proactive programs for preparedness, risk management and other senior management functions.

the cube represents a particular level of a particular service provided to a given category of user. Presenting these three dimensions in one illustration helps one to visualize the possibilities and to identify opportunities for growth.

Each level of service can be matched with each service type in Figure 20.3. The medical services may deal, for example, with treatment of individual cases or preventive services to groups of workers. These are the most common types of medical services, but opportunities to provide consultative and educational services are often overlooked. While physicians' expertise may not be well utilized on a cost-effective basis by providing only educational programs, highly professional programs designed with physicians' input can be provided at reasonable cost by health educators or nurses and are very popular among some types of employers and groups of workers. Industrial hygiene services are usually provided on the case management or consultation level, but a market can be created for periodic assessments for purposes of prevention and to ensure compliance with government regulations.

The users of the services, shown along the base of the cube in the front-back dimension in Figure 20.3, may include larger businesses, small business, public agencies, and, potentially, labor unions. Individual workers do not constitute a market for OHSs in the same way that they and their families are a market for personal healthcare. The "consumers" of healthcare are those who use the system and make the choices. In the occupational healthcare system, it is usually the

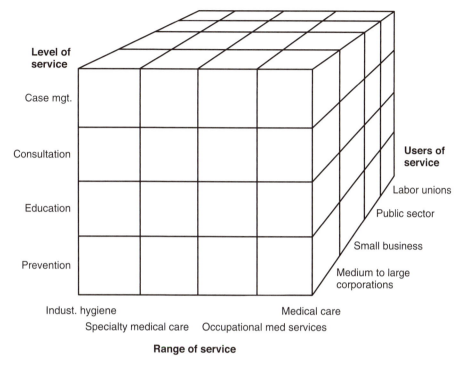

Figure 20.3. Marketing "cube" for OHSs.

employer who makes the initial choice and who purchases (directly or through workers' compensation) health services on behalf of the worker. Even when an individual worker changes physicians or seeks care for an occupational health problem from his or her own doctor, the system constrains the choice by allowing only a limited number of charges and refusing to pay for unauthorized referrals. In marketing OHSs, therefore, the essential target is usually the employer. As a practical matter, the workers' needs must always be met, but the employer's needs must also be reasonably satisfied or the relationship between provider and client may be brief.

The level of services, on the vertical axis, represents a continuum from direct case management to prevention. Diagnosis, treatment, rehabilitation, and follow-up are familiar as the medical model, but the approach of direct intervention also applies to the management of specific problems that arise in the workplace, such as hazards that have been identified or clusters of health problems suggesting that a hazard must be searched for. Consultation is problem evaluation and solving that requires less direct intervention but particular insight and expertise, not only into the problem but also into the needs, motivations, and resources of those asking for the assistance. Education includes not only formal training sessions but opportunities to increase the awareness and sophistication of clients so that the services used are more highly valued. Most fundamentally, prevention is the foundation of sound occupational health practice.

The range of services, presented in the horizontal dimension, is the easiest to conceptualize. "Medical care" includes routine health services, including acute care, periodic health surveillance, and possibly services performed on-site in the employers' facilities. "Occupational medicine services" in this context refers to the specific services such as periodic health surveillance and workers' compensation management that require knowledge and understanding of the occupational healthcare system. "Specialty medical services" refers to an advanced level of care in medical diagnosis and treatment, such as dermatology or toxicology. "Industrial (or occupational) hygiene" is the recognition, evaluation, and control of hazards in the workplace and is performed by industrial (or occupational) hygienists, a specialized profession, as described elsewhere in this chapter.

The most basic level of care is within the capability of most primary care physicians and clinics and is marketable to local area employers. A clinical practice will compete on this level primarily on price (because employers assume that basic medical care can be provided by any qualified medical practitioner), convenience, short waiting times, and prompt completion of paperwork. Figure 20.4 illustrates the marketing cube for this primary level of care. From a business point of view, this is a high-throughput, relatively low-margin operation, and its growth potential depends on local employers and the profile of industry.

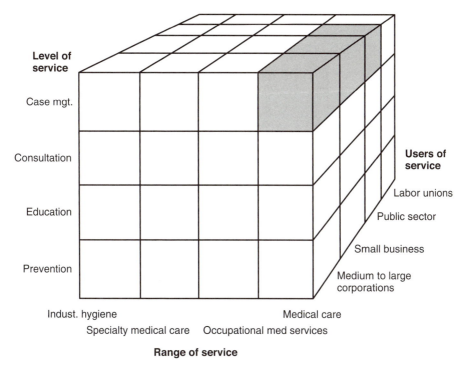

Figure 20.4. Marketing cube for basic clinical services, such as might be provided by a physician's office or clinic without an OEM physician.

"Occupational medicine services" include specialty care provided by occupational physicians, usually emphasizing occupational disease management, toxicology, independent medical evaluations (IMEs), consultation by referral, and medicolegal services. Specialty medical care is rendered on a referral basis for special problems. These higher-level services are marketable to a wider range of clients and sometimes, especially in the case of medicolegal services, to insurance carriers, workers, and employers out of the immediate area. These are services that, in a business sense, add value and lead to a practice that may have lower through-put but equal or greater revenue because of higher fees commensurate with the higher level of service. To sustain such an operation, however, requires qualifications and credentials, such as board-certification in occupational medicine, that indicate

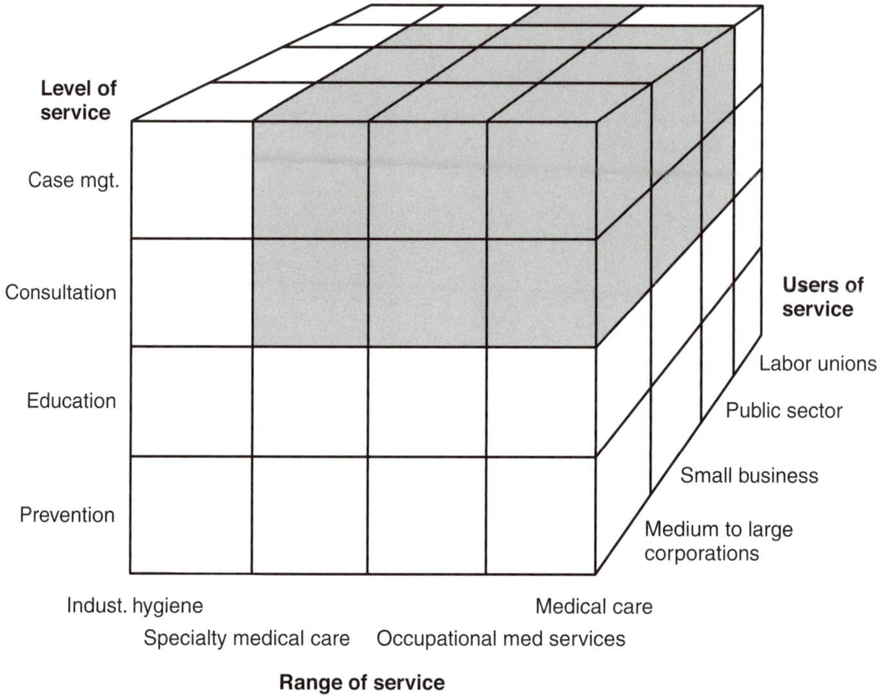

Figure 20.5. Marketing cube for primary care and specialty services in OEM.

competence and, especially for IME and medicolegal work, that establish medical credibility when there is a dispute, which is always. Figure 20.5 illustrates the marketing cube for a well-established occupational medicine specialty practice.

"Integrated OHSs" combine medical practice with occupational hygiene or other support services in order to evaluate the workplace and to assist in problem solving. They are necessarily team operations. Occupational (or industrial) hygiene services must be provided on the employer's site (usually with a laboratory as a base of operations elsewhere) but are not provided by physicians. There are fewer examples of this type of practice than others, but they are especially appealing to large employers. Occupational (industrial) hygiene services are usually provided by consultants hired for the purpose by

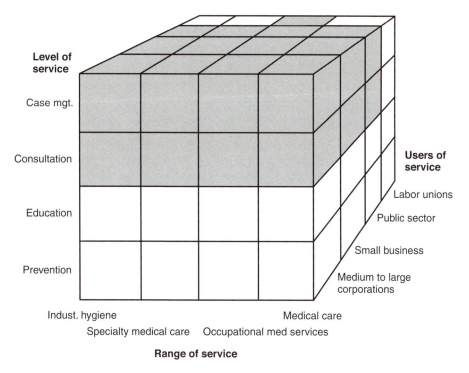

Figure 20.6. Marketing cube for integrated OHSs, including occupational hygiene.

the employer if they are not available in-house. This split between medical and engineering services may not be logical from the standpoint of resolving the problem, but it reflects the different professional roles of the physician and the engineer. Where industrial hygiene services have been offered by clinics, they have often been undervalued or subordinated to the medical services despite their critical role in evaluating and controlling hazards.

Because they require more people and specialized equipment, integrated OHSs carry a higher overhead than other forms of occupational medicine practice. An advantage is that such practices can expand the scope of their operations without adding more physicians. Figure 20.6 illustrates the marketing cube for an integrated occupational medicine and hygiene.

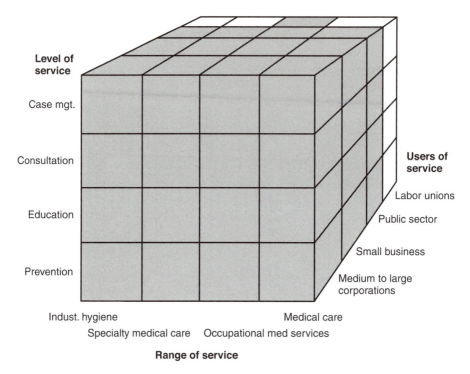

Figure 20.7. Marketing cube for comprehensive OHSs.

"Comprehensive OHSs," as illustrated in the marketing cube in Figure 20.7, are full-service practices, usually consulting operations with close ties to clinics or academic groups (such as member clinics of the Association of Occupational and Environmental Clinics), that can provide employers with prevention, education, and health promotion programs as well as hygiene and clinical services. The trend in such operations in the private sector is to establish national presence and visibility and in all sectors to work through networks rather than to house all functions in one office.

Occupational health clinics providing services for multiple employers usually emphasize basic medical care and occupational medicine services. Large group practices are also in a strong position to provide specialty medical care.

Outreach to employers is not necessarily reassuring to injured workers, who may fear that the relationship between employer and healthcare provider is too close. There should be a concomitant effort to demonstrate to the injured worker that the service is accessible, caring, worker-centered, and respectful of privacy. This is only right, but it is also good business. If they have any alternative, employers are unlikely to continue to utilize an OHS if they get complaints from their workers or hear stories about inefficiency and wasted time. Thus, although the primary marketing target has to be employers, every effort should be made to ensure that workers are satisfied with their care and feel well treated.

Labor unions sometimes have their own insurance plans and sometimes have their own medical consultants or services. They are also potentially sources of referrals, often for disputed or difficult cases. Members tend to rely on unions for advice on medical referrals for occupational problems more than on their personal physicians. Unions sometimes contract for educational and preventive services for their members but usually prefer to work with academic or nonprofit organizations.

Marketing is a particular problem among OHSs sponsored by hospitals and large group practices because the marketing effort is almost always subordinated to an overall institutional marketing plan. Hospitals and group practices obviously want to maximize the yield of their overall marketing budget. They are usually not enthusiastic about a separate marketing campaign for their occupational health referral clinics. However, advertising in the community for personal healthcare services is not the same as persuading workers' compensation carriers and employers that an OHS is the best place to send difficult cases, will expedite delivery of care, and will reduce waiting time to a minimum. This cannot be achieved if the OHS is combined with primary care or other specialties (especially pediatrics) and shares a waiting room with general patients (and especially children with contagious upper respiratory tract infections). Most administrators, however, expect the OHS to start small and cheap and upgrade only as it demonstrates its viability from a business perspective.

The OHS in Hospitals and Large Groups

OHSs that are sponsored by hospitals, large multispecialty medical groups, managed care organizations, and integrated healthcare systems have common problems.

Most hospitals and group practices do not allow acute or primary care OHSs to develop properly. There are several reasons for this. Most hospital administrators have similar attitudes:

- They expect a high-volume, high-revenue-generating clinical service but will not design facilities nor staff, automate, or streamline procedures to support efficient operation. (This failing is most common in hospitals.)

- They expect the occupational medicine service to conform to a familiar model of service delivery, such as a high-value consultation practice (e.g., cardiology). (This failing is most common in group practices.)

- They do not recognize or acknowledge occupational medicine credentials, the nature of the specialized occupational medicine services, or the need for support services involving hazard assessment and control.

- They want to protect their existing emergency room or urgent care facilities from competition.

- They see paperwork flow as a secondary issue rather than a primary, essential, deal-making or deal-breaking part of occupational healthcare service.

- They are reluctant to set up a special administrative system for case management for OEM practice.

- They resist purchasing software because they want their in-house system to be used. (General healthcare software is poorly suited to occupational healthcare services, which specialized packages to be efficient and productive. There are several good products available.)

- They choose not to make an investment because they have been led to believe that occupational medicine is a cash cow that can fund itself from revenues.

- They price healthcare services so that they won't undercut their fees for general healthcare, thus pricing these services out of the market for employers.

- They do not market the OHS, or they do so only in combination with their general marketing, which is not aimed at employers and is mostly irrelevant to them.

Hospitals and large group practices are usually reluctant to hire staff on the basis of experience in workers' compensation, or those who are qualified for special occupational health services, such as "medical review officers" (MROs) or provision of commercial driver examination services (following United States Department of Transportation requirements; see Chapter 18), or staff with the specialized skills to manage workers' compensation cases well. Instead, they usually assign untrained clerical staff or nurses and resist efforts for them to be trained to a high level of expertise. This is not just to contain costs. It is also so that the staff can be reassigned again in the future without resistance and because using higher levels of expertise would lead to expectations for increased pay. Hospitals and group practices also expect that trauma care will generate referrals to surgery as much as possible—which most occupational injuries, involving soft tissue, do not need—and will use in-house rehabilitation, which may not be convenient for the injured worker.

The essence of responsive occupational medicine practice is case management and navigating the patient through the process (setting goals, coordinating care, tracking, monitoring progress, assessing fitness for duty). Hospitals are very reluctant to invest in the systems, software, and personnel to do this because there is no counterpart in other parts of their system and because it would require investment in up-front costs, before revenue is recovered. Hospitals and group practices almost invariably expect the OHS to fund its growth from the balance of revenues after overhead and almost never invest in it.

Hospitals and groups are reluctant to grant discounts in pricing clinical services such as audiometric examinations and chest films, in part because they do not want to set a precedent of departing from the fee schedule for other clinical services and in part because they want to maximize their overall revenue. However, a diagnostic test is not a screening test, and the cost is usually unacceptable to employers for pre-placement evaluations, periodic health evaluations, and screening. The result is that employers will usually go elsewhere and not return, if they have an alternative. Similarly, overhead does not reflect the realities of occupational health practice. Overhead calculations are made on the basis of expenses incurred by the entire hospital medical staff or the whole group practice, and the multiplier that is calculated from it (for example, a clinician may be expected to bring in three times as much in billings as his or her salary or "draw" for the year) takes into account many expenses for equipment and support services that the OHS almost never uses. The result is an overhead burden that often makes the OHS noncompetitive with other providers for anything other than acute injury care.

Healthcare administrators often try to force the referral clinic into an inappropriate model of specialist care, such as cardiology. This is a particular problem for practice plans at teaching institutions, hospital systems with outpatient facilities, and multispecialty group practices, where managers think they know what a specialty clinic looks like and expect the OHS to fit into that model, which does not serve occupational medicine well. The typical case referred to a consultant specialist for clinical evaluation in occupational medicine is extremely time-consuming, and billing fees for clinical services often cover only a fraction of the overhead and personnel cost. The best an OHS emulating this model can usually achieve is to be self-sustaining on the basis of revenue generated from a mixture of cases that includes a large fraction of patients requiring low-intensity screening and preventive services that cost little to provide. However, unless the consultant is well known, high-value cases usually will not come to the OHS in the first place.

Although referral clinics and academic occupational medicine specialty clinics have these inherent problems, they confer advantages to the institutions and providers that can far outweigh their economic disadvantages if they are used strategically. The clinic may be the cornerstone of a practice that brings in much more revenue from "high-value" cases, such as independent medical evaluations and medicolegal cases. However, these cannot be supported unless there is an outlet for clinical practice. Unfortunately, the accounting and tracking systems of hospitals and group practices, being service code driven rather than invoice driven, do not recognize this income stream and so it is invisible to hospital and group administrators.

Hospitals and group practices expect that specialty clinics will spin off large billings in procedures, clinical tests, and consultations. Occupational health referral clinics rarely can do this because patients have often been seen by many physicians and have been extensively worked up before they are referred to clinic and by then the primary challenge is not treatment but causation analysis, impairment, and case management. OEM physicians do not perform expensive procedures, but they do bill at relatively high rates per hour for specialized services, which the hospital or clinic, again, cannot recognize through a conventional billing system. These fiscal constraints can be overcome by developing a mix of cases, basing such services at institutions such as teaching hospitals where physicians are on salary and overhead is subsidized, and associating a specialty clinic with a medical facility that also deals with occupational injuries at the primary care level.

Hospitals and large groups are logical homes for OHSs, but the services may not do well unless the hospital or group allows them to develop and grow according their own logic and in response to occupational medicine, not by conforming to a generalized template for healthcare.

SERVICES TO SMALL ENTERPRISES

Small enterprises are employers that operate with a small number of employees relative to their industry sector. Small business represents by far the largest number of companies in the private sector and as a sector employs the most Americans and Canadians. The U.S.

Small Business Administration reported in 2008 that by its definition of small business, such enterprises constituted 98.2 percent of American businesses, employing over half the nonfarm workforce, paying 45 percent of the total payroll, generating up to 80 percent of new jobs and 28 percent of export value, and employing 40 percent of engineers, scientists, and other highly technical personnel. This is true not only for the United States and Canada but in every economy around the world, regardless of economic system. Of course, these statistics, while emphasizing the scale of the enterprise, mask the great diversity of small enterprises, from high-technology start-ups, to franchises of fast food retailers, to the corner dry cleaners. The defining issue in common among these enterprises is that, whatever other business advantage they may have, they are too small to achieve economies of scale in support services that are peripheral to their main product or service line, such as occupational health and safety.

For small companies, of fewer than 50 employees, the cost of regulatory compliance (occupational, environmental, and socioeconomic) is estimated to be seven to ten times as great per employee as for larger firms of 50 to 250 employees. A similar but lesser differential probably applies to companies with fewer than 500 employees compared to companies with more than 500. Industries with fewer than 100 employees rarely employ full-time occupational health professionals and depend instead on either part-time healthcare providers (physicians or occupational health nurses) or on community-based services. Many of the smallest companies are owned and operated by families or are vehicles for a single individual. Companies with 20–250 employees have a higher injury rate than either smaller or larger corporations. Thus small enterprises have a particularly acute need for occupational medicine services delivered at reasonable cost.

Large corporations have several advantages over most small firms in complying with good occupational safety and health practices, among them a much larger pool of technical talent to correct hazards, established in-house medical programs, favorable cash-flow and capital margins allowing resources to be put into occupational health and safety, and the capacity to assign responsibility for full-time management of safety and health programs to specific employees. The small firm is almost invariably working on a much narrower margin and by definition has far fewer resources in capital, personnel, and facilities at its command. Because of its obvious disadvantages, the small enterprise requires special attention if it is to attain improvement in occupational injury and illness rates.

The direct benefits of prevention-oriented OHSs for small enterprises are also proportionately greater than for large concerns. Few small enterprises can absorb the consequences of absence or disability of a trained employee or manager without the loss being reflected in performance. In very small enterprises the workforce may be made up mostly or entirely of family members. One might think that small enterprises would demand preventive services up to the limit they could afford. In practice, this is rarely the case.

The decentralized nature of small enterprises makes it difficult to serve their needs in a coordinated fashion. Practical limits on cost and local accessibility make serving small enterprises logistically difficult at a consistent standard.

In the United States, services to small enterprises are incompletely covered, both geographically and in terms of service mix, but are more readily accessible than elsewhere because of widespread outsourcing of occupational services in the 1980s. This seeded communities with providers and facilities that were previously available only in-house at larger companies. Most of these services, including both medical and hygiene services, supported themselves primarily but not entirely with contracts to larger employers, leaving enough capacity and creating a financial incentive to provide services to small enterprises.

At various times, governments have supported pilot projects to provide small enterprises with centralized OHSs. The best known of these demonstration projects is the Slough Industrial Health Service, established in 1948 in the United Kingdom to serve the smaller enterprises clustered in an industrial park called Slough Estates, in Berkshire. This prototype was highly successful in its day but required an ongoing subsidy to maintain a full range of services, including occupational hygiene. It continues today under the name Corporate

Health. Sweden developed a network of occupational health centers covering the entire country as a result of a labor-management agreement. In the early 1990s, the entire system was a political casualty of a more conservative government. In many countries, such as Kuwait, occupational health clinics are supported by the government. Government-sponsored occupational health centers have not been developed in the United States or Canada except in Quebec, where they are incorporated in the community health center network and OHCOW in Ontario, which is more often used for consultation than primary services.

The logistical problems of providing consistent service to small enterprises are formidable, but the potential rewards more than justify the effort. Most of society's economic activity and employment is to be found in small enterprises. Developing services for small-scale industry is therefore an important strategy to improve occupational health standards in general, and the effect of even small improvements consistently applied will be multiplied by the larger numbers of workers involved. Small industry must now cope as best it can and usually must turn to resources in the community to provide assistance in solving its problems.

Small enterprises have many competing priorities and often perceive occupational health and safety as a regulatory burden imposed on them rather than as an integral part of operating a business. Many managers in small enterprises have no clear idea of the hazards of their workplace or think only of one or a few highly visible hazards. This should not be surprising, because their interest and expertise is in business, not health. Invisible threats, such as cancer-causing chemicals, tend to be lost among urgent day-to-day matters of business. A handful of these managers, especially owner-managers, take the attitude that acceptance of some risk is a necessary part of success in their business and that if they have taken risks themselves, their employees should be prepared to do so as well. The great majority, however, are simply not knowledgeable about the cost-effective prevention of injury and illness in the workplace and would have little time to learn if they were aware. Provision of sound occupational medicine services to small enterprises requires the easy availability of effective consultation to solve problems and education regarding the value and appropriate utilization of such services by small enterprise managers. It is not reasonable to expect all managers of small enterprises to solve their own problems in their own way. They must have help based nearby in their own community.

Managers and owners of small enterprises tend to be conservative in their use of OHSs, limiting use to the care of injured or ill employees or screening activities required by law. There is usually more ready acceptance of treatment and rehabilitative services than preventive-oriented services. Most perceive preventive or health promotion services with some skepticism, but the depth of this attitude depends in large part on the nature of the industry and the attitudes in the community. Occupational (industrial) hygiene, the evaluation of hazards in the workplace and the design of controls, is not a familiar concept to many small enterprises managers, who assume that they will incur an excessive cost. It should be a function of all services available to small enterprises to educate and guide managers in achieving greater cost-effectiveness through selective utilization of medical and hygiene services.

To the owner or plant manager, occupational health coverage is a consumptive rather than an investment cost, as it might be seen from the overall perspective of society. A heavy involvement in prevention or hazard control or health promotion may or may not forestall a future event from occurring; the cost is tangible, but the benefit is not. Furthermore, employees come and go, and a heavy investment one year may be lost with personnel turnover the next, particularly since the benefits are usually apparent only in the long term. In larger companies costs associated with disability and absenteeism may be reduced by company medical programs, but to a small company the costs of maintaining health services is usually out of proportion to the visible benefits. Although intensive safety control applied to companies with high injury rates does appear to reduce downtime, lower insurance premiums and workers' compensation levies, and improve morale, it is doubtful that managers of small enterprises that perceive them to be low in risk to begin with can be motivated to institute expensive in-house programs except when these are used as benefits to attract exceptionally talented employees. Costs must therefore be kept as low as practicable when marketing to small enterprises.

There exists a severe shortage of the skilled professionals in occupational health and safety who are available to supply services, especially to small enterprises. Four specific measures have been proposed to overcome this problem:

- Increased training in occupational safety and health in medical school and expanded postgraduate continuing medical education in occupational medicine in order to increase the expertise of practicing primary care physicians
- Provision of clinic-based occupational safety and health services serving many employers
- Expanded use of nonphysician health professionals, particularly nurse practitioners
- Simplification of procedures such as standardized medical examinations for fitness-to-work evaluations appropriate to particular occupations or workers exposed to specific hazards to be performed by a physician untrained in occupational medicine

Outpatient clinical services for small enterprises have been provided for decades by private practitioners and more recently by group practices. These services have been largely inconspicuous, however, since they constitute only a small part of the activities of such practices.

MANAGED CARE IN OCCUPATIONAL MEDICINE

Increasingly, primary medical care in the United States is provided by managed care organizations (MCOs), professionally managed groups of physicians and other healthcare professionals organized into corporate entities to achieve coordination and economies of scale. Physicians are subject to controls and restrictions on their practices imposed by institutional procedures, clinical guidelines, limited pharmacopoeia, prior authorization, and utilization review. Increasingly as well, MCOs market their services to groups of patients defined by residence, employer, or other common characteristics.

Today, even services delivered outside of an MCO are likely to be reimbursed below billing on a fee schedule based on median rates or by a capitation allowance, with the financial risk accepted by the provider rather than the third-party payer. Because of intensifying competition and the increasingly risky financial situation in which medical practitioners and health providers such as clinics and hospitals find themselves, occupational medicine services are often used as a way to attract large groups of employees and their dependents as a patient base to enhance the financial stability of a captive health maintenance organization or preferred provider association.

Occupational medicine services, however, are not as driven by managed care as general medical care. Reimbursement rates for workers' compensation, for example, are now quite competitive with fee schedules for general medical services. The OEM physician also has the opportunity to engage in other, high-value services that have no equivalent in general medicine.

Fee-for-service, in theory, favors overutilization of services because the more services provided, the more fees the provider collects; in most cases, it is the physician who recommends a treatment, not the patient. Prepaid practice, in theory, favors underutilization because the less the provider must expend in costs to provide services, the more the provider saves from the prepaid amount. That is why third-party payers have increasingly introduced utilization review procedures to ensure that the care given is medically indicated and why health maintenance organizations, which are prepaid, conduct quality assurance reviews to ensure that patients are not going without needed care. In workers' compensation, the physician is compensated on a fee-for-service basis according to a fee schedule fixed by the workers' compensation board. The interests of the employer, the carrier, and usually the patient favor a speedy return to work. The idea is to further the interests of all parties by returning the patient to work promptly, thereby reducing the losses to the employer from absence, returning the patient to his previous earning potential, and settling outstanding claims on the part of the carrier.

A basic difference between general and occupational healthcare is appropriate utilization. Frequent return visits and heavy use of rehabilitative services such as physical therapy, to a degree that would seem to constitute overutilization in general healthcare, may be quite appropriate in occupational medicine practice as long as they contribute to returning the patient to work as soon as the patient is able. The intensity of care is intended to further the interests of all parties: to return the patient to work promptly, to reduce losses to the employer from absence, to promote prompt settlement of claims, and to reduce long-term expense on the part of the carrier.

Liability Position of OEM Physicians

Most coverage for OEM physicians is provided by the employer. For physicians in private practice, individual policies are available through the American College of Occupational and Environmental Medicine, which provides coverage for both liability for clinical services and errors and omissions for nonclinical services, such as consulting and medicolegal work.

Insurance companies in the United States and in Canada (specifically the Canadian Medical Protective Association) categorize physicians into risk categories, with as few as three and as many as nine classes. OEM physicians tend to be treated very differently by different companies. OEM physicians, almost uniquely, fall into either the highest or the lowest risk categories depending on their particular situation and their degree of formal training. The factors that are most often cited in determining whether an OEM physician would be considered low-risk are board certification in occupational medicine, whether one's activities are primarily of an administrative nature, the emphasis on preventive medicine in the practice, and whether the practice is included within a large organization. Factors cited as determining a high-risk classification include the lack of specialty credentials, a preponderance of patient care responsibilities, emphasis on surgery or on trauma cases, and solo practice.

The most suitable type of coverage for an OEM physician depends, in large part, on whether one's practice involves clinical care in high-risk situations and to some degree on whether one is in solo practice (and thus relatively unprotected) or in an institutional setting.

RESOURCES

Guidotti TL, Cowell JWF, Jamieson GG. *OHSs: A Practical Approach*. Chicago: American Medical Association; 1989. [Reprinted as a "classic" in occupational medicine by Blackburn Press, http://www.blackburnpress.com/]

Moser R Jr. *Effective Management of Health and Safety Programs: A Practical Guide*. 3rd ed. Beverley Farms, MA: OEM Press; 2008.

NOTEWORTHY READINGS

Cullen MR. Occupational medicine: a new focus for general internal medicine. *Arch Intern Med*. 1985;145:511–515.

De Hart RL. *Guidelines for Establishing an Occupational Medical Program*. Chicago: American Occupational Medical Association; 1987.

Felton JS. *Occupational Medical Management: A Guide to the Organization and Operation of In-Plant OHSs*. Boston: OEM Health Information; 1989.

Guidotti TL. The general internist and occupational medicine. *J Gen Intern Med*. 1986;1:201–202.

Guidotti TL, Cowell JWF, Jamieson GG. *OHSs: A Practical Approach*. Chicago: American Medical Association, 1989.

Murray R, Schilling RSF. Functions of an OHS. In: *Occupational Health Practice*. London: Butterworths; 1981: 145–158.

Newkirk WL, Jones LD. *OHSs: A Guide to Program Planning and Management*. Chicago: American Hospital Publishing; 1989.

Rest K, Ed. How to begin an occupational health program—administrative and ethical issues (entire issue). *Semin Occup Med*. 1986;1(1):1–96.

Smith I. *Occupational Health: A Practical Guide for Managers*. London: Taylor and Francis; 2007.

21 WORKERS' COMPENSATION

Workers' compensation is a cornerstone of occupational medicine. The occupational and environmental medicine (OEM) physician should therefore invest considerable time and effort in understanding the principles of workers' compensation and learn as much about the system in which one practices as one possibly can. (There is no counterpart in environmental medicine.) At the outset, it should be noted that the correct form is "workers' compensation" (plural possessive), not "worker's compensation" (singular possessive), and that "workman's" or "workmen's" compensation is an obsolete, historical term that survives today in the names and texts of legislation passed in earlier times, when all workers were assumed to be men.

Eligibility for the insurance benefit is based on an injury or illness that "arises from work" or that "arises out of and in the course of employment," in the most common language. Causation and relationship to work is therefore an important, if implicit, part of every workers' compensation case. Issues of causation become complicated in occupational disease cases and require a systematic approach to evidence, aspects of which are discussed in Chapters 3 and 23.

Workers' compensation is a social insurance system, one of the earliest. It provides injured workers with two essential services: income replacement and payment of medical and rehabilitation expenses. Workers' compensation began in Europe in the mid-nineteenth century and was first put into practice in Germany in 1884 in its modern form. It began as a great reform. Workers' compensation pioneered no-fault insurance, introduced alternative dispute resolution, created a counterweight to abusive power of employers, created incentives for safety and injury prevention, and saved countless families from sudden impoverishment. Workers' compensation was not introduced into North America until 1911, during the historic but eclectic movement for social reform known as the Progressive Era. Over time, inequities and abuses crept back into the system, which became rigid and parochial. The state-level organization of workers' compensation led to fragmentation, inconsistency between states, and heterogeneous policies. The system as a whole came to be seen as corrupt and unresponsive, dominated by lawyers who had reintroduced the litigiousness and delays that workers' compensation had originally sought to overcome. Over the last two decades, however, a great reform movement has reenergized workers' compensation. Now, workers' compensation systems are laboratories of experimentation and innovation in managed care.

Virtually all OEM physicians work at least in part within the workers' compensation system (colloquially and universally called "workers' comp"). Workers' compensation is one of three pillars of occupational health practice, the others being the occupational healthcare system and medicolegal practice, including independent medical examiner services. It is a parallel healthcare system sharing providers with the general healthcare system but funded and managed very differently. Workers' compensation is much older than managed care, arose from and was a response to the adversarial tort litigation system, and is not covered by much current legislation, such as provisions regarding confidentiality and access to information in general healthcare. These features have given workers' compensation different characteristics from other healthcare systems.

Today, workers' compensation reform can be read as a compromise between interests who would have preferred the status quo but realize that it was unsustainable and those who would prefer a more thoroughgoing transformation but know that there is no political will for it. It has become the country's second largest healthcare system (about $55 billion in 2003), coming after the general healthcare system (about $1.7 trillion in 2005) and ahead of the military's Defense Health Program (about $18 billion in 2005).

DESIGN AND PRINCIPLES

Workers' compensation is a "no-fault" insurance plan designed to pay for medical care and to compensate the injured worker for wages lost during periods of temporary or permanent disability and rehabilitation due to injury or illness resulting from work. Critics of the no-fault aspect of workers' compensation point out that the absence of a means of identifying fault or a motive for doing so removes a check on the commitment of employers to run a safe workplace. Defenders point out that that is more properly the function of a regulatory agency and that the experience rating system is a means of penalizing employers that demonstrate poor performance.

An important principle of modern workers' compensation systems is that it is necessary to demonstrate that the injury arose out of work, but it is not necessary to find that an employer was at fault for a worker to receive benefits. Likewise, negligence or fault on the part of a worker does not disqualify him or her from entitlement to benefits. Causation analysis is essential in workers' compensation claims but is properly limited to establishing the relationship to work. This is usually obvious in an injury. The challenge of establishing causation in occupation disease is much greater, and at times the standard of persuasion that is needed requires much more detail on the circumstances of the injury than should be required to answer the essential question of whether the condition arose from work.

The general standard for adjudication in workers' compensation is the "weight of evidence," which derives from the tort system that gave birth to workers' compensation. Most workers' compensation acts tip the scale deliberately by specifying that when the balance of probabilities is even, the benefit of the doubt should be given to the claimant. (Vermont does not.) Some states, such as California, and systems such as the Railroad Workers Act require the demonstration of a "substantial contribution" of work factors to the injury but do not require that the injury be completely the result of workplace hazards.

Workers' compensation pays benefits for wage replacement and medical care as a primary responsibility. The objective is to compensate the injured worker for wages lost during periods of temporary or permanent disability and to pay for treatment and rehabilitation required to recover from injury or illness resulting from work. Retraining benefits are sometimes available. Incidental costs, such as transportation to and from treatment and for workers' compensation board interviews or evaluations are sometimes provided. Benefits are also paid to survivors after fatalities.

Workers' compensation introduced a new legal remedy in which the "industrial relationship" between employer and employee would be considered to be deeper than work in exchange for pay. The cost of healthcare for on-the-job injuries would be treated as an operating expense to be shared on an industry-wide basis. The worker would be guaranteed a fair and rapid adjudication of claims and sufficient compensation. (This, at least, was the ideal.)

Workers' compensation is based on what is often called "an historic compromise." The injured worker gave up the right to sue the employer and the employer gave up the right to reject the claim or to defend themselves in court. Under workers' compensation legislation, the employer is required by law (except in Texas, where it is voluntary) to carry insurance to cover on-the-job injuries and compensation for disability. The employee, on the other hand, is not permitted to sue the employer for medical costs or compensation. The employee trades the uncertainty and delay of a court proceeding, which could possibly result in a large judgment, for prompt payment of predictably more limited benefits. The employer gives up the right to argue against a penalty but benefits by avoiding expensiv litigation. This, at least, is how the system is supposed to work.

Workers' compensation is organized at the state and provincial level (with separate systems for federal employees in both the United States and Canada), and there is much variation in process and benefits. It was originally designed for industrial workers and so has large gaps in coverage, for example excluding agricultural workers in most states. It operates strictly on an insurance model, mostly through private commercial carriers, and is not a welfare or entitlement program. Workers' compensation is financed by a payroll premium levied on employers, not financed by taxes.

The essential services provided by workers' compensation are (1) income replacement for workers who cannot do their job because of injury or disease arising out of their work and (2) coverage for medical and rehabilitation expenses for the treatment of work-related injury and illness. Benefits are also provided to the dependents of workers in case of fatality. Individual workers' compensation carriers and boards may provide additional services, such as job retraining, but these two services are the foundation of the system. It follows logically, then, that the first decision in a workers' compensation claim is whether the injury or illness did in fact arise out of work. For most injuries, this is not in question. For diseases, including musculoskeletal disorders (which are treated as diseases in workers' compensation), the connection to work is not always obvious and may be disputed. As a consequence, there is always an appeals mechanism in the workers' compensation system.

Intensive management of care is another effective approach. Requesting regular progress reports, advising on management where appropriate, offering employee's facilities for rehabilitation, frequent visits to the occupational health department, and encouraging second opinions for major surgical interventions all tend to promote appropriate management of the case and provide opportunities for monitoring and evaluating progress. The procedure for evaluating fitness to work (see Chapter 18) can then be followed in order to return the worker to the job as soon as he or she is ready, minimizing unproductive time on compensation, and avoiding a return too early, when re-injury may occur.

The level of benefits varies greatly by jurisdiction. Within the United States, West Virginia, Maine, Montana, the Federal Employees system, Hawaii, Oklahoma, Washington, Alaska, and California pay the highest benefits per $100 of covered wages, in that order. Comparisons may easily be misleading, however. Criteria and policies vary markedly, introducing great disparities in equity. States with heavy employment in high-risk industries, such as mining, may pay more. States with a large representation of more highly paid workers may pay less as a ratio to payroll.

The workers' compensation system is the sole legal recourse for injured workers that it covers. This means that a worker cannot sue, or be sued by, an employer. This is referred to as "exclusive remedy" and is written into workers' compensation acts. Although the exclusive remedy has been challenged in the courts, it has always held on appeal, if not in the initial ruling. Most of the challenges have been brought on the grounds that the "exclusive remedy" provision denies workers "due process" in having their cases heard. Also, lapses in the process itself, such as arbitrary actions or failures to comply with regulations on the part of the administrative judge or hearing officer, can themselves be grounds for legal action under some circumstances.

One opening for workers and employers is that the right to sue a third party is preserved to both. If a product used in the workplace is faulty and causes an injury during normal use or if the manufacturer or distributor did not effectively or honestly represent or communicate the hazard ("failure to warn"), there may be grounds for legal action. Likewise, if a chemical formulation causes an occupational health problem that should have been known and that potential problem was not communicated to the purchaser, grounds may exist for a lawsuit against the third party, usually the manufacturer or distributor. Third party suits have been heavily used in asbestos litigation. Ordinarily, judgments won against a third party are first applied to reimburse the employer or carrier for the value of benefits already paid to the worker, with the balance going to the worker directly. Third-party litigation is complicated, and expert legal counsel is advisable before proceeding with action under this or any other legal premise.

Workers compensation carriers also sue third parties and sometimes sue one another to obtain reimbursement for extraordinary claims. This is called "subrogation." For example, the province of Alberta experienced a large number of claims for asbestos-associated disease in oil refinery workers who had also worked in Texas in jobs that also involved handling asbestos. The Workers' Compensation Board of Alberta paid the benefits and then sued carriers in Texas for the share that would have been apportioned to the Texas companies and was able to recover millions of dollars.

In the United States, various state agencies, which may be industrial relations department, insurance commissions, or departments of banking or insurance, house offices of workers' compensation regulation that mandate consistent adjudication processes, regulate insurance premiums, and provide an appeals process separate from the carrier, usually a tribunal system using an administrative law judge or a hearing officer. Appeals are considered to be a form of alternate dispute resolution rather than modeled after courtroom procedures and so the rules of evidence are relaxed. Certain "presumptions" are legislated in many states. Presumption means that certain claims are presumed to be meritorious unless proven otherwise because the disease in question is known to be associated with an occupation, requiring carriers to accept claims unless there is evidence to rebut the claim.

In Canada, workers' compensation boards (WCBs) are provincial bodies created by law to operate the workers' compensation system and workers' compensation tribunals (in Québec, *la Commission des lesions professionelles*) are autonomous agencies that exist to provide a fair appeals mechanism in resolving disputed claim. Workers' compensation boards are empowered to set fees for compensation and medical reimbursement and guidelines for assessing disability. The "board" is the governing body of the WCB, variably appointed or selected but usually balanced among representatives of labor and industry as well as public servants. The WCB itself usually maintains its own staff of medical consultants as well as retaining authority to refer claimants to outside expert medical examiners and advisers when the claim warrants. Some WCBs also provide direct medical and social services to injured workers, such as rehabilitation and vocational training, either in-house or by contracting out for delivery of these services.

Workers' compensation procedures have become exceedingly complex. Workers' compensation laws and rates are set by each state and province, with separate systems for federal employees and certain designated groups, such as longshoremen in the United States. There are seventy separate workers' compensation programs in North America, each with different procedures and levels of benefits. The system does not universally cover agricultural workers, self-employed persons, business owners, workplaces with less than a minimum number of employees in particular industries, domestic workers, or workers who are providing services on a contract basis as individuals. Volunteers, such as volunteer firefighters, are not covered. These omissions result in a substantial fraction of the workforce remaining unprotected and forced to rely on their general health insurance, welfare, or unemployment insurance as their safety nets.

Seamen in the U.S. Merchant Marine, Longshoremen (Longshore and Harbor Workers' Compensation Act), railroad workers (Railroad Workers Injury and Federal Employers Liability Act), federal employees (Federal Employees Compensation Act), maritime workers (Jones Act), coal miners (Black Lung Benefits Act), and federal vendors and federal-contractor energy workers in the nuclear industry (Energy Employees Occupational Illness Compensation Program, EEOICP) are covered by other systems in the United States, with special rules. The oldest of these systems predate the state workers' compensation acts. They are governed by federal acts in most cases because they involve workers in interstate trade or transportation. In general, they reset the burden of evidence such that injuries are compensable if there has been any substantial contribution to impairment, and they do not require the full weight of evidence to prove causation. The Longshoreman and Harbor Workers' Act of 1927, administered by the U.S. Department of Labor, created an insurance plan for shore-based maritime workers. EEOICP was initiated in 2001 to cover former employees of vendors and contractors at nuclear facilities for which the Atomic Energy Commission and then the Department of Energy were responsible and who may be at increased risk for illness from chemical exposure. Administration of EEOICP was recently moved from the Department of Energy to the Department of Labor.

Physicians sometimes resist dealing with workers' compensation cases because the forms are tedious and the cases get complicated. Workers' compensation does require paperwork and administrative detail on the part of the clinician, but the system meets a serious social need and under current fee schedules usually reimburses the physician at a rate for the time spent that is better than many other cognitive (nonprocedural) healthcare services.

HISTORY

Workers' compensation was the first social insurance plan to be introduced into North America, preceding unemployment insurance, as a cornerstone of protection for workers. It was a direct response to the social crisis that developed during the Industrial Revolution and the rising rates of injury and disability among workers in unsafe factories, mines, and workshops. Until workers' compensation was introduced, the injured worker had to sue his or her employer for compensation for an injury on the job.

Before workers' compensation, employees were considered under the law to have entered into an unwritten contract with the employer, in which they accepted all risk associated with their work as a condition of employment. Workers assumed legal responsibility for their own safety, even for measures beyond their control, and could sue employers only on grounds of criminal intent or criminal negligence, both of which were nearly impossible to prove.

During most of the nineteenth century, the United States and Canada were both developing countries with a chronic labor shortage (although not necessarily later and in the big cities) and dependent for growth on foreign direct investment (from London, in both cases). Law courts deliberately tried to protect the interest of employers in order to promote economic development, keep wages low, and make entrepreneurship attractive. The legal theories of the day stacked the deck against the worker.

Employers could readily defend themselves by invoking the prevailing legal doctrines or by confusing the picture of what happened. Originally, at the beginning of the eighteenth century, there was a doctrine in British common law (which applied to the colonies) called "the law of vicarious responsibility." It held that the master was responsible for the acts of the servant and by extension the employer was responsible for the acts of the employee. However, this doctrine was largely blunted in the early 1800s by the "fellow servant" doctrine, which held that employers were not responsible for acts of their employees that resulted in injury to themselves or other employees. Before workers' compensation, employees were considered under the law to have entered into an unwritten contract with the employer ("assumption of risk"), in which they accepted all risk associated with their work as a condition of employment. If a worker were injured by the action of another employee, the employer was not responsible (under the "fellow servant doctrine"). If any action by the injured worker could be construed to have contributed to the risk, it was defensible under the doctrine of "contributory negligence." Sometimes juries sided with the injured worker anyway, but usually the legal defenses for employers were insurmountable.

By the late nineteenth century in Europe and later the United States, the Industrial Revolution had caused serious social discontent. The new industrial economy was based on hourly wage rates, production, and (especially in Europe) a labor surplus in cities (and, for several countries, their colonies) that caused competition among workers that kept wages low. Although wages in the United States and Canada were higher than in Europe during this period, workers were often divided, immigration caused short-term labor surpluses in the new industrial cities, and in the absence of unions workers could not act collectively to demand higher wages. In both North America and Europe technology threatened job security for workers who could be replaced by a machine and kept wages lower than they would have been otherwise, while at the same time keeping the prices of commodities low so that workers could live on them. In the United States, especially, technology and energy resources (water at first, fossil fuels later) were used on a large scale to replace relatively scarce labor, somewhat offsetting the labor shortage, but these technological innovations were often very dangerous: open belts and gears, unguarded blades, inadequate ventilation, unprotected exposure to lead and acid fumes, and poor working conditions were the norm. Technology (initially borrowed from Britain) gave the rapidly growing American economy an early edge in industrial production, which it used to great advantage in the twentieth century. In Europe there had been revolutions in many countries around 1850, and there was a great fear of social and political instability. In the United States and Canada, there were periodic displays of rebellion and early labor unions were organizing, which raised similar fears. Labor insecurity was at the root of the discontent, although even at the time occupational health and safety was considered a side issue.

Employers hired workers "at will" and could fire them without cause. Social safety nets only existed through charity and mutual assistance pacts, which in the United States were usually based on ethnicity among immigrants and were considered suspiciously socialistic. The result was often a sense of desperation about finding and keeping a job. Work was often dangerous, fast-paced, and easy to lose if the worker could not keep up. When a worker was injured on the job, income for the family stopped, and if the injury resulted in permanent impairment, it could thrust the family from relative comfort into poverty almost immediately.

Occupational injuries, especially fatalities, were cheap in the nineteenth century because healthcare, which was not very good anyway, cost little and life expectancy was short. Employers occasionally recognized their responsibility and paid compensation or gave what they considered to be a charitable contribution to the family but usually paid nothing at all.

Workers' compensation introduced a new legal remedy in which employer and employee were considered to have a special "industrial" relationship more complex than a simple contract for work in exchange for pay. It was based on a new theory that recognized that at least as an ideal both sides would have to give something up in order to get something in return. The theory implicitly recognized that as owners of the facilities and means of production, employers are in control of the workplace and have a responsibility to workers who are injured or made ill in their employ. The outlines of a historic compromise took place, negotiated in part by early unions and workers' representatives but also by some employers who saw it as a way of reducing class conflict and introducing more stability into the workplace. The outline of the compromise was that workers would give up the right to sue their employers and employers would give up the right to refuse claims for injury. In return, the workers would receive a guarantee of reimbursement for lost wages and their medical expenses would be covered. The system would be run as an insurance business, using actuarial methods, which contained costs for the employers and avoided the risk of generous juries. Industrial sectors would have collective responsibility for their sector, because they would be insured on a group basis, which was thought to be an incentive to bring poorly performing employers in line. The system would be managed, or at least overseen, by government. Because it would cover all industrial workers and because fault or liability would not be at issue, the system would operate as no-fault insurance. Politically, the concept was irresistible because it received backing from both capital and labor and addressed a serious problem that was threatening social stability. The same unsettled social and economic conditions in the United States gave rise to the Progressive Era, a period of reform at the beginning of the twentieth century during which workers' compensation perfectly fit the political agenda.

Workers' compensation started in Europe in the mid-nineteenth century and was first put into practice in Germany in 1884 in something like its modern form (both workers and employers contributed to the fund, however). It was part of a package of reforms introduced by Chancellor Otto von Bismarck that was intended to quell political unrest and to head off revolution. (Other reforms included mandatory national healthcare insurance and the retirement pension.) Within a few years, other countries in Europe adopted similar systems, notably the Austro-Hungarian Empire, where many early innovations occurred and where it became a big business. (Franz Kafka was employed in Prague by a workers' compensation carrier.) Workers' compensation was adopted in England in 1897 and operated until 1948, when the National Health Service was developed and a modified tort system for occupational injury and illness replaced it.

Workers' compensation was not introduced into North America until 1911, first in Wisconsin, Washington, and Ohio, when it arose as a reform movement during the Progressive Era of American politics. Most states adopted some form of workers' compensation on the English model (with less state management) by 1920 with the last being Hawaii in 1963. This history led to the present patchwork of programs and policies.

The German model (more centralization with state management) was introduced into Canada by way of Ontario by Chief Justice William Meredith in a highly influential report in 1913 that quickly shaped national policy and made workers' compensation policies more consistent across the country than in the United States. The essential principles articulated by Meredith were no-fault compensation, collective liability (within industrial sectors), security of payment (reliable and timely benefits delivered to workers), exclusive jurisdiction (keeping claims out of the courts), and an independent board to govern the system (to shield the system from political influence). The Canadian system thereafter developed along its own path with strong and large provincial "workers' compensation boards" organized as crown corporations, which serve as monopoly insurance carriers.

In the United States, the evolution of the system was different and emphasized the free and competitive insurance market in most states. The workers' compensation system worked in tandem with increased interest in occupational safety and had a stronger preventive component. Adjustments could be made in the "experience rating," which helped determine premiums paid by employers within a particular industry class, which created incentives to reduce the injury rate. However, as time went on, healthcare became more expensive and premiums became higher, the differential in payment that was governed by the experience rating became less significant as a cost. At the same time, regulation ensured that the full increase in cost would not be transmitted to employers in disruptive jumps in premiums.

During the 1920s, workers' compensation expanded in coverage and programs and became the major social support system for working Americans. There was no other social insurance program at the time. Workers' compensation programs managed large pots of money and, unlike Canada, were not shielded from political influence.

During the Depression, workers' compensation was an incomplete but necessary safety net for many injured workers. However, perceptions of employment and safety changed. The dominant attitude was that workers were lucky to have jobs at all. Safety became more expensive to struggling employers than absorbing the cost in workers' compensation premiums. Federal efforts to impose requirements for uniform and effective occupational safety regulations on states were resisted. Workers' compensation systems faced a huge challenge in occupational disease claims, particular for silicosis, which imposed huge unfunded liabilities. In 1939, the U.S. federal government bailed out failing state workers' compensation systems nationally in order to keep the entire system from collapsing. One effect of this was to create more uniformity among programs than had existed before, especially in terms of standards and impairment ratings. However, the system remained fragmentary and controlled by state priorities and politics.

World War II, expenditures for which ended the Depression, led to more claims activity in workers' compensation, and protection of injured workers was perceived, at least to some extent, as patriotic because it supported the war effort. The postwar era was a period of general decline in efficiency and integrity of the system. The New Deal had introduced other important social insurance programs and employment benefits that made workers' compensation less economically important even while it expanded in assets and coverage. The country was preoccupied in the early 1950s with the debate over national health insurance, and there may have been a general assumption that such a plan would absorb workers' compensation, as had occurred in the United Kingdom, although the National Health Service was very different from the insurance plans under discussion in the United States at the time. The workers' compensation system, marginalized and left to its own devices, became a political backwater, degenerating over time into special interest pleading, local fiefdoms, corruption, and political games played with money.

By 1972, the situation with state workers' compensation systems had reached the point of generating political pressure for reform at the federal level. In that year, a National Commission on State Workmens' Compensation Laws delivered a report that recommended mandatory standards for state systems. It did not explicitly recommend federalizing the workers' compensation system, but that would have been the logical next step if state programs did not comply with the recommendations. State programs did respond, however, and dramatically raised benefits to workers.

The 1980s saw the beginning of rapidly rising medical care costs and escalating premiums for employers. Caught in the middle because rates were regulated, the workers' compensation insurance industry lost money during this period. The pendulum swung back and led to a reduction in level of benefits, efforts to control costs, and the beginning of managed care models in workers' compensation. The industry became very profitable again.

The 1990s saw the beginning of major reform efforts, pioneered in states such as Florida and Massachusetts, and culminating in 2004 with thoroughgoing changes in California, the largest workers' compensation system.

What happened in California was a political phenomenon of the first order. In 2003, a sitting governor was recalled and Arnold Schwarzenegger, a movie actor, was elected to replace him in the recall election. Reforming workers' compensation became, uniquely, not just a matter of practical politics, as it always had been, but a demonstration of political will by the new governor, a means of establishing control, and obtaining buy-in from every important economic constituency (employers, injured workers, insurance carriers, providers, economic interests concerned with competitiveness, and firms considering a move into or out of California). With the possible exception of West Virginia, there is no other example in recent years in which workers' compensation assumed such a central role in a state's political agenda.

The vehicle for workers' compensation reform in California was Senate Bill 899, which was passed in 2004. SB 899 allows workers up to $10,000 in medical expenses paid for by employers while the claim is pending (before it is accepted or denied), requires that if injured workers wish to be treated by a physician other than the one selected by the employer they must do so within ten days and choose from a preapproved panel, allows closed healthcare provider networks for providing care, defines the qualifications of independent medical examiners (IMEs), caps access to rehabilitation services, replaces vocational rehabilitation benefits with a "supplemental job displacement benefit" if the injured worker could not return to his or her job, caps the duration of temporary disability to two years, creates incentives for returning workers with permanent disabilities to work, codifies the agreed medical examiner (AME) system, provides new avenues for dispute resolution, and allows system innovation under state supervision. In the world of workers' compensation, these are revolutionary changes. SB 899 also made evidence-based management the presumptive standard of care by imposing a new requirement for apportionment by cause in causation analysis (discussed later) and the adoption of evidence-based criteria for impairment assessment, treatment guidelines (using the *ACOEM Practice Guidelines*, which are discussed in Chapter 16), and utilization review.

Although the changes in workers' compensation have been invigorating and bold, the economic crisis of 2008–2009 initially threatens to upset everything. Whether it was at last achieving sustainability or not, the workers' compensation system in virtually every jurisdiction will face new and unanticipated challenges that will force even more radical changes.

The current or some future severe economic recession may force a crisis similar to 1939. It is not inconceivable that workers' compensation may require a federal bailout, which would create an opportunity to rationalize the system. Although for years there was no political will for a federal system of workers' compensation, the political landscape has abruptly changed, and it might become feasible again. Alternatively, renewed movement toward a comprehensive healthcare insurance plan, although sidelined at the moment by the economic situation, might create circumstances similar to 1950 when workers' compensation could have been incorporated into a national healthcare insurance plan. The trajectory of current economic and political change guarantees that the issue of what to do with workers' compensation will be revisited in coming years.

CLAIMS MANAGEMENT

A worker injured on the job is initially sent for medical care. In half of the states (such as Wisconsin) and the District of Columbia, the worker has his or her choice of which physician to see, but in other states (including Virginia and California) the employer makes the initial choice, although the worker can change physicians later if he or she desires. Some states (such as California) allow the worker to choose if they notify the employer before the injury of their physician of choice and increasingly often impose the restriction that the physician has to be on a list of approved providers. If the worker sees another physician, the cost of the encounter may not be covered by workers' compensation. In some cases, the insurance carrier may disqualify a particular physician or insist on another choice, particularly when there has been a pattern of suspected abuse or inadequate or ill-informed management of workers' compensation cases. The board or insurance carrier may also require periodic evaluation by another physician, sometimes called an "expert medical examiner" or "independent medical examiner," either on its own staff or an outside consultant. The purpose is to monitor progress and to have another set of eyes observing the treatment and recovery process.

The first visit to a physician for an occupational injury or illness does not require authorization from the workers' compensation carrier. For subsequent visits to be covered or for referral to a specialist to be reimbursed, care must be approved by the carrier in advance. The physician must file a "physician's first report" form within a certain time limit once an occupationally associated injury or illness is recognized. This is a provision of law and is as legally binding as the requirement to notify the health department of a communicable disease. The workers' compensation carrier pays the physician a fixed fee set by the state for the report.

The physician's first report form initiates the claim. (Claims can also be initiated by employee's or employer's first reports, which are separate forms.) The first report automatically triggers a disability benefits review if the worker is off work more than a few days and establishes the injury as possibly work related.

The claim is initially reviewed by a case manager, who makes the decision to accept or reject the claim in the first instance. The case manager may accept or reject the claim on the basis of the first report, which is the means by which it is notified that a claim has been made, but seldom contests cases that are straightforward. The great majority of cases are not disputed.

The process of compensating the worker for wages lost because of disability is called indemnification. The intent is to compensate the injured worker for that proportion of future earnings lost due to the disability arising from the injury. Income benefits are triggered by the physician's or the employer's first report, which opens a file on the case. The benefits calculations are complex and are based on a formula that derives a disability rating, not on the level of impairment alone. Payment of temporary disability benefits begins after a brief waiting period (usually seven days) and continues until the worker has either recovered completely or has improved as much as he or she is likely to. In the former case, the payments cease. In the latter case, permanent partial disability payments are based on the disability rating that derives from residual impairment and other factors. (See Chapter 18.)

Until the worker can return to work, the carrier also pays for interim visits, consultations, and rehabilitation as long as the services are approved by the carrier in advance. If the disability is permanent, it is rated (see Chapter 18) and a weekly payment is made up to a maximum amount depending on the worker's capacity to work. Workers' compensation benefits cover only work-related disability. A person who is also impaired for some other reason must seek other sources of income maintenance for the non–work-related component.

After follow-up visits, written supplemental reports from the physician are provided to the carrier in order to monitor the course of recovery, control the continuation of benefits, and initiate payment for medical and rehabilitative services. Because progress reports by the physician are the means by which the carrier is kept informed of the case, it is critical that reports be submitted on a timely basis and that they be complete and accurate. The insurance carrier and the employer usually have the right to require an examination by a physician of their choice in order to monitor the progress of the patient-worker to determine when he or she is fit to return to work.

Complications of a work-related injury are treated as work related. Therefore misadventures in surgery, drug side effects, and medical complications are all covered by the medical treatment reimbursement provided by workers' compensation. However, incidental illness, second injuries that are not directly related to the initial injury and are not work related, or conditions that arise from personal health problems are not covered, even if they contribute to impairment and disability. These are assumed to be covered by other social insurance programs, such as Social Security. Some workers' compensation jurisdictions arrange offset payments coordinated with private insurance or social insurance programs, but most do not. No workers' compensation and few private insurance plans allow double collection of benefits for the same disability.

The final report terminates the case in the files of the carrier, establishes fitness to work (see Chapter 18), and establishes for the record any permanent disability that remains.

The workers' compensation carrier may choose to address questions of fact or opinions regarding diagnosis, impairment evaluation, and medical management by retaining an "independent medical examiner" (IME), whose function it is to resolve medical uncertainties. The IME may review the file and examine the injured worker but does not engage in treatment or assume care of the injured worker. The IME forms no physician-patient relationship with the injured worker; his or her sole responsibility is to render a disinterested and objective report on matters of fact and, if asked, to render an opinion. In California, a variant of the IME system is used in which both claimants and the carrier agree on one physician, called the "agreed medical examiner" (AME) to perform the independent medical examination (which is also called an IME).

As in any benefits program, some level of abuse occurs in workers' compensation. Usually, this takes the form of a worker claiming that an injury occurred on the job when it did not or of an employer concealing the frequency of injuries on the site by fraudulent or censored reporting. Sometimes, the degree of disability claimed is exaggerated by the worker or minimized by the employer. Outright malingering by workers appears to be relatively rare overall. More common is for a nonmeritorious claim to be put forward to see how far it will go by a claimant who may or may not be convinced of its merit but who has decided to let the system sort it out.

Mistaken claims, submitted in good faith by workers who feel that they have been injured but who are incorrect in this assumption, should not be considered abuse. They are part of the discrimination and evaluation problem, and it is the responsibility of the system to resolve them.

APPEALS

The carrier may contest the claim on the grounds that it probably is not work related or that the level of impairment is not as great as described. A second level of review takes place within the workers' compensation carrier, usually conducted by a staff or consultant physician or senior case manager. Either the worker or the carrier may appeal the second ruling or contest the amount of disability to a special board or tribunal that reviews such cases.

The tribunal is an autonomous body separate from the workers' compensation carrier. It functions like an administrative law court, but the rules of evidence are relaxed and the process is less formal. The case is reviewed by an administrative judge or hearing officer and sometimes by a panel, with the support of consultants and dedicated staff, who are usually health professionals with prior experience within the workers' compensation system. Hearings are often held, allowing oral presentation of arguments and examination of witnesses. Because of the quasi-juridical form of the hearing, most claimants feel the need for advocates to state their case and may hire lawyers or obtain representation from a union.

Decisions follow deliberation on the case and are based on the weight of evidence. The rationale behind the decision is explained in a report that is not unlike a court opinion but less formal. Unlike courts, however, workers' compensation tribunals are not bound by precedent. The reason is that claims are required, in most legislative acts, to be made on the basis of the facts of the individual case, not on other considerations or legal authority.

Disputed cases are usually those in which causation is not obvious. Workers' compensation systems were primarily designed to handle occupational injuries (which by definition in workers' compensation arise from a single event) and do not function very well in dealing with occupational diseases, repetitive strain injury (which is deemed a "disease" in workers' compensation because it does not arise from a single event and is therefore evaluated under the theory of "cumulative injury"), "mental mental" cases (a term of art meaning mental stress resulting in mental symptoms or impairment, which might otherwise be called psychogenic stress outcomes, as discussed in Chapter 13), unusual outcomes, or any condition that is also common in the general population or associated with smoking. In relatively rare cases, there may be a suspicion of malingering or the circumstances surrounding the injury may be complicated or suspicious (in other words, there is evidence that the worker may not have been injured on the job and may have sustained the injury elsewhere).

Cases in which there is no objective finding, such as low back pain, are especially difficult because symptoms reported by the patient have a strong subjective and emotional component, especially pain. Pain is subject to "symptom magnification" or "symptom amplification" (unconsciously increasing in perceived intensity due to anxiety or attention focused on the problem), "symptom exaggeration" (overinterpretation when the symptom is actually there), and malingering (fraudulent representation). As a whole, the workers' compensation is seldom persuaded unless there is some evidence of an objective finding in a case. Because subjective complaints lend themselves more easily to false or self-serving representation than disorders with objective, documentable findings, case managers usually have a higher threshold for acceptance for back pain or chronic pain. While doubtless this helps to weed out nonmeritorious claims, it places a considerable and occasionally unattainable burden of proof on the claimant with a meritorious but subjective claim, such as regional complex pain syndrome.

Although workers' compensation carriers are reluctant to admit it, claims that are difficult to resolve or understand are usually rejected in the first instance. The appeals level is better suited to review and deal with them, but some claimants accept their initial rejection and never pursue the matter. Other claimants, particularly those who are aged, retired, or seriously disabled, may have little motivation to go through a long, drawn-out appeals process. Some may settle for other disability payments, through Social Security or Canada Pension (see Chapter 18) or not file a claim at all. This is thought to be the reason that the number of claims for asbestos-related disease is far less than would be predicted on the basis of the prevalence in working populations exposed to asbestos. Some workers' compensation carriers have special units for such difficult cases or cases that are likely to be disputed or may provide specialized technical support and consultation for the case managers in such cases.

Claims are normally reviewed first by a case manager in the role of an "adjudicator." This is an employee of the insurance carrier, which in Canada is the Workers' Compensation Board itself. The adjudicator is empowered to make a decision accepting or rejecting the claim on the basis of the evidence provided or to request further information. Most claims are easily adjudicated because they reflect obvious injuries and are not disputed by the employer. A small fraction, however, are ambiguous, incomplete, doubtful, unfamiliar to the adjudicator, or disputed by the employer. These are the problem cases that consume the time and attention of the WCB system as a whole.

When a claim is rejected or a disability rating is not to the satisfaction of an injured worker, an appeals mechanism is provided for review of the case. In the United States, this often takes the form of an administrative hearing, following a courtroom procedure. Often, however, the appeals hearings are rather informal and involve a minimum of procedural rules. The appeal may involve review of the documents only or an appearance before an administrative tribunal. Often, legal counsel is present, although advocates for the claimant do not have to be lawyers and some WCBs provide advocates on behalf of the claimants on a system much like that of public defenders in the courtroom. Decisions by this tribunal are usually binding but may be reviewed at a higher level on a discretionary basis, often by appearance before the board itself.

Two problems arise frequently in disputed cases. The first occurs when the workers' compensation carrier and a personal health insurance carrier both dispute a claim. This leaves the claimant without compensation and, after the workers' compensation appeals mechanism is exhausted, often leads to a lawsuit against the insurance company. The other is when temporary disability benefits expire but the workers' compensation carrier denies responsibility for permanent disability. The claimant must then apply for long-term disability (LTD) and is at risk that the claim will be denied. The transition from short-term disability to LTD is often a time when claims are re-evaluated and further opinions are sought.

DISABILITY EVALUATION

Disability evaluation, in general, is a measure of how permanent impairment affects the capacity to participate in activities of life and work. Within workers' compensation, the grounds for evaluating impairment in workers' compensation are narrow and tied closely to employability. Disability based on the impairment is driven primarily by projections of the future job market for the worker and is prepared by actuaries, as it would be in other insurance.

On the basis of the information obtained, the adjudicator must make a judgment on whether to accept the claim and, if accepted, at what rating of disability. A disability rating is a complex, weighted percentage figure that relates the degree of functional impairment (as determined medically, as discussed in Chapter 18) and employability given the worker's level of education and training and the local or regional market for such skills. A disability rating may be temporary or permanent. Benefit payments for temporary disability are a set fraction of the worker's earnings before the injury (such as 80 percent of pre-injury income), which takes into account that expenses directly related to work, such as transportation, are reduced during the period of disability. Permanent disability causes most of the problems because it is the basis for either long-term payment or a lump sum reflecting diminished employment capability for the rest of the claimant's life.

Chapter 18 discusses impairment evaluation and the relationship between impairment and disability. Disability evaluation takes into account three basic elements:

- The impairment model (A): Impairment assessment and how it relates to disability evaluation is discussed in Chapter 18. Impairment in a given case may be evaluated against guidelines (such as the *AMA Guides to the Evaluation of Permanent Impairment*), schedules (awarding a fixed amount or assuming total disability in a particular condition), or job requirements.
- The wage loss formula (B): This element calculates the actual loss of wages as a direct result of the injury.
- Loss of earnings capacity (C): This model projects future loss of earnings as a result of the impairment (A), based on actuarial models.

Thus, the formula for rating disability is the sum of B and C (which is a function of A). Because disability evaluations start from the impairment evaluation, the level of impairment is often a central issue that requires clarification by an IME.

INSURANCE OPERATIONS

Workers' compensation insurance carriers are insurance companies that write policies for employers for workers' compensation coverage. In the United States, they are usually private. The industry is highly concentrated with only a few companies writing the majority of policies nationwide in the United States (CAN, Fireman's Fund, Liberty Mutual, The Hartford, and Travelers). In twenty states, as in California, there are special state-administered insurance pools for companies that are not acceptable to private carriers, as an insurer of "last resort"; their premiums are expensive. In twenty-four states and the District of Columbia, there are only private insurance carriers. Self-insurance is allowed for large private firms in all but two states and is usually done by capitalizing a fund set up with a contractor to manage claims. In all Canadian provinces and in five American states (North Dakota, Ohio, Washington, West Virginia, and Wyoming) and two dependencies (Puerto Rico and the U.S. Virgin Islands), there are single-payer, publicly administered monopoly workers' compensation boards. The Federal Employees Compensation Act in the United States and the Government Workers' Compensation Act Labour Program in Canada are publicly funded through taxes. In British Columbia, uniquely, the Workers' Compensation Board is also the regulatory agency for occupational health.

Participation in workers' compensation is required by law for employers that qualify, except in Texas, where it is voluntary. Rates are assessed on the basis of the total payroll of the employer. The employer pays an annual assessment to the carrier for coverage, based on a standard rate to cover the frequency and amount of claims in the employer's industry, modified according to the number of occupational injury claims actually experienced by that employer in the years immediately preceding. The "experience rating" of an employer, as it is called, represents a means of providing an incentive to employers to improve their performance as well as protecting conscientious employers in the industry from the poor performance of their competitors.

Workers' compensation carriers have a variety of funds and reserve mechanisms to cover special situations. Reserves are often set aside for special categories of claims that are likely to result in expensive benefits. Asbestos-related disease is one such category.

"Second injury funds" are special funds or pools set aside under common or government regulatory management to cover claims for exacerbation by a subsequent injury after the first has left a worker with a disability. They reimburse the employer's workers' compensation carrier for the benefits for the differential in impairment between the initial and the later injuries and are not counted against the record of the employer in the experience rating. The reason they exist is to remove barriers to hiring disabled workers, one of which is that employers are often reluctant to hire workers with previous work-related injury on the grounds that they are more likely to injure themselves or are unsafe workers. Second injury funds relieve the employer and the carrier of financial risk for new impairment that arises because the second injury does not count against the employer's insurance rating.

"Unfunded liabilities" are projected future claims that may occur for which the carrier has not set aside funds. Some potential liabilities are unfunded because they may not occur and the carrier is assuming a risk. However, often unfunded liabilities were not appreciated or recognized, and the carrier is financially unprepared. Asbestos-related claims, for example, were a surprise to some carriers, who did not set aside enough in reserves to cover the anticipated costs.

Costs tend to be shifted between workers' compensation and unemployment insurance (UI), personal health insurance, long-term disability insurance (LTD) or Social Security, and welfare benefits. Workers who are injured off the job are not entitled to workers' compensation benefits but may apply for personal health insurance benefits and, if permanently disabled, for LTD. Many costs of occupational disease, for example, are never recognized or claimed, particularly when the worker is retired, and so are hidden in the costs of Medicare or Social Security Disability Insurance. Long-term care insurance and workers' compensation should be complementary, but too often the claimant falls between the cracks if both of them disallow the claim. There is a strong incentive to file a claim for workers' compensation even when the claim is tenuous at best because the benefits are longer term, no copayment or deductible is charged to the patient, and there may be no or fewer restrictions regarding subsequent employment. Workers whose claims under workers' compensation are denied but who feel that they cannot work often apply for UI and for LTD (if they are eligible) and subsequently, when eligibility expires, welfare or Social Security Disability Insurance if they have no other source of income.

There are several ways within the complexities of the workers' compensation system that employers can minimize escalating workers' compensation system assessments. The best way, of course, is to improve performance by reducing the frequency of work-related injuries and illnesses by controlling hazards and training employees. A bad way is to fail to report relatively minor injuries, a distortion of the system which keeps the workers' compensation system, the regulatory system, occupational health and safety regulatory agencies, and the employer in the dark about a potentially serious problem and a violation of the law. Underreporting of minor injuries (in workers' compensation and in the OSHA 300 log) is very common. The worst way, however, is to fire or threaten to fire employees that are injured or report injuries. This is a reprehensible practice and collusion with it violates the ethics of occupational medicine. Unfortunately it is a common tactic of unscrupulous employers.

APPORTIONMENT

In California in 2004, OEM and other physicians were required for the first time to apportion causation in workers' compensation reports. This was a truly revolutionary requirement. It reversed conventional thinking in workers' compensation, which was that apportionment may be applied to harm, impairment, or disability but never cause. However, it depends fundamentally on the judgment of clinicians, not on verifiable science.

Apportionment by cause is, in essence, an attempt to assess what percentage of a given level of impairment was caused by one causal factor compared to another. In principle, this would be very much like apportioning impairment, which workers' compensation carriers do routinely, except that the underlying cause of the disorder would be considered rather than how much impairment a second injury caused or a work-related injury on top of a pre-existing nonoccupational impairment. Apportionment of "harm" or "fault" is commonly used in tort law after a judgment to determine the share of damages that must be paid by each defendant. However, workers' compensation is a no-fault insurance plan, so apportionment of damages or by fault cannot be used.

The benefits of apportionment, if it could be done accurately and usefully, are obvious: adjudication would be simpler (especially if formulae could be worked out for relative proportions under certain assumptions), adjudication would be fairer to employers and some injured workers, financial resources would not be diverted away from injured workers and toward compensating for nonoccupational disease, incentives might be created for workers to take responsibility for their own health, the burden of disease would be more fairly shared among workers' compensation carriers and health insurers, and the relative contribution to disability benefits for permanent impairment could be divided up and allocated to different payers, such as pension plans and private long-term disability insurance.

Apportionment by cause is only useful across a narrow range of the total spectrum of causation. A particular cause may, conceptually, be apportioned as a sole cause, a sufficient cause, a substantial contributing factor, or a barely substantial but contributing factor, or not a significant factor. If an occupational cause is responsible for more than 50 percent of causation, then it would normally be treated as the sole cause. If causation is less than some nominal amount that represents a substantial contribution, say 10 percent, then it is not really significant in terms of its main effect, and the real question is whether it was the straw that broke the camel's back. In other words, whether "but for" that small contribution the injury or disease would have occurred. Apportionment by cause therefore only operates meaningfully over less than half of the spectrum of causation.

Apportionment should not be confused with attribution, as the term is used in epidemiology (see Chapter 2). Attribution is a statistical approach, which applies only to populations. The attributable risk is the risk, and attributable risk fraction the proportion, of cases of a particular injury or disease that can be attributed to a particular risk factor. However, these estimates do not apply to individuals. Unless the individual belongs to a well-defined subgroup (in which case the confidence intervals are usually wide), the population risk estimate in an epidemiological study only represents a best estimate of what the risk would be for members of the group, chosen at random. Workers' compensation acts require that adjudication be based on the individual's circumstances, not on generalities. Furthermore, estimates of attributable risk fraction (the percentage of a disease associated with a certain risk or putatively causal factor) are hardly ever available for many risk factors in a single, relevant study. Picking and choosing estimates from different studies and then comparing them is methodologically suspect.

These problems essentially preclude the use of epidemiologic findings to make fine distinctions and careful calculations of apportionment by cause. Epidemiological findings provide best estimates and rough guides and cannot go much beyond an imprecise ranking of causes. (This discussion may be considered heresy among epidemiologists.)

On the other hand, epidemiological findings inform apportionment by providing insight in a general way and providing guidance on the magnitude of risk in the past. Knowledge of past risk for groups does help the physician in thinking about comparative risks for an individual but in an indirect way through individualized risk estimates.

The individual approach to apportionment is to take into account all the factors relevant to the individual claimant and to compare them with respect to their known relative strength (as reflected in epidemiological studies) and how much influence they are likely to have had in the individual case. This approach can be done in two ways by (1) attempting to isolate the best applicable epidemiological risk estimate by looking at subgroups that most closely match the claimant's personal characteristics or (2) identifying personal risk factors and building a case for or against them being sufficiently substantial in magnitude to influence the outcome.

Building a risk profile from individual characteristics of the claimant is more difficult. The most important personal characteristic is usually age, especially for cancer and heart disease, and age-specific risk estimates are available for most common diseases. The age-specific risks associated with cigarette smoking are also available for many common diseases. Risk estimates associated with occupational exposures may be available from relevant epidemiological studies. One must then factor in family history, lifestyle, and other pertinent characteristics, for which risk estimates are not knowable. In practice, this means a judgment call in adjusting risk up or down in the individual case and in comparing relative contributions to the outcome.

The result is an uncertain mix of defensible quantitative risk estimates and subjective judgments with respect to risk patterns. Clinicians may be better able to adjust a risk estimate up or down compared to a known epidemiologically derived risk than they are in guessing the absolute risk with a "knowledge peg" (a term in cognitive psychology that refers to a prompt that starts speculation from a point of relative certainty). This does not mean guessing. It means applying the judgment of a clinician to a "post hoc" probability that takes into account prior knowledge and risk levels in the community but is difficult to calculate and communicate.

Although it is attractive to place greater emphasis on quantitative risk estimates, there is a good reason not to. That is because the application of conventional statistics to events in the past is not correct. (See Chapter 2 for the same argument as applied to cluster analysis.) Conventional, "frequentist" statistics are designed to describe events in the past and to predict the probability of events in the future (assuming no change in underlying factors). They are not designed to predict probabilities in the past. In other words, they do not accurately describe the probability that a particular outcome would have happened in the past, from the point of view of an observer before the event occurred. This is the domain of Bayesian statistics, a methodology developed for clinical studies and other situations in which one is looking backward to see how likely it was that certain things happened. Bayesian statistics are much more complicated than frequentist statistics and are almost never used in medicolegal or workers' compensation.

Because of all these drawbacks, a more qualitative or subjective individualized risk apportionment may paradoxically be a more reasonable approach to the problem than a misleadingly sophisticated analysis using frequentist (conventional) statistics. In practice, apportionment by cause is inexact and often difficult. These limitations are acceptable, however, if they provided at least a rough and defensible guide for apportionment, as crude as halves, quarters, and bits rather than unattainable accuracy to the second decimal.

OCCUPATIONAL DISEASE

In workers' compensation terminology, the term "disease" is applied to conditions that do not arise from a single event. Conditions such as noise-induced hearing loss, repetitive strain injury, chronic low back pain that did not start with a defined event, and other chronic disorders are classified as "diseases" rather than injuries because they are not associated with a single event, whether or not they involve the musculoskeletal system and whether or not they involve physical hazards and the release of energy (as discussed in Chapters 9 and 16). Occupational diseases present a particular challenge for workers' compensation.

Occupational disease cases are particularly difficult to manage in the workers' compensation system. They are greatly underreported and underrepresented in claims. As noted, there may be little motivation for retired workers, especially, to pursue a claim knowing that it will be disputed and that the benefits may not be great. There is no incentive on the part of carriers to go out and find cases. Occupational disease may be difficult or even impossible to prove, especially if the latency period is long, there is no exposure data, and the disease could arise from factors outside of work.

The workers' compensation system developed with the implicit assumption that all or most occupational injuries could be recognized. When a visible injury occurs at work, the system tends to function well. When diagnostic criteria, subjective complaints, and chronic illness come into the picture, the system has much more difficulty dealing with the claim. This differential response to injury and disease has shaped the system so much that it can fairly be described as a mechanism oriented to the injury incident and unresponsive to the health status of the worker.

Three mechanisms have emerged as a means of dealing with the problem: the concept of cumulative injury or trauma, schedules of designated work-related diseases, and rebuttable presumptions.

Some chronic diseases and health conditions that cannot be attributed to just one event or the responsibility of one employer are evaluated under the legal doctrine of "cumulative injury," which assumes that the condition arose as the result of countless tiny injuries on the job that collectively added up to a single impairment. The theory of cumulative injury is applied to both noise-induced hearing loss and repetitive strain injury and assumes that the ultimate outcome arose from numerous small, even infinitesimal injuries. The concept of cumulative injury approaches this problem by assuming that the injury is the cumulative result of numerous small, discrete injuries of roughly equal magnitude that occurred at every opportunity for exposure. The doctrine sidesteps the need to demonstrate a single incident of injury, which is deeply embedded in the initial claims evaluation process. It allows apportionment of responsibility by time among various employers if the worker has had a mobile employment history. The doctrine allows the board to sidestep the difficult issue of apportioning causation and instead to apportion responsibility for its share of the cumulative effect to employers on the basis of the duration of exposure that occurred in each workplace, on the theory that each exposure opportunity provided a setting for injury.

For example, impairment from noise-induced hearing loss can be apportioned based on the relative loudness (if data are available) and duration of assignment to various loud workplaces under different employers. This makes it possible to assess the relative proportion of benefits between carriers insuring different employers. This concept works best for noise-induced hearing loss, in which it approximates the real situation, and less well for repetitive strain injuries, in which the relative timing, ergonomic issues, and specific circumstances play a greater role.

Slowly developing disorders that do not fit the cumulative event doctrine pose greater problems for workers' compensation. The injury is not immediately apparent and often gets worse with continued exposure, in the case of respiratory disorders. An individual may change jobs numerous times before the disorder becomes clinically apparent. In the case of long-term, developed health effects, such as cancer, the worker may even have retired before the disorder is recognized. There are usually technical and logistical problems to demonstrating causation. For example, for cases of occupational cancer, latency periods may be variable in length, recent exposures are relatively less important, and exposure data on earlier exposures are almost never available. As well, many occupational diseases, such as lung cancer, have nonoccupational causes such as smoking, and are known to be occupational only because they are statistically elevated in frequency compared to the general population.

There are two related approaches to the problem of occupational disease that can be used for disorders that do not fit the doctrine of cumulative injury. One is the "schedule," or designated list, and the other is the rebuttable presumption. "Presumption" refers to the policy that certain types of claims should normally be accepted because the disease risk is presumed.

A schedule is a list of designated compensable work-related diseases and is a form of presumption. They normally include disorders that are well established to be occupational in origin. The diseases are usually relatively rare and closely associated with a certain occupation. Examples include mesothelioma and asbestos exposure, acute myelogenous leukemia and benzene, and nasal cancer and woodworkers. Such lists are in common use in some North American jurisdictions, such as Ontario and British Columbia, and in many other countries, such as Germany. The Black Lung Benefits Act is the best example in the United States: The test is simply to prove that the claimant has the disease and is a coal miner because only coal miners get it. The evidentiary burden to establish a schedule is to document that a particular illness is work related and should be added to the list. Thereafter, the burden on the claimant is to demonstrate that the disorder is, indeed, the diagnosis in question. Thus, schedules tend to grow very slowly. A criticism of scheduling of compensable disorders is that it is usually very difficult to add disorders to the list until the scientific evidence is so complete that many workers will have foregone compensation for years and may well have died before their eligibility is accepted. This is most often the case for newly unrecognized disorders and was well illustrated by the initial reluctance to recognize asbestosis for what it was.

"Rebuttable presumption" is, simply, the policy that claims should be normally but not always accepted when, all other things being equal, a claim received from a worker in a certain occupation is more likely than not to have arisen out of work, whether or not it is possible to prove the association in the individual case. This is demonstrated epidemiologically when the risk for the group is at least doubled compared to a reference population, which satisfies the legal criterion of weight of evidence, or "as or more likely than not." A doubling of risk is equivalent to even odds, which is a mathematical statement that the risk arising out of work is equal to the risk of all other factors and corresponds to the adjudication standard of the weight of evidence. An example is the widespread presumption for certain cancers in firefighters, which is based on rarity and elevated risk (kidney cancer) or assumptions made on risk that are burdensome to prove (lung cancer).

Presumptions are normally rebuttable, meaning that the adjudicating body may also examine evidence in the individual case that supports or calls into question the individual claimant's risk profile (such as the personal smoking history) and the relationship to work (such as duration of employment). From the standpoint of social policy, a policy of rebuttable presumptions accepts that some nonmeritorious cases will inevitably be compensated in the interest of the greater good of ensuring that all meritorious cases are compensated. Presumptions lift a substantial burden of documentation and advocacy from the claimant and expedite management of claims. They are often legislated and consciously made less burdensome and more accessible for certain groups as a matter of social policy, such as presumptions for public safety personnel who take an uncommon level of personal risk in their work.

REFORM

At a time when it is showing signs of renewal and reinvention, the workers' compensation system in the United States is, at the time of this writing (2009), under severe financial stress due to the current economic crisis. It remains to be seen whether reforms will continue or accelerate, or whether the system as a whole will become unsustainable. (The Canadian system may respond differently.)

The issues most prominent today in discussions regarding the workers' compensation system include the following:

- Financial solvency: The economic recession is bound to affect workers' compensation dramatically. Historically, injury rates drop during a recession because of reduced business activity. However, claim rates may rise because workers who are about to be laid off often submit workers' compensation claims, hoping for an income supplement for a partial disability that was previously tolerable. Carriers are likely to be pushed out of business through a combination of rising claims, reduced investment income, and chronic business losses. Until recently, workers' compensation was a profitable line of business. Since about 2000, however, workers compensation carriers have lost money, especially in California, and several carriers have withdrawn from states in which they did not have a competitive advantage. This has reduced competition, which in turn tended to push premiums higher, but because the carriers are regulated, the upward pressure has not been passed on in full to employers. One business problem is that administrative expenses for workers' compensation policies are high compared to other forms of insurance.

- Managed care: As the California experience demonstrates, workers' compensation has emerged after a late start as a highly managed healthcare system. Provider panels, utilization review, practice guidelines, and electronic medical records are incorporated into workers' compensation case management, and carriers tend to be much more directive than in the past. Unfortunately, this does not necessarily lead to proactive integration and coordination of care. Much of the management of workers' compensation is a logistical issue of getting various providers to a common understanding, tracking referrals and opinions, monitoring progress, and setting goals. There remains a disconnect that includes the treating physician and other parts of the system that reflects fragmentation in the general healthcare system.

- Increasing severity: Over twenty years there has been a trend toward increasing severity of disability among cases. This, of course, drives higher costs.

- Timely and sufficient benefits: In theory, the system was designed to provide payment much faster than would be the case if the worker had to sue the employer. For routine injuries, payment is reasonably prompt in most cases. However, any claim that is unusual, disputed, or requires further documentation is at risk for delay in processing and may require appeal. This often delays payment of benefits by months.

- Benefits: Benefits paid to injured workers tend to be low compared to other forms of insurance. They are calculated as a percentage of wages (typically two-thirds) and capped, so that high earners do not receive a proportionally greater benefit. Some states index benefits to current wages in the state. None take into account out-of-pocket expenses, indirect costs, or social costs of disability.

- Fee schedules: Until recently, medical fees were usually compensated at or below reasonable and customary charges, but in recent years the fee schedule has risen, and changes in the medical care system seem to have slowed the rise in payments for general care. As a result, there is now little difference in some fee schedules between payment from workers' compensation and from other sources; workers' compensation payment is also generally more reliable than collections from some other sources. Some jurisdictions still lag behind, however, and the history of inadequate compensation has influenced the attitudes of physicians, particularly those who are older, toward the system as a whole.

- Prevention of permanent disability: From a human perspective, permanent disability reduces the person's capacity to participate in society and, with it, earning potential. Improving the outcome of treatment and recovery after injury benefits the injured worker, reduces the level of residual disability, and reduces costs. Two-thirds of payments for disability benefits are for permanent disability, and it is a truism in workers' compensation that a relatively small number of high-cost claims, particularly back pain, drive the majority of the benefit total.

- Integration: Because occupational diseases are often difficult to recognize and because it is human nature to attempt to get the highest benefit to which one may feel one is entitled, there is considerable trading and cross-subsidy among workers' compensation, personal health insurance, Social Security, and LTD. As these all represent insurance schemes, as opposed to welfare, which is a transfer payment mechanism, the proposal has frequently been put forward that they should be unified into a single system. New Zealand did something along these lines in 1974 by creating a streamlined, unitary no-fault personal injury compensation system that treated work-related and non-work-related claims similarly (for example, automotive injuries, medical misadventures, unintentional injury, and occupational injuries are all treated the same). The system is widely considered successful in achieving equity for workers, controlling costs, and operating efficiently and simply, but it had a rocky beginning.

- Panels: The establishment of national or regional boards of experts to agree on causation and level of impairment by consensus might significantly improve the quality and consistency of adjudication. This is standard procedure in Germany.

- Institutes and centers: In Canada, government entities have been created that conduct research, investigate theories of causation, and document evidence for important adjudication decisions. The reports are publicly available and may be peer reviewed. Ontario has organized this function within the broader Workplace Safety and Insurance Board (WSIB). Québec has organized centers of excellence within the adjudicating body (*la Commission de la santé et securité du travail,* CSST), and supports a research institute (*Institut de recherché Robert Sauvé en santé et en securité du travail,* IRSST).

- Federalization: Federalization of the workers' compensation system in the United States is not being discussed currently, but the option is likely to return to the national agenda as a consequence of the current economic crisis, especially if there is a need for a bailout. It is difficult to imagine the political constellation that would force it, since states are likely to oppose such a move, but there has not been an economic challenge to the system of this magnitude since 1939. The experience of 1972 suggests that the widespread perception of system failure was not enough to trigger federalization, at least in that political era. On the other hand, the return of healthcare insurance to the national agenda, combined with conditions imposed by the federal government for financial assistance, might result in a national system (perhaps resembling that for federal workers), absorption into a broader healthcare insurance system (as in the United Kingdom), or some alternative as yet unknown.

The tort system continues to have its defenders, who point out that for all the perceived abuse, the tort system provides a mechanism to determine liability and therefore works toward justice and a fairer level of compensation to individual cases. The workers' compensation system, on the other hand, was created in a simpler era in which the tort process was not working to the advantage of the claimant but has become highly bureaucratic and unresponsive. By this thinking, the tort system should be kept intact as the ultimate resort for the claimant, because in the absence of the threat of tort action, employers are far less likely to be cooperative. Employers in this era are thought to fear court action more than workers do because of the unpredictability in awards inherent in the tort action. This is very much a minority view.

In the future, fundamental reform might return to the geographical origins of workers' compensation and consider as a model the current German system (the *Berufgenoßschaften*), in which workers' compensation insurance is organized regionally as a nonprofit public utility controlled by governing boards to which are appointed representatives of labor, industry, and the public. (This is already the case in Canada.) The German insurance bodies occupy a much more central role in the healthcare system and exert stronger incentives toward prevention.

In 1998, the American College of Occupational and Environmental Medicine published "The Eight Best Ideas for Workers' Compensation Reform." They are worth revisiting:

1. View workplace injuries and illnesses as evidence of prevention failure and use them to target safety and enforcement programs.

2. Require active linkages between injury and illness care services, prevention strategies, and disability reduction programs.

3. Make sure that job-related health decisions are made by health-care professionals with appropriate training and expertise.

4. Expect active participation by both employers and injured workers.

5. Begin management of job and life disruption as soon as disability begins.

6. Use evaluation and ratings systems based on objective, standardized methods as the basis for awards for both physical impairment and vocational disability.

7. Encourage workers' compensation managed care organizations to innovate; when provider choice is limited, require proof of quality.

8. Demand better and more standardized data and use them to guide medical care, to direct reforms, and to inform purchasers.

RESOURCES

Guidotti TL, Rose SG. *Science on the Witness Stand: Evaluating Scientific Evidence in Law, Adjudication, and Policy.* Beverley Farms, MA: OEM Press; 2001.

Sall RE. *Strategies in Workers' Compensation.* Lanham, MD: Hamilton Books; 2004.

Strunin L, Boden LI. The workers' compensation system: worker friend or foe? *Am J Ind Med.* 2004;45:338–345.

NOTEWORTHY READINGS

American College of Occupational and Environmental Medicine. ACOEM's eight best ideas for workers' compensation reforms. *J Occup Environ Med.* 1998;40(3):207–208.

Dembe AE, Fox SE, Himmelstein J. *Improving Workers' Compensation Medical Care: A National Challenge.* Beverley Farms, MA: OEM Press; 2003.

Guidotti TL. Considering apportionment by cause: its methods and limitations. *J Workers Comp.* 1998;7(4):55–71.

Guidotti TL. The Big Bang? An eventful year in workers' compensation. *Annu Rev Pub Health.* 2005;27:153–166.

Guidotti TL, Cowell JWF, eds. Worker's compensation. *Occup Med: State Art Rev.* 1998;13(2):241–459. [*Occupational Medicine: State of the Art Reviews* was a monograph series. This issue was devoted to workers' compensation and has many articles of continuing interest.]

Neumark D. The workers' compensation crisis in California: A primer. California Economic Policy (Public Policy Institute of California), San Francisco, January 2005. Available at www.ppic.org/content/pubs/EP_105DNEP.pdf.

Nuckols TK, Wunn BO, Lim Y-W, Shaw R, Mattke S, et al. *Evaluating Medical Treatment Guideline Sets for Injured Workers in California.* Santa Monica, CA: Institute for Civil Justice, Rand Corporation; 2004.

Pace NM, Reville RT, Galway L, Geller AB, Hayden O, Hill LA, et al. *Improving Dispute Resolution for California's Injured Workers.* Santa Monica, CA: Institute for Civil Justice, Rand Corporation; 2003.

Peele PB, Tollerud DJ. Managed care in workers' compensation plans. *Annu Rev Pub Health.* 2001:22:1–13.

Williams CT, Rena VP, Burton JF Jr. 2004. *Workers' Compensation: Benefits, Coverage, and Costs, 2002.* Washington, DC: National Academy of Social Insurance; August 2004.

22 EMERGENCY MANAGEMENT

The occupational and environmental medicine (OEM) physician is increasingly valuable to employers for his or her potential to contribute to the survival of the enterprise, not just its efficient operation. After several years of highly visible disasters, some employers, especially in critical industry sectors, have come to a new realization of the criticality of OEM functions to business continuity. Awareness is spreading in the corporate sector, stirred by recognition of the profound threat to continuity of operations and the survival of key personnel presented by natural disasters, major industrial incidents, and intentional assaults.

OEM physicians are now called upon to act in response to public and management concern over threats from intentional assaults (including terrorism), unintentional incidents that may result in mass casualties, and natural disasters. The occupational health system has similar, and in some cases more robust, capabilities than the general public health system. The scope of responsibility of OEM physicians and the demand for expertise and instant response has grew from dealing with workplace-specific hazards and injuries to being prepared to confront mass-casualty events and other large-scale threats to the workplace. Occupational physicians now have an opportunity to contribute as expert advisors on emergency management, including naturally occurring disasters, emerging and reemerging infectious diseases, and security issues involving chemical, biological, and radiological threats.

Employers in critical industries and government agencies have become deeply concerned with continuity of operations and the security of their personnel. The imperatives of corporate security and homeland defense since 2001 have, in turn, invigorated and expanded the mission of OEM for disaster planning and emergency management.

At many enterprises, employers and their employees rely on occupational health providers for health information and care with a focus on the threats, hazards, and injuries unique to workplace organizations. To be effective, the OEM physician must work as a partner in a coordinated effort by an emergency management team that includes managers, technical personnel, and emergency responders.

HISTORY

The role of the occupational physician in emergency management evolved from the historic involvement of occupational physicians in disaster planning, workforce protection, and prevention of disease and injury.

Roots

Since the Industrial Revolution, practitioners of occupational medicine have had to treat victims of mass casualties and industrial misadventures. The "industrial surgeon" was sometimes called upon to manage the consequences of injuries on a mass scale, such as railroad accidents. This expanded the scope of occupational medicine practice and led to a role for the physician in "accident prevention," which at the time did not distinguish between prevention of individual injuries and mass casualties. Later, particularly as corporate medical departments were established and expanded in the early twentieth century, the occupational physician became a recognized resource for disaster planning and emergency response.

During the Second World War, the occupational physician played a valuable and respected role in ensuring safe and secure operation of critical industries. Interest in disaster planning and emergency response declined after the war except in hazardous industries, especially after the Bhopal catastrophe in 1984, when thousands of local residents in India died after release of a toxic gas from a local chemical plant owned by an American company. The response to the Bhopal disaster in the United States was the Emergency Planning and Community Right to Know Act (1986), which focused on the community's right to know of local hazards and not on prevention, security, and mitigation. For the most part, the role of OEM physicians in emergency management was marginalized. Even so the American College of Occupational and Environmental Medicine (ACOEM) continued to provide opportunities for its members to learn practical skills in disaster planning and emergency management. Anticipating the future threat, in 2000 ACOEM was among the first medical specialty organizations to train its members in practical issues in bioterrorism and homeland security.

Events at the Turn of the Century

The OEM physician's role in disaster planning and emergency management returned to center stage after the tragic events of "9/11" (September 11, in shorthand American usage, of 2001) and especially the anthrax assaults in its aftermath. The terrorist assault using hijacked airplanes in an attempt to destroy the Pentagon was a strike at military power, but the assault on the twin towers of the World Trade Center in New York was directed at the financial system of the United States and targeted employees working in the financial district, as did the earlier bombing there in 1993. Following the catastrophe, a huge relocation effort moved the employees and executives of financial institutions to temporary locations in New Jersey, where business continuity was quickly restored. OEM physicians at these financial institutions played a key role in managing health problems that arose, especially among older executives who were not well. (This story has not been told but should be in due time.)

During the immediate response to the emergency, many workers did not use personal protective equipment and ignored safe work practices in their desperation to rescue victims. The Occupational Health and Safety Administration (OSHA), the National Institute for Occupational Safety and Health (NIOSH), and New York state officials were not supported in efforts to encourage the use of safe work practices and personal protection among responders, although OSHA brought equipment to the scene. The immediate result may have been a much larger number of injuries than would otherwise have occurred (5,222 incidents), including one fatality and many eye disorders, which probably impeded the rescue and recovery effort significantly. Several years later, a high rate of chronic respiratory symptoms has been documented among responders. OEM physicians at area academic institutions have played a critical role in documenting these health effects.

In the aftermath of 9/11, anthrax assaults—almost certainly perpetrated by a biological warfare expert with unknown motives—specifically targeted workers in the communications industry, both print journalism (in the first attack) and television (on the ABC studios in New York), as well as politicians and employees at the U.S. Capitol. There was an obvious connection between the workplace and the anthrax threat in issues involving exposure of postal employees, two of whom died. OEM physicians in Washington, D.C., handled much of the care of workers who had been or could have been exposed. Immediately following the tragedy of 9/11, an ACOEM task force produced a guide to the management of mental health issues among survivors of mass assaults, disseminated it to all members and posted it on the College Web site—all within four days. This achievement was unique and widely admired among medical specialty organizations.

The SARS outbreak of 2003 stimulated an organized response among several OEM physicians who formed a network to share information and recommendations for the protection of employees under their responsibility. This network, guided by information received by companies operating in the affected region, especially an airline, helped corporate medical directors to decide on policies for travel, whether to suspend local operations, and measures for worker protection. The safety of health care workers was also a major issue during the epidemic, especially in Toronto. Documentation of the outbreaks in Toronto, Hong Kong, and Singapore has relied heavily on research by academic OEM physicians in those places.

In 2003, ACOEM developed the Occupational Health Advisory Committee (OH-AC) as a resource for coordinating responses, accessing management resources, and sharing information in times of crisis. The OH-AC was a part of a larger health care and public health sector coordinating council for the purpose of information sharing, analysis, and coordination (ISAC), organized at the request of the U.S. Department of Homeland Security. Subsequently, ACOEM developed and supported the Occupational Health and Disaster Expert Network (OHDEN) as a support tool for occupational health professionals faced with the challenge of emergency management. Its mission was to provide occupational health professionals with what they need when they need it in time of crisis. ACOEM and OHDEN briefly played a role in the aftermath of Hurricane Katrina in 2005, as described in the next subsection, facilitating early return to work. Unfortunately, the effort could not be sustained due to lack of funding.

The potential role of the OEM physician was also highlighted by several highly visible plant incidents during the decade (such as the Texas BP refinery explosion in 2004) and the civilian smallpox vaccination preparedness campaign in 2003, which predated the modern vaccine and was unsuccessful in meeting its objectives.

Lessons from Hurricanes Katrina and Rita

Hurricanes Katrina and Rita, both in 2005, and their aftermath had a profound effect on perceptions of OEM and emergency preparedness.

Three distinct and important lessons were learned as a result of these natural disasters:

- Natural disasters are no less a threat to national security than intentional assaults
- In an emergency, employers may be on their own for extended periods of time
- Occupational health professionals can help mitigate an emergency

The first lesson that Katrina and Rita taught is that natural disasters and public health crises are as much threats to national security as intentional assaults. The effects of Katrina exceeded that of 9/11 in causing widespread destruction and dislocating American life. An entire region that played a vital role in the American economy, and still played a unique role in the country's culture, ground to a halt after its devastation by a storm that was not only predictable but had been predicted for years. A hurricane of that magnitude and in that location had, in fact, been the scenario for a training exercise for agencies in the region just the year before.

During Katrina and Rita, about 19 percent of the nation's oil refining capacity and 25 percent of its oil producing capacity became unavailable. The country temporarily lost 13 percent of its natural gas capacity. Together, the storms destroyed 113 offshore oil and gas platforms. The Port of New Orleans, the major cargo transportation hub of the southeast United States, was closed to operations. Consequences of such magnitude are beyond the reach of conventional terrorist acts (excepting possibly a nuclear threat) and equally or more disruptive to our society, economy, and ability to respond to subsequent threats.

The failure of the federal response in the days following Katrina compounded any shortcomings of the state and local governments. It forced all Americans, including employers, to realize that in a serious event, they are likely to be on their own for much longer than they might have supposed.

Obviously, in such a situation major employers would be well advised to protect themselves from the most likely disasters with redundant or private protective measures but could not reasonably be expected to sustain a catastrophic loss of a magnitude to destabilize an entire region. The rationale for business continuity is not only to keep the enterprise viable (and workers employed) but to carry out critical economic functions and to supply essential services. An example of this was the rapid response of Wal-Mart in supplying food and essential goods within the region struck by Katrina within a few days of the hurricane, far exceeding the capacity of federal and local emergency agencies.

The third lesson from Katrina and Rita is that occupational health and safety professionals can and did play a constructive role in emergency management, as did public health professionals generally. Rescuers took personal risks to save the stranded citizens of New Orleans. Less dramatically, public health agencies quickly identified and documented the risks of water contamination, warned of risks from carbon monoxide from portable generators, identified dermatitis and wound infections as major health risks, and identified outbreaks of norovirus-induced gastroenteritis. The role of public health professionals was widely, if insufficiently, recognized as essential and constructive. However, occupational health professionals, who play a public health role for the employed population, also played a constructive role, although it was largely invisible at the time and played-out mostly within the private sector or dispersed in communities.

Occupational health clinics and OEM physicians and nurses treated the injured, from wherever they came. Occupational health professionals returned critical personnel to work as soon as it was possible, to hasten economic recovery and rebuilding. Occupational Safety and Health Administration professionals warned against hazards in the floodwaters and the destroyed, abandoned houses, but were stymied because supplies for personal protection were nowhere to be found. The many stories of what occupational health professionals achieved in the aftermath of Katrina need to be collected and documented.

The Occupational Health and Disaster Expert Network (OHDEN) was a Web-based support system for occupational health professionals in emergency management developed in 2003 and supported by ACOEM. At the time of Katrina, OHDEN was still a prototype, with about two dozen participants. During the worst week, immediately following the hurricane, OHDEN briefly became operational, providing occupational health professionals in the region, their managers elsewhere in the country, and experienced consultants and advisors with a place to go for useful information, best practices, frequent updates, and shared information. Much of this information was actually used in the field, for example recommendations were downloaded, evaluated, and incorporated into one oil company's emergency corporate policy on worker protection for their refinery employees. Two weeks later, drawing on the OHDEN experience and the questions that arose, the same team developed a one-hour seminar by teleconference sponsored by ACOEM. On September 13, 2006, 200 occupational health professionals heard recommendations and had their questions answered on how best to return workers in the region to their jobs safely and how to monitor returning workers for possible physical and mental disorders. The ISAC/OH-AC and OHDEN experience during Katrina can be interpreted as "proof of concept," demonstrating that occupational health professionals can play a constructive role in planning, consequence management, and recovery.

A third phase in the recent evolution of emergency management occurred with the recognition of "distributed emergencies" as a different class of event. Epidemics initiated by intentional release of commicable biological agents (thought most likely to be smallpox, should it occur) had stimulated contingency planning for protecting civilian populations against emergencies that play out over time, as in the case of epidemics, rather than as catastrophic events. However, the initial response tended to be focused on setting up special-purpose monitoring and rapid response systems, rather than a broader systems approach and reinforcement of the existing but resource-starved public health system. SARS, as noted, gave immediacy to these concerns and demonstrated that in the event, the first line of defense is the public health system and employers, most obviously in the healthcare system. By 2007, the risk of an pandemic of avian influenza was the most prominent issue for planners and involved many OEM physicians outside of healthcare institutions, particularly in establishing policies and contingency planning for their employers. As it happened, the pandemic that came, in 2009, was of Influenza A H1N1, however many of the same precautions and plans applied. The H1N1 event, which is still playing out at the time of this writing, demonstrated the value of sound occupational health practice, in this case respiratory protection, and also revealed new problems, such as unexpected resistance to vaccination based on irrational beliefs and distrust of authority, and the need to deal with circulating rumors, for example the false idea that N95 respirators were dangerous for pregnant women.

These emergencies demonstrated that the capacity of occupational health professionals to act decisively and effectively to mitigate the consequences of a disaster is not just theoretical. It is real and proven.

ROLE OF OCCUPATIONAL HEALTH SERVICES

Employers face a quandary in preparing for emergencies. On a small scale, they would want to be able to manage an emergency within the organization, in order to confine the damage and keep it from being too disruptive to the continuity of business. "Business continuity" is a major concern not only for the employer's benefit but because employers in critical industries many need to furnish essential goods and services for the community without interruption. However, there is a practical limit to what they can prepare for. As companies consider emergencies of increasing magnitude, employers must rely on external assistance, such as fire departments and local health care providers. Beyond a certain point, when an emergency becomes so great that it disrupts the community on which the employer would depend for support, planning for emergency response may cease to be viable. Sort of that catastrophic point, however, there is much that an employer can do to mitigate the effects of an emergency, through preparation, planning, and properly strengthening the occupational health service.

An occupational health service cannot, alone, deal with a disaster. Any definition of disaster, and there are many, emphasizes that it is a sudden event with severe adverse consequences that outstrips the capacity of local resources and requires external assistance. However, a strong and well-trained occupational health service can significantly enhance the chances of successful management and survival of a disaster and protect business continuity by managing health issues and serving as liaison with public health agencies. Larger, on-site services may even have the capacity to assist in the community response.

Disasters have a recognized "cycle" with distinct phases:

- Pre-event (during which planning and preparation may be occurring)
- The "prodromal phase" (in which there may be a warning)
- Impact (in which the most important factor is resilience)
- Rescue (when emergency management is most critical)
- Recovery (which involves reconstruction)

Business continuity, especially in critical industries, may be important to resupply and sustain the community during rescue efforts and is essential to recovery, either because of critical goods (such as food) and services (such as transportation) or by providing the basis for financial recovery in the affected region through employment and restoring the circulation of money.

Many concepts familiar to physicians from emergency medicine are useful in emergency management, such as triage. However, "emergency management" is broader than emergency medical care and fundamentally involves planning, coordination, communication, and integration at the level of the organization, not the provision of medical services. The OEM physician may or may not render emergency medical assistance in the response phase but should play a central role in the preparedness, recovery, and mitigation phases of emergency management in any organization in which they are placed.

Occupational Health Services

Occupational health services represent a workplace health system with similar, and in some cases, more robust capabilities than the general public health system. In the wake of a series of terrorist actions and natural disasters since the fall of 2001, the demands on and expectations of occupational physicians to play a central role in disaster preparedness and response have grown dramatically. Their scope of responsibility and the requirements for their expertise and instant response grew from dealing with workplace-specific hazards and injuries to being prepared to confront mass-casualty weapons and other large-scale threats to the workplace.

To perform these duties effectively requires committed time for preparedness activities and a unit that is structured and whose providers are trained to play such a role in time of crisis. However, it is costly and inefficient for even large corporations to dedicate a full staff and support structure for the management of an event that may or may not materialize. This is why adaptation of the existing occupational health service makes sense for many employers, especially those in critical or hazardous industries. Perhaps most attractive to cost-conscious managers, investment in expanding the emergency management capacity within an occupational health service is not "lost" if an event never occurs. The same systems support and enhance the traditional occupational health services that industry and government employees require and may lead to cost savings, increased productivity, and reduced liability in their own right.

Employers already have in place a structure on which to build to protect their operations and personnel in the form of their occupational health services. Adaptation of the existing occupational health service makes sense for many employers, especially those in critical or hazardous industries. Expanding the mission of the occupational health service builds new efficiencies into the emergency response system. The same resources used for tracking employees' health can be used for surveillance to detect potential disease outbreaks due to bioterrorism. The technology of hazard identification and measurement can be applied to detect chemical or radiation threats. The medical staff on duty primarily to monitor health and to provide timely clinical care to workers can provide surge capacity to the community in time of crisis. Clinical health services can be applied to keep key personnel on the job and safe, especially when they are moved to new locations or are operating under conditions of stress and extreme risk.

The usefulness of a trained, well-informed, prequalified medical resource for dealing with incidents on site is obvious. These may include, but are certainly not limited to, sending infectious material through the mail to company personnel (anthrax and the much more common anthrax threat, or anonymous "white powder"), the threat of company equipment (such as chemical storage facilities) used as instruments of assault, and managing the psychological consequences of an assault. The OEM physician, who is trained in hazard assessment, may also assume the responsibility of determining when a site is safe to reenter or a facility to be reopened.

An enterprise may be in a better position to control its liability and potential loss if it develops a flexible, effective emergency management capability within its occupational health services. The employer would also be able to show due diligence in anticipating and preparing for plausible threats. This could reduce its exposure for punitive awards or claims based on negligence or omission, if despite its best efforts something does occur. A company that is seen to be prepared is less likely to be accused after the fact of ignoring a foreseeable threat.

Less obvious, but equally valuable, is the role that occupational health services may play in managing the consequences of widespread disruption of business operations due to major threats and of protecting the business, the product, and the brand against catastrophe in cases in which a company's products, facilities, or operations are used to deliver a threat or as targets for terrorist activity. In time of crisis, the occupational health service may help get community back on its feet by helping to keep an employer open or critical infrastructure functioning. Within the occupational health service, the OEM physician may be called upon to manage the corporate response to serious health-related issues, such as travel to areas in emerging infections are a risk, rapid investigation of suspicious outbreaks of disease or following exposure to potential hazards, and to determine when reentry and re-occupancy is possible in contaminated facilities, such as occurred after the decontamination of post office facilities contaminated with anthrax.

Role of the OEM Physician

The OEM physician has a critical role to play in disaster preparedness and emergency management. The role includes, but is not limited to, protecting the workforce, preserving business continuity, preventing plant- or facility-specific incidents, planning for the mobilization of resources in the event of a community-wide catastrophe, vulnerability assessment, risk communication, and collaborating with community resources and authorities, such as public health departments and regulatory agencies.

The OEM physician is well prepared to work with management and technical personnel at the plant, enterprise, or corporate level in preparing for plausible incidents, planning for an effective response, identifying resources that will be required, and advising on their deployment.

The role of the OEM physician in emergency management is distinct from those of emergency medicine and emergency management personnel. The typical occupational physician is not a specialist in emergency medicine, an expert in emergency management and incident command, or a safety engineer, notwithstanding that many individual occupational physicians do have special expertise in these areas.

The role of the OEM physician in disaster preparedness is also distinct from those of safety engineering and risk managers. The occupational physician is generally well-prepared to work with other professionals, which may include occupational health nurses, engineers, industrial hygienists, emergency medicine specialists, or emergency management professionals, on a team focused on the response to an incident. The skills brought to the table by OEM physicians are complementary and reflect the unique value of both public health and clinical training.

The OEM physician is well equipped to manage many aspects of disaster planning and emergency management because relevant knowledge and skills are already core competencies in occupational and environmental medicine, including:

- Knowledge of specific threats, including a broad range of chemical, biological, and physical hazards
- Knowledge of personal protection and other applied approaches to health protection and the skills to evaluate the adequacy of protection at the individual level
- A systematic approach to monitoring and protecting the health of populations, that is, people in groups
- A systematic approach to monitoring and protecting the health of workers and other persons at risk, that is, people as individuals
- Skills in managing behavioral factors associated with the workplace and stressful events
- Detailed knowledge of individual plants, working populations, communities, and resources within their areas of responsibility
- Managerial skills and the skills to effect change through policies and management of information
- Clinical skills and an understanding of appropriate utilization
- Working knowledge of regulations, regulatory compliance, and the structure of government agencies responsible for health protection at most relevant levels
- Experience in evaluating individuals for fitness to work, which may be applied in emergency situations
- Experience in evaluating workplaces for safety and health protection, which may be applied in emergency situations

- Expertise in risk management, including risk communication in an emergency
- Occupational health management for first responders

First Responders

Details on the management of occupational health for first responders are beyond the scope of this book, but this subsection will outline some general principles. The term "first responder" has been extended (by the homeland security community) to include those who are first to receive the victims in the emergency room. First responders in a workplace situation are usually corporate security personnel who arrive on the scene before public safety personnel have time to get there. Many employers, particularly in the mining and oil and gas industries, have their own firefighters, rescue teams, and hazmat teams.

The overriding priority of first responders is to protect the victims and to secure the location. They rescue or otherwise protect others who are not able to save themselves. If the personal risk is acceptable, they have as a secondary objective that of protecting property from destruction or damage. To achieve these priorities, first responders allow themselves to be exposed to hazards that are unusual for anyone else in the community and that would not be tolerated in other occupations.

The occupations normally considered among first responders include the following:

- Police
- Fire fighters (often cross-trained as EMS and hazmat personnel)
- Emergency medical service (EMS) personnel
- Rescue personnel
- Volunteers (who should be appropriately supervised)

The occupational risks of first responders include the same hazards that threaten the victims. Because they often arrive before the site has been secured, decontaminated, or thoroughly searched, first responders themselves face threatening situations on arrival. For example, the first arrivals at the site of a terrorist bombing must face the real possibility of a second explosive device intended for them. Even after the site is secured, first responders are confronted with events and circumstances outside the usual experience of human beings in their daily lives.

The occupational hazards experienced by first responders depend on their role at the scene. Physical hazards predominate, since first responders are often working in unsafe, unknown conditions. Police are more likely to experience intentional injury through violence, whether directed at them or as a consequence of controlling and restraining others. Firefighters are particularly subject to thermal stress and ergonomic stress. Hazmat workers may be adequately protected from chemical hazards by their protective suits and gear but experience thermal stress working with that same gear in hot weather conditions or near fires. Because of the many ways and frequency with which heat stress occurs as a problem in emergency situations, the provision of clean water and breaks for hydration is an important aspect of sustaining the overall response.

There are many physical dangers at scenes of explosions, earthquakes, or natural surface disasters. These include unstable structures, live wires, jagged surfaces and sharp edges, and fire hazard from ruptured gas lines. Injuries can be minimized by intensive training, job experience, strict pre-placement screening, and physical fitness, but personal protection and safe work procedures are also required. There is an understandable tendency to ignore personal safety in the rush to save another, but all too often the result is an avoidable casualty. An injured first responder on the scene not only becomes unavailable to do his or her job but imposes a burden on a rescue and first response system that needs to reserve its full effort for the victims.

Psychological adjustment factors are important in all public safety occupations. The nature of the work, involving extraordinary risk and experiences of danger beyond that is normal life, place first responders at risk for post-traumatic stress disorder, especially if they are involved in incidents in which victims cannot be saved or a team member dies.

Within the field there is an on-going debate over the effectiveness of "postincident debriefing," a procedure in which responders talk in groups about what happened and their feelings about the events. This intervention used to be promoted extensively in public safety departments, but many responders disliked it. It is now much less often used. Recent research suggests that "reliving" traumatic events is highly stressful and that this intervention does not help. A strong support network and an invitation for those who want to talk about the past to do so in a safe environment may be superior.

Although each of the occupations that constitute first responders has its own set of hazards, risks, and traditions, first responders share several features in common including:

- An awareness of personal danger, often accompanied by coping mechanisms that may include denial;
- Long periods of relative quiet or routine interrupted abruptly by periods of intense activity often accompanied by psychological stress;
- Rigid codes of behavior and high expectations for performance, often accompanied by complicated job responsibilities and guidelines and high penalties for failure;
- A strong ethic of teamwork and comradery, always with a strong sense of mutual reliance and social penalties for letting down one's co-workers; and
- A rigid hierarchy or "chain of command," which is necessary in order to reduce uncertainty and to make sure that procedures are followed correctly.

These characteristics shape the culture of first responders and may make it difficult for them to "open up" psychologically. They also create a strong social support system that strengthens the responder community and makes it psychologically resilient.

Services and Functions in Emergency Management

The most essential function of the OEM physician and other health professionals is planning. Planning for foreseeable industrial disasters can inform and refine the response to unforeseen threats, given that sophisticated disaster planning is a matter of identifying resources and contingencies for all threats, not deriving detailed plans for single-threat incidents. Planning must be done across the organization, with participation from all relevant management groups (including human resources, operations, maintenance, security, inventory, finance, legal affairs, and, of course, occupational health and safety). Planning must be coordinated with local public health agencies, hospitals, insurance carriers, and health care providers and may require involvement of suppliers, transportation carriers, and local utilities.

Planning for contingencies at a particular site should take into account the layout of the site, natural and constructed barriers, threats and hazards on the site, and routes for evacuation, means to secure the premises while preserving access for ambulances and first responders for operational response (for example, for staging rescue operations, triage, stabilizing casualties, decontamination, and "incident command" activities). Even locations without special hazards may benefit from such contingency planning in the event of an external threat. For example, the first anthrax assault was in the office of a newspaper, not normally a high-risk location. Decontamination may have to be continued at the hospital or a second location away from the industrial incident.

Traditionally, the corporate medical director usually assumed responsibility within the organization for planning the medical response to emergencies, identifying facilities and resources for dealing with serious injuries and mass casualties, and providing health protection for key personnel if required. Although outsourcing has reduced the direct involvement of occupational physicians in planning emergency management in many organizations, particularly in the service sector, this important function has not been replaced by external consultants because it requires a practitioner with intimate knowledge of the operations, hazards, workforce, and policies of the organization.

The OEM physician can also add value to the management of catastrophic consequences in other ways. These include:

- Representing the employer to public safety and health agencies during the event (and cultivating relationships with them beforehand)
- Survival of key personnel in a catastrophic event
- Continuity of business following a catastrophic event
- Obtaining resources for assistance in a health-related emergency
- Surveillance of the workforce and the early detection of an outbreak
- Integration of emergency response with public health agencies
- Surge capacity in the event of a local event requiring mobilization of all available medical resources
- Vaccination programs and other protective measures
- Establishing on-site consequence management and mitigation programs
- Developing decontamination plans
- Creation effective personal protective equipment (PPE)
- Clearance for reentry to facilities, such as contaminated sites
- Liaison with "local emergency planning committees," which are councils for emergency planning for chemical disasters, pre-hospital care providers, and local hospitals
- Continuing education and training on-site and in the community of indigenous risks inherent to the operation
- Access to MSDSs (material safety data sheets; see Chapter 14) for hazardous chemicals and other hazard information
- Advising public health agencies on particular hazards, their risk, and appropriate treatment (for example, hydrofluoric acid, which

is used in industrial settings but is not generally familiar to public health officials)

- Lead any after-action discussion to effect process and system improvement

- Triage, dealing with the "worried well," persons with health concerns, and ruling out health problems so that attention can be focused on urgent issues

BUILDING CAPACITY

The key to building capacity to manage emergencies within the occupational health service is to build an effective and efficient team. Teamwork comes from training and planning but also from regular personal contact and cooperation. A team that functions well in the complex duties of an occupational health services and that already knows the operations, workforce, and facilities is more likely to function well in an emergency than an outside provider—who may not be around in a crisis.

Training is the way in which effective teams are built. In emergency management, training places a heavy emphasis on simulations and on "table-top exercises," which are more or less realistic scenarios that are worked through in real time, with participants playing various roles as responders. The usefulness of these exercises depends in large part on how realistic the scenario is and how the situation is made to change over time as it unfolds, in order to simulate unpredictable events. Training is critical to readiness and effective response, but it is not completely innocuous. Recent research suggests that people who role-play during simulations may experience some of the same psychological stress reactions as those who experience an actual event.

Acquiring the necessary expertise is obviously required. The occupational health staff may require special training to take on the additional functions, but this is not much of a stretch from current duties. County emergency managers are eager to share training opportunities through grants and other programs within the public domain. The expense for preparedness may be justified by potential reductions in insurance premiums.

Establishing networks and agreements for mutual assistance may be critical. Here the occupational health staff can coordinate arrangements with local hospitals, specialist practitioners, public health agencies, and first responders in advance and maintain personal relationships required for smooth operation in the event of a crisis. The occupational health service may be able to provide surge capacity to the community in times of extreme need.

Certain routine functions can be anticipated and planned for. For example, if anthrax or some other threat is suspected in the mailroom, procedures (in the case of anthrax, quite simple) can be put in place in advance to protect employees, limit disruption, and rapidly evaluate evolving situations. This last function is particularly important to deter inevitable hoaxes and to prevent disruptions to business from ill-defined or unknown hazards. For example, the common scenario of an unknown "white powder" appearing on a loading dock or in an office can shut down operations for a day or more until a toxic substance is ruled out. Having the capacity on hand to show that it is harmless saves time and anxiety.

Likewise, dealing with panic among employees from rumors or incidental illness occurring at the worksite requires skill in rapid assessment and in risk communication (see Chapter 7) but can save an enterprise from devastating loss of confidence and the potential loss from employees who may refuse to come to work.

OEM physicians engaged in emergency management should be familiar with the "incident command system" (ICS), which is used by most public safety organizations, is being adopted by public health agencies, and is the conceptual basis for the U.S. National Emergency Management Plan. The ICS was developed in order to eliminate confusion in terminology, roles, and authority during emergencies. It is designed to be "interoperable" (operational regardless of the agency or setting), unambiguous, accountable, and scalable (it can be increased to the level of entire organizations or decreased to describe the different

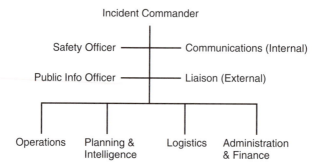

Figure 22.1. The incident command system at its most basic.

tasks of a single person). The basic structure of an ICS is illustrated in Figure 22.1. When a public safety or health unit arrives on the scene or takes control of a situation, command authority is automatically given, all other things being equal, to the person with the most experience handling that type of problem, regardless of rank. The responders are divided into four line units, all under the direction of the incident commander: operations, planning and intelligence, logistics, and administration and finance. "Operations" deals with implementing the response, which in the case of a fire would be the unit responding, and in a broad and serious emergency may coordinate several public safety agencies (for example, police, fire, hazmat response, emergency medical services, and public health agencies). "Planning and intelligence" handles incoming information and plans the next step in the response, providing the incident commander with guidance on strategy and tactics. "Logistics" coordinates the movement of staff and supplies, to ensure that the right assets are available and deployed. "Administration and finance" keeps track of expenses and keeps a log of what is done, so that reimbursement for costs can be settled later. The incident commander is supported by four staff functions: one is responsible for maintaining internal communications among the responders (today this would often be an IT function); a safety officer who is tasked with protecting the health and safety of the responders; a liaison officer with government agencies, public safety units responding on request because of mutual assistance agreements, and other stakeholders, such as local employers; and a public information officer who serves as sole spokesperson and the single source for external communications with media local residents, callers and outside inquiries.

CHEMICAL HAZARDS

Among the worst plausible scenarios in industrial accident prevention and management are fires and explosions in chemical facilities. The worst chemical disaster in history from a fixed site was the famous incident in Bhopal, India, in 1984, which killed at least 3,800 people. In recent years, industrial communities have also needed to face the threat of intentional assaults using stationary sites as commandeered weapons (see section on terrorism). Most uncontrolled chemical releases occur during transportation incidents, such as derailed railroad tanker cars or trucking accidents.

"Chemical safety" is the general term for managing the hazards and risk associated with chemicals in order to protect workers and community residents from incidents of uncontrolled release or exposure. Chemical safety primarily means risk management, reducing the chance of an incident in the first place, reducing the release of chemicals if something does happen, and reducing the damage that the chemicals can do if they are released.

The increased concern over chemical safety has motivated changes to reduce the vulnerability of the entire supply and transportation system as well as increasing security for facilities on site such as stronger and safer tanks, greater control and monitoring of chemical production, and particularly substitution of more hazardous chemicals with less hazardous alternatives.

Moving toward increasing chemical safety and security is a strategy for "no regrets," meaning that the investment in a safer system is not lost, even if nothing untoward occurs. Effective interventions change the vulnerability of the entire supply and transportation system as well as facilities on site. Historically, transportation systems have been even more vulnerable to incidents than plant sites and storage facilities.

When substitutions are made of less hazardous chemical substances, the supply chain and transportation system—the tankers, pipelines, and barges carrying the materials—also become safer.

Since 1985, with the initiation of an industry-wide program called Responsible Care®, the emphasis in chemical safety has been on anticipating and mitigating the risk of unintentional incidents and releases, particularly to neighboring communities and along transportation corridors. Chemical safety since 2001 has emphasized prevention of opportunistic acts of terrorism on site or the commandeering of hazardous materials for intentional assaults.

The primary concerns associated with particular chemicals are:

- Explosion
- Flammability
- Acute toxicity
- Exothermy (release of heat)
- Corrosiveness.

Responsible Care® requires participating companies to practice stewardship of chemicals throughout the product lifecycle. The essential elements of Responsible Care® are community participation, planning for emergencies, emissions reduction, occupational safety, and environmental sustainability. It is now worldwide.

Another program, mandated by the U.S. Environmental Protection Agency, requires community consultation on chemical facilities and the formation of a Local Emergency Planning Committee (LECP) where chemicals are manufactured, stored, or shipped. The LECP provides a forum for developing emergency response plans and disseminating information.

Chemical incidents have strict reporting requirements. They must be reported and may be investigated by the Chemical Safety and Hazard Investigation Board in the United States.

PANDEMIC INFLUENZA AND
DISTRIBUTED EMERGENCIES

Some emergency situations develop over time and not in one place; these have been called "distributed emergencies." Global pandemics of infectious disease are the prototype for such emergencies, and their management provides a general model for dealing with emergencies that unfold more in time rather than space. These emergencies are not confined to infectious disease, however. The same model may apply to new drugs of abuse as they become popular in community after community, catastrophic changes in longevity (such as occurred in the central republics of the former Soviet Union after its dissolution), and famine. Infectious disease, however, is a present threat as well as clearer model for thinking about distributed emergencies.

At the time of writing (2009), the most credible immediate threat of widespread serious illness remains the H5N1 strain of influenza, an avian disease that has already crossed the species barrier and has caused several human outbreaks. (The novel influenza A H1N1 is the current pandemic. but mortality is not heavy.) The major risk is that a substantial number of people around the world will die or become incapacitated for a time, disrupting essential services. Employers in critical sectors, such as transportation, food production, water treatment, public safety, and especially health care, have to be concerned about how well they will manage when as many as 40 percent of workers may be incapacitated at the same time (the U.S. federal government's scenario for planning).

The World Health Organization (WHO) and Centers for Disease Control and Prevention (CDC) are following the situation closely but depend on national and local health departments to monitor the progress of bird infections and to identify human outbreaks. The recent experience with SARS suggests that reporting is not always complete or timely.

The risk is that an outbreak of influenza will become a "pandemic" (worldwide epidemic) with the same or comparable virulence as the 1918 influenza pandemic, which caused millions of deaths worldwide and was unusual in that the influenza pneumonia it caused was most severe in the young and fit. Influenza outbreaks do occur every few decades, although not of that severity, and the world is overdue. It is not clear what the characteristics of a future pandemic might be or what specific antigenic determinants the virus will have that will affect vaccine development.

In the event of a pandemic, WHO, CDC, and Canadian agencies will provide extensive guidance on their Web sites, as they do now for pandemic preparedness. The WHO Web site (http://www.who.int/csr/resources/publications/influenza/WHO_CDS_CSR_GIP_2005_4/en/) is at the level of national planning. The U.S. government has an interagency Web site that relies heavily on the CDC (http://www.pandemicflu.gov/), provides links to state and local Web sites, and would be augmented during a crisis. Similarly, the Government of Canada maintains an interagency Web site (http://www.influenza.gc.ca/index_e.html) that relies heavily on Health Canada and the Public Health Agency of Canada.

Whatever the ultimate shape of the response to pandemic influenza, it will have the following elements, which should be part of any pandemic plan for employers:

- Social isolation. Efforts will be made to reduce the frequency of face-to-face contact among employees in order to slow transmission. Distance learning, telecommuting, and work at home will be encouraged.

- Risk and crisis communication. Efforts to inform and educate the public will be essential. (See Chapter 7.)

- Prioritization. Nonessential activities requiring human contact may be curtailed.

- Surveillance. The outbreak will be tracked by local public health agencies and internationally by WHO and CDC.

- Home care and triage. Persons showing symptoms of influenza will be encouraged to stay at home if their symptoms are low-grade, may be cared for at designated intermediate care centers (which will be set up in schools and churches) if they require supportive care that they cannot get at home, and only admitted to hospital when severely ill. As in the case of SARS, H5N1 influenza cases may initially be concentrated in a small number of hospitals in order to limit exposure if the outbreak appears small.

- Vaccine development. The vaccine will be developed as soon as the antigenic determinants are known but will take months to produce in quantity.

- Immunization. Immunization rests on three strategies. The primary strategy is that as soon as a specific vaccine is available, it will be administered as widely as possible, with priority given to certain groups (such as health care workers) for the earliest batches. The secondary strategy will be a polyvalent influenza vaccine that is designed on a probabilistic basis to cross-react with the strains of H5N1 most likely to be present in the pandemic. The supportive strategy is to encourage near-universal immunization against seasonal influenza, so that during a pandemic the natural background of seasonal influenza can be minimized, removing a burden to the health care system and minimizing confusion. It should be possible to arrange mass immunizations for employees. The staff of the occupational health service may also be asked by local public health authorities to participate in community immunization campaigns if needed and if liability can be managed.

- Antiviral medication. There may be a limited role for oseltamivir (Tamiflu®) and possibly zanamivir (Relenza®) in a pandemic outbreak, especially for the seriously ill. Zanamivir must be taken by inhaler because it is not bioavailable orally, which limits its market acceptability. Supplies of both drugs are finite, and treatment inhibits the development of immunity, so that patients remain at risk for recurrent viral infection. Unfortunately, some avian strains are already resistant to oseltamivir.

Whether or not there will be a pandemic remains to be seen, although it seems likely. The value of pandemic preparedness however, is not limited to one threat. The principles are broadly applicable to other highly contagious emerging infections (such as SARS) and to bioterrorist threats (such as smallpox). The general lessons (the importance of surveillance, information, and interruption of the chain of transmission) may have application in other types of distributed emergencies.

The response to pandemic influenza has been criticized as disproportionate to the real threat. Given the disruption and mortality of pandemics in the past, however, failure to plan seems foolhardy. Shortly before 2000, in what was called the "Y2K" scare, many responsible professionals believed that the information systems of the world were at risk of paralysis because 2000 would be confused with 1900 in old programming formats. Although nothing happened, the desperate preparations for Y2K had the effect of replacing and upgrading infrastructure and making business IT systems, and the Internet, more resilient in advance of the emergencies of 2001 and more resistant to hackers. Similarly, pandemic preparedness will motivate and concentrate efforts in emergency management.

TERRORISM

The threat of a terrorist attack on a private facility seemed remote until 2001 but since then has grown more plausible.

Terrorism has emerged as a threat largely as the result of converging issues of security, international relations, and public health. These include the following:

- Changes in the international order
- Changes in the ideology and practice of terrorism
- Changes in the capacity of the system to cope

Terrorism is a response to asymmetry of strength. Terrorists will attempt to use whatever tactics they can to make up the difference in force in order to get what they want. Terrorist groups have been changing tactics away from the traditional reliance on causing fear toward more "direct action." This strategy seeks to deliberately incapacitate or seriously harm major institutions, such as financial system in New York in 1993 and 2001, rather than primarily to "send a message." This is not to say that fear and terror do not still figure into the strategy, but terrorists are changing their strategies from fear and terror as primary objectives to one of using fear and terror as enhancement factors. Critical economic sectors and infrastructure are likely to be at higher risk than in the past, whether they are public or private. The potential for terrorism to become an occupational hazard has become significant.

Weapons of mass destruction have become a viable tool for well-organized international terrorist networks. The major reason to use them would be to do harm, to inflict injury, and to paralyze economic systems in ways that a conventional explosive, with its limited blast area, could not achieve. In addition weapons of mass destruction, particularly the ones that are most feared—chemical, certain biological agents, and radioactivity—increase the psychological impact. The public is more likely to stay intimidated if people perceive that they may be a victim of a mass casualty at any time rather than the unlikely victim who happens to be in the wrong place at the wrong time in a bombing.

Weapons of mass destruction are of five types:

- Chemical
- Biological
- Radiological
- Nuclear
- Explosive

Chemical agents have technical limitations that make them less effective for sophisticated terrorist operations. If the perpetrators have the expertise and access, they will undoubtedly use them, but they have limitations. The technical difficulties with using chemical agents largely reflect problems of dispersing them and rapid dilution in the atmosphere. Chemical agents are most effective in confined spaces and are unreliable even there. (The sarin gas attack on the Tokyo subway by the Japanese cult Aum Shinrikyo in 1995 only killed twelve people.) Once a chemical assault is over, it is largely over—chemical residues tend to degrade, adhere to surfaces, or dissipate quickly with time. The suddenness of the attack and the technical issues associated with dispersal (which requires the perpetrator to manipulate the device up to the last minute) also make it difficult for the perpetrator to escape.

Biological agents have a major advantage in cost, adaptability, flexibility, ease of concealment, and the impact on the population when they are dispersed. As a consequence they have emerged along with chemical weapons as one of the categories of choice for well-organized terrorist groups. Biological agents also have some potential disadvantages. There are sufficient technical problems in dispersing the agents to make bioterrorism difficult for most perpetrators. Clues may also be abundant in biological attacks because of the genetic material of the organism, which ultimately led to identification of the perpetrator of the anthrax assaults in the United States in 2001. Anthrax remains the most likely agent for a biological assault because of its favorable biological properties and stability of the spores.

Radiological agents contain radionuclides that during an explosion with a conventional charge contaminate an area with radioactivity. This is called a dirty bomb. The effects of a dirty bomb would actually be limited and mostly psychological. The immediate damage would be the result of the explosion, not the radioactive material, and would be limited to the blast zone. There would be no immediate health effects or acute symptoms because the radiation would be dispersed and so radiation poisoning would be unlikely. People in the area and downwind would be at risk for radiation health effects over the long term, including elevated cancer risk, but the effect would not be seen for many years, and by then many people would have died of other causes.

Nuclear explosions, on the other hand, would be devastating and almost impossible to manage within the blast zone. Radiation fallout would be much more intense, and the blast effects would be far greater. There is no question that a nuclear threat is the most serious of the weapons of mass destruction.

Conventional explosives are often overlooked as weapons of mass destruction, but they can be serious threats to large buildings and public spaces. As a practical matter, when a blast occurs it is important to move away from windows and face the other way to avoid flying glass. It is also important to remember that perpetrators often place second bombs in order to catch the unwary, injure first responders (mostly police), and amplify the psychological effect.

A more detailed discussion of terrorist threats is beyond the scope of this book.

RESOURCES

Ciottone GR, Anderson PD, Auf Der Heide E, Darling RG, Jacoby I, Noji E, Suner S. *Disaster Medicine*. Philadelphia: Elsevier Mosby; 2006.

Haddow GD, Bullock JA. *Introduction to Emergency Management*. Boston: Butterworth Heinemann; 2003: 37–47.

NOTEWORTHY READINGS

Brinkley D. *The Great Deluge: Hurricane Katrina, New Orleans, and the Mississippi Gulf Coast*. New York: William Morrow; 2006.

Barry JM. *The Great Influenza*. New York, Penguin, 2004.

Cahill K. *Emergency Relief Operations*. New York: Fordham University Press; 2003.

Guidotti, T.L. (1986). Managing incidents involving hazardous substances. *Am J Prev Med*. (2): 14–154.

Guidotti TL. Occupational medicine in time of crisis. *J Homeland Secur Emerg Manage*. 2005;2(3):art. 4. Available at http://www.bepress.com/jhsem/vol2/iss3/4/. Accessed September 30, 2005.

Guidotti TL. Managing incidents involving hazardous substances. *Am J Preventive Med.* 1986;2:14–154.

Guidotti TL, Hoffman H. Terrorism and the civilian response. In: Upfal MJ, Krieger GR, Phillips SD, Guidotti TL, Weissman D. Terrorism: biological, chemical, and nuclear. *Clin Occup Environ Med.* 2003;2(2):169–180.

Hogan DE, Burstein JL. *Disaster Medicine.* Philadelphia: Lippincott Williams & Wilkins; 2002: 108–109.

Hudson TW, Roberts M. Corporate response to terrorism. In: Upfal MJ, Krieger GR, Phillips SD, Guidotti TL, Weissman D. Terrorism: biological, chemical, and nuclear. *Clin Occup Environ Med.* 2003;2(2):389–404.

Keyes, Burstein JL, Schwartz Swienton, eds. *Medical Response to Terrorism: Preparedness and Clinical Practice.* Baltimore: Lippincott Williams & Wilkins; 2005.

Landesman LY. *Public Health Management of Disasters: The Practice Guide.* Washington, DC: American Public Health Association; 2001: 145.

Leas RD. Cleveland East Ohio Gas Company shows value of well-organized emergency medical program. *Ohio State Med J.* 1944;40:1172–1174.

Levy BS, Sidel VW. *War and Public Health.* 2nd ed. New York: Oxford University Press; 2008.

McLellan RK, Deitchman SD. Role of the occupational and environmental medicine physician. In: Upfal MJ, Krieger GR, Phillips SD, Guidotti TL, Weissman D. Terrorism: biological, chemical, and nuclear. *Clin Occup Environ Med.* 2003;2(2):181–190.

Panamerican Health Organization. *Management of Dead Bodies in Disaster Situations.* Washington, DC: PHO; 2004.

Vogt BM, Sorensen JH. How clean is safe? Improving the effectiveness of decontamination of structures and people following chemical and biological incidents. Oak Ridge, TN: Oak Ridge National Laboratory; 2002. ORNL/TM-2002/178

23 MEDICOLEGAL SERVICES

The specialized health and medical knowledge in occupational and environmental medicine (OEM) are essential to the resolution of many health-related disputes in law and adjudication (such as workers' compensation) and provide essential input into public policy decisions, such as standards setting. OEM physicians often play an important role in evaluating scientific knowledge and defining the medical facts and interpretation of a particular case in law. This is a proper role for the qualified physician and a necessary part of OEM practice at an advanced level. Providing sound advice in legal disputes and administrative judgments is one of the most important services OEM physicians offer society.

This chapter is not intended to provide legal advice and was not written by a lawyer. Law and the rules of evidence, which govern what the court will accept or reject as valid to take into consideration, change over time and vary from jurisdiction to jurisdiction. It is essential that any OEM physician or any other expert be guided by the laws and rules of evidence in the jurisdiction where they are working or will be providing testimony. That means listening to the lawyer who is steering the case and not relying on nonlegal sources, including this chapter, as specific guidance.

In the United States and Canada, OEM physicians are involved in litigation as expert witnesses mostly in personal injury (tort) cases and occasionally in criminal cases (usually involving toxic exposures). Even more often, OEM physicians are involved as experts in the deliberations of adjudication systems derived from personal-injury law; such deliberations substitute the judgments of a panel, judge, or tribunal for those of a trial. They are called "alternative dispute resolution" systems. The most important and the oldest such system, certainly in North America, is the workers' compensation system, which is at the center of OEM practice.

On a practical level, the legal system lacks the technical capacity to evaluate the validity of knowledge as evidence and therefore relies heavily on expert opinion. Much expert-witness testimony is disputed and controversial, and some experts are accused of crossing ethical lines and offering up "junk science." However, the court depends on expert witnesses to help them interpret the facts of the case: it cannot function without them.

Expert knowledge—especially health and medical knowledge—is essential to the resolution of many disputes in law (such as tort litigation) and administrative adjudication (such as workers' compensation). The medical or health expert provides essential input into public policy decisions. How to use this knowledge is not always clear. There are no broadly agreed-upon rules for the application of this knowledge, except those recognized by the law. In the United States, the culture of scientific investigation and the legal privileges given expert witnesses are reflected in legal precedents (cases that have already been decided by higher courts) and in the Federal Rules of Evidence. Although physicians are subordinate to the requirements of the legal system when they serve as expert witnesses, the law recognizes professional standards and the norms of medicine and, increasingly, epidemiology. The law allows testimony on professional standards to be treated as matters of fact rather than opinion, exempts the expert witness from the usual prohibition against "hearsay" evidence (when the witness did not directly and personally observe what happened), places great weight on the qualifications of an expert, and is heavily influenced (definitively in states with the "Frye rule") by the collective opinion of professionals. On the other hand, the law increasingly demands documentation and logic rather than opinion, and expects the expert to use the legal principle of the "weight of evidence" rather than the much more conservative scientific standard of certainty in interpreting the evidence.

THE SOCIAL FUNCTIONS OF LITIGATION

Experts play a critical role in the resolution of some of society's most taxing problems of equity and justice. The expert OEM physician is usually involved in complicated cases involving uncertainty, questions of causation, and arcane knowledge in medicine and toxicology. That is because the simple cases do not require such expertise. It is useful to review just why the OEM expert is doing this and what constructive social role is achieved.

For well over a century, people in the English-speaking world have thought that litigation is excessive and too expensive, as represented in Dickens's novel *Bleak House*. The long, drawn-out lawsuit that is at the center of the novel takes place in a Victorian England that was rapidly becoming the first modern country: a mercantile, technology-driven, and commercially expansive contemporary superpower with new communities arising from the breakdown and formation of social classes, immigration, and internal population movement. Today's times are similar, especially with respect to globalization and technological development; but the pace is much faster now, and disputes have to be resolved more quickly. The legal system is the ultimate venue where disputes are worked out, and if there is an expectation that a matter will land in court anyway, there is an incentive to litigate to get a definitive answer and skip efforts to negotiate.

The fundamental and ultimate set of rules for resolving disputes in a pluralistic society is the law. Litigation, the resort to law to resolve conflicts, is to be expected in a complicated, pluralistic, often-transient society. Societies that are homogeneous have other ways to settle their differences. Within traditional communities, there are accepted informal means of dispute resolution, such as the intervention of village or tribal elders, religious figures, senior family members, "strong men" (government and business figures who have the power to impose a decision), private adjudication or arbitration procedures (increasingly popular in the United States), and public consensus ("the court of public opinion"). On the other hand, different communities do not necessarily agree about norms and acceptable behavior. In a pluralistic society where no one community dominates, the generally respected institutions for resolving disputes within one community do not apply to the others or to the majority. Some external means of dispute resolution is required. Mechanisms of dispute resolution that once existed within traditional communities also eventually break down in pluralistic societies, as cultures become more open, immigrants become assimilated, and society changes.

Even when people share the same culture and values, they may perceive the stakes as far too high to resolve disputes in a provisional fashion. The law is the final arbiter, and its decisions can be enforced. Why not go straight for the definitive resolution and save time?

Litigation also serves a deterrent function. Through anticipation and fear of an adverse judgment or a very expensive court battle, it deters the actor from actions that are likely to infringe on the rights or interests of others. It does so without being an absolute impediment, so some "gray areas" may be explored and risks can be taken within a narrow range. Compared to criminal law and to government regulation, neither of which are very adaptable or flexible—for good reason—tort liability emerges as the most flexible and potentially the most effective form of dispute resolution in law that our society has to offer, despite its high cost and inconvenience. If society is dissatisfied with it, at least part of that dissatisfaction can be blamed on the failure to support other ways of resolving problems.

Litigants contribute to a resolution of social problems related to responsibility and liability, contribute (occasionally) to setting precedents, and support the deterrent effect, all in the process of resolving their own cases. The litigants also bear the cost for this socially useful function and, in some cases, the risk of catastrophic judgments. One problem with the social role of tort liability is therefore that the costs of providing a social function for all are borne by the litigants individually. The cost of this system is essentially underwritten by the losers in the actions and by the public, which maintains the judicial system. The costs may be large and unpredictable, and by the nature of litigation an action precipitated by one party may result in disastrous expenses for the other party, as well as collateral damage such as loss of reputation or business, even if they are not found culpable.

TORT LITIGATION

The area of law that deals with personal injury—when one person or entity has caused harm to another—is called "tort law" in the American and Commonwealth legal systems. The injury may be a physical injury, an economic loss, a failure to fulfill a duty owed, or some other privation. This injury is called a "tort" in English. The French word from which "tort" derives is the same as the root for the word "torture" and the word "tortuous." Many people think that this is highly appropriate, because tort law has often been difficult, painful, and convoluted, especially in the United States.

In recent years, class action suits have raised litigation to new levels of intensity and magnitude. Actions taken against asbestos manufacturers, the tobacco industry, and gun manufacturers have conferred a major social benefit, both by compensating the injured and by deterring further abuses. The huge judgments rendered and the legal fees paid have subsidized exploratory litigation by entrepreneurial law firms to open new grounds for tort litigation. The threat of a big lawsuit is a deterring factor against irresponsible or reckless behavior. At a time when the prevailing political sentiment was against regulation, and regulatory activity by OSHA and the FDA was restricted by Congressional intervention, this litigation may have served as the backstop to ensure that public health gains were not lost. Other cases have led to unfortunate results, such as the alleged fraud committed in high-profile class action lawsuits involving silicosis in 2004 and 2005. Such cases not only abuse the legal system; they also compromise the chances of justice for legitimate cases and damage the credibility of OEM.

The application of medical knowledge in tort litigation has had successes and failures. Litigation over the legacy of asbestos exposure remains highly controversial: arguments over criteria for recognizing asbestos-related diseases are at the heart of the controversy, despite decades of high-quality research. Several efforts have been made in the United States Congress to set up an adjudication system, most recently in 2007. One particularly controversial issue has been the formulation of fair criteria for accepting claims. Litigation over silicone breast implants and the risk of autoimmune disease came to a halt after it was finally decided that the scientific evidence did not support claims of injury. Litigation over the safety of Bendectin (an antiemetic used in pregnancy) forced the drug off the market despite its proven efficacy and good safety record. The key case led to a major decision on the treatment of scientific evidence in federal courts. The common factor in these sets of cases has to do with opinions regarding causation, where these issues are particularly evident.

Much of tort law in the United States as it is applied to the risk of disease, rather than traumatic injury, arose from litigation before and during the 1920s. Plaintiff's counsel often attempted to relate cancer and other chronic health problems to physical trauma. A common example was the claim that cancer was the result of a recent blow or injury to a body part. The rationale invariably was one of *post hoc, ergo propter hoc*, meaning that because the outcome came after the incident, the incident must have been causal. As the science of the day became more sophisticated, courts soon threw out this argument as specious because there was no plausible mechanism relating the injury to cancer risk.

Occupational health- and injury-related tort litigation has a special burden. The workers' compensation system handles the vast majority of occupational cases—with varying degrees of success—for injury and for occupational disease. Because workers' compensation is an alternative dispute-resolution mechanism that constitutes an "exclusive remedy," with levels of appeal within the system but no appeal outside it, legal actions can only be undertaken on the grounds that the workers' compensation process was unfairly applied (which is hard to prove in a quasi-judicial system that does not recognize precedent or follow the rules of evidence) or is unconstitutional to begin with (hard to argue given settled law and almost a century of acceptance). Needless to say, these legal actions are exceedingly rare. As a consequence, legal actions in occupational health usually involve "third-party liability," in which the manufacturer or distributor is sued for failure to provide a safe product or to warn of hazards. Very rarely, cases of egregious neglect or willful disregard for workers' safety will be prosecuted as criminal cases or even murder.

Environmental tort litigation is broader and highly diverse. A fuller elaboration is beyond the scope of this chapter.

In all matters related to procedure and timing, the expert should rely on legal counsel in the case to describe the steps in the process and the timetable. The sequence of events in American and Commonwealth legal cases normally involves filing a complaint, discovery, preparation of opinions, and depositions. Once the strength of evidence on both sides is apparent, there is a period of pretrial preparation, during which the possibility of settlement is usually raised. Very few cases actually go to trial. A decision to offer or accept a settlement may have nothing to do with the strength of the case, and the expert should never become emotionally invested in presenting his or her testimony at trial. It is not the expert's case. Adjudication procedures are simpler and usually involve preparation of an opinion and possibly an administrative hearing.

Frye and *Daubert*

For many years, the judicial standard for expert testimony across the United States was the Frye rule (articulated in a 1923 decision in *Frye v. United States*, 93 F. 1013). The Frye rule was interpreted as admitting the conventional or consensus view of a particular field or discipline, such as medicine, and discouraging admission of innovative or novel theories. This rule was based on wording from the opinion that stated, "the thing from which the deduction is made must be sufficiently established to have gained general recognition in the particular field in which it belongs." Over time, the application of the Frye rule is believed by many to have drifted into admitting professional opinions that could be found to have some basis in some field, however narrow or self-defined. For others, however, the Frye rule, if rigorously applied, is a correction against individualistic or poorly supported opinion and a means of grounding testimony in the mainstream of the expert's field of practice. The Frye rule remains the basis of evaluating or allowing expert testimony in many states, including California, but its application depends importantly on state law and precedent.

In the United States, a 1993 Supreme Court decision attempted to clarify the standard for applying scientific information to dispute resolution in federal courts and in many states that apply the Federal Rules of Evidence. The decision in *Daubert v. Merrell Dow Pharmaceuticals, Inc.* (507 U.S. 579) set forth a new and higher standard for federal courts in reviewing scientific evidence. (This was the decision in the Bendectin case.) The effect of this decision was that judges presiding over technically complicated cases were instructed to serve as "gatekeepers" and were required to evaluate the admissibility of evidence proffered by experts. This requires evaluating and monitoring scientific evidence, evidence that judges cannot be expected to have mastered. This decision was later reflected in the decisions of many state supreme courts, including that of Texas (which reached similar conclusions in the form of two mutually supportive opinions, usually called *Havner-Robinson*).

In keeping with an earlier trend in some state appellate courts and in general trends in adjudication bodies, *Daubert* requires federal courts to examine the quality and methodology underlying testimony in arriving at their admissibility decisions and thus to apply the standards of science to scientific testimony. Its influence has been felt throughout the legal system, resulting in higher expectations for rigor and persuasiveness in the opinions offered by expert witnesses, even when the local standard is the Frye rule or some variation of it. A consequence of the *Daubert* decision is that it is now much harder to demonstrate sufficient admissible evidence to support a "first case" when a hazard is new or an association has not previously been recognized.

The *Daubert* decision imposed a great burden on courts. Few judges and clerks are prepared to assess scientific data independently and few have staffs equipped to do this knowledgeably. Most lawyers will agree that law school was never designed to prepare them for technical issues in science. In practice, decisions on whether to admit expert testimony in a case may require a special evidentiary hearing to determine whether the expert has met the standards of *Daubert* or the applicable state rules of evidence.

Since *Daubert*, courts have required more documentation of the evidence and have set a higher standard. Peer review is now accepted as meeting this legal standard, and experts are often asked on the stand if the evidence they cite and the opinions, or theory of the case, they espouse have been peer-reviewed. Theories that are specific to a particular case have no opportunity to be peer-reviewed. The assessment of whether a scientific theory is worth hearing therefore takes place before the jury ever hears it or the judge allows it to become part of the record.

Other legal systems have taken other approaches. For example, in Canada the emphasis in the courts is not on excluding or evaluating scientific evidence when it is introduced. The emphasis is on weighing the testimony for scientific validity after it has been given. The jury, with instructions from the judge, decides whether what they have already heard was worth hearing.

THE EXPERT WITNESS

Expert testimony is an old and venerable function of health professionals. In general, the law respects the opinion of physicians and other expert witnesses, but the role of the expert witness has changed from providing an authoritative opinion alone. In past years, the informed judgment of health professionals, without reference to the evidence, carried greater weight than it does today. Junk science and the spectacle of "dueling experts" who seem to fight without firm grounds for their positions have provoked a backlash. Since the *Daubert* decision, courts have put much greater emphasis on defensible arguments based on empirical data and less emphasis on expert judgment. The ability to base testimony on evidence, and to fit the evidence together in a way that appears objective, is far more important in today's courtroom. A personal, subjective, or idiosyncratic interpretation of the facts contributes little and may even undermine one's professional credibility.

The role of the expert witness is to establish and interpret issues of fact. There are five essential responsibilities for the expert witness:

- To establish pertinent facts
- To place them in a context
- To explain the theory of the case in terms that are comprehensible to the lay court
- To render quantitative assessments in qualitative terms
- To derive an assessment of the degree of injury in terms that can be dealt with by the court

The role of the expert witness in civil cases is normally to provide testimony and informed opinion to establish or define issues of fact in a tort. The medical expert witness is also usually called upon in these settings to testify as to causation and damages related to health and physical impairment. Opinion is not enough, but it is allowed. This is one of the few situations in legal proceedings when witnesses are allowed to testify on the basis of personal opinion rather than knowledge. An adjudication proceeding, such as an appeal of a workers' compensation claim, is similar.

The first responsibility is to present pertinent facts in a meaningful context. It is now more important than ever to show that these facts are pertinent to the case and reflect the best scientific information available. It is also critical to integrate the facts of the discipline (such as cancer rates for various occupations and exposures) with the facts of the case so that the testimony is not an abstract discussion, but directly pertinent to the individual circumstances of the case. This also means careful attention when the profile of a particular plaintiff or claimant does not fit the average of characteristics or the overall profile of a population in an epidemiological study—for example, if a plaintiff developed cancer at an unusually young age. It is not enough to testify that there is an association between exposures characteristic of an occupation and the risk of cancer, for example. It is now important to specify that for workers of a certain age and background risk profile there is persuasive evidence that the risk is elevated to an extent that for this group it is more likely than not the cause of the site-specific outcome in any particular case. This is the same logic as a "rebuttable presumption," which will be described later in this chapter.

Explaining the context is the second responsibility. The meaningful context for these facts is just as important as the facts themselves. The facts must be related by scientific interpretation in the expert witness's treatment, just as the elements of the case are related by legal principles in the lawyer's analysis. The expert witness has always been expected to express a sound opinion in a comprehensible fashion. However, the expert is now expected to provide solid grounds and a coherent chain of logic for the opinion expressed, and to place it in a context that assists the adjudicator in arriving at an informed decision. The expert is expected to reflect either a professional consensus or a well-supported minority opinion with evidence of backing in the scientific community.

This interpretation must be explicit and convincing. The expert needs to explain why an exposure probably caused the outcome in the particular case, establishing what is called "causation," described in greater detail below. This may mean presenting the mechanisms of carcinogenesis in more or less detail to make the link clearly. It is necessary to establish the clear chain of logic and to base the interpretation of the case on the best available facts and estimates, but unless these scientific considerations eventually lead to a qualitative assessment of "more likely than not," they are going to be more confusing than helpful. Thus, the expert witness still must render an informed, qualitative opinion, but it must be preceded by and grounded upon a defensible scientific argument. The expert has a responsibility to provide a clear rationale behind the opinion and to articulate it in a manner that is useful to the adjudicating body.

The third responsibility is to communicate the theory of the case in terms that the judge or jury has no trouble grasping. The cliché is that judges, like most lawyers, went into law because they did not do well in science at school, and sometimes this is true. Finding a theory that makes sense is not enough. The theory of the case must also be communicated clearly and simply. In court, even a reasonable theory developed to fit the particulars of a highly unusual case may appear idiosyncratic, even bizarre, when distorted by the "other side." "Framing" is a term of art for reviewing the facts of the case, developing a theory of what happened, and explaining what happened as a coherent narrative. A robust theory should stand up to more than one interpretation of events and does not depend on too many assumptions; it should never depend on just a single fact. This is not easy, but if a theory of a case is likely to be true, it should be able to explain all of the essential facts of the case and predict other facts as well.

A common mistake on the part of plaintiffs' experts is to focus narrowly on proving the case and then to go no further when a reasonable theory has been formulated. Experienced experts focus on disproving the case and finding what is wrong with the theory, whether they are advising the plaintiff or defense. For the plaintiff expert, it is essential to put the theory to the test before the opposition does so in court. For the defense, the task is much easier. The defense expert only needs to poke holes in the plaintiff's theory and raise the possibility of other explanations, not prove them.

An apparently rational but complicated theory of a case may easily require so many contingent steps that the final odds that the theory resembles what happened are much less than even; in other words, the more elaborate a theory, the more likely that part or all of it is wrong. Explaining a theory that complicated to a jury is also not easy. The simpler the theory and the fewer the steps, the more likely it is that the entire sequence of events is true, and the easier it is to explain. (This principle is called "Occam's razor.") So the essence of framing a theory of a case is to identify the key facts, put them together simply, challenge the theory to explain anomalous or unexpected facts (before the opposition does this in court), and gather the supporting evidence to document the theory.

A critical part of clear communication, and the fourth responsibility, is to render quantitative information in qualitative terms. Numbers should be kept to a minimum in expert testimony, especially in a jury trial, but whenever possible they should be described with examples. A probability of 50 percent is an abstraction; the balance of probabilities is a metaphor; a coin toss is a vivid example everyone can understand. It is not enough to speak of a probability of 10^{-6}. The concept of one in a million has to be made graphically, such as by referring to one person in the whole population of Denver or Calgary or some other comparison that will mean something to a person without technical training. A part per billion has to be compared to ten drops of water in a swimming pool, not expressed as 10^{-9}.

In some tort cases and in many workers' compensation adjudication proceedings, the expert also has the role of evaluating damages, describing future health risks, and rating disability. Evaluating the degree of injury in terms that the court or tribunal can understand may be of greater or lesser importance depending on the case and the qualifications of the expert witness. For medical experts, this may involve an assessment of permanent impairment or long-term disability and future risk of developing a complication. On the defense side, it may involve a rebuttal. This aspect of the expert witness's role is highly individualized and reflects the circumstances of the particular case and the expert witness's specific role as determined by counsel.

The adversarial structure of the American and Commonwealth legal systems encourages extreme interpretations. This has given space for junk science and bogus experts. One might ask why the court does not use its own experts. Something like this has been attempted by judges who have set up expert panels to advise them in class action lawsuits, but such examples are very rare. In the rare instances when a judge has had access to a consultant capable of rendering an independent assessment, there have been concerns that the in-house expert could unduly affect the decision by manipulating the assessment and by inadvertently supplanting the role of the judge in deciding on the admissibility of scientific testimony.

The foundation of a trial in the American or Commonwealth system of law is advocacy on behalf of two opposing sides that have a duty to present their own best case. It would be inimical to the operation of the legal system if, for example, plaintiff and defense experts, or claimants and adjudicators, let their experts meet in conference to decide among themselves which scientific interpretation is correct.

CAUSATION

Most cases in which an OEM physician is likely to be engaged involve causation. Properly speaking, causation is the causal event, and causality is the relationship between cause and effect: one is specific and the other is general. However, they are often used interchangeably, with "causality" being preferred in the United Kingdom and "causation" in North America. The systematic process leading to the determination, to a reasonable approximation, of the most likely cause is called "causation analysis." For the OEM physician, causation analysis requires a familiarity with the methodologies of epidemiology, toxicology, clinical medicine, and, increasingly, risk science. (Causation and causality in epidemiology are discussed in Chapter 3.)

"Causation" refers, in this context, to the risk factors or exposures that initiate the process leading to the health outcome. The concept is akin to that of etiology in clinical medicine, but without the implication that there must be only a single cause. The concept of causation in epidemiology assumes that the risk factors bear a "causal" relationship in that they either establish a necessary condition that allows the outcome, or set into motion a mechanism that results in the outcome. There is no assumption, as there is in common language and in the work of some epistemologists, that a cause must be "sufficient" in itself to produce an effect.

A cause, in the sense that is used in most toxic tort cases (especially when cancer risk is involved), is a factor that contributes to the likelihood that an outcome will occur. This is a stochastic, or probabilistic, definition, not strictly a mechanistic definition. There is a certain probability, or odds, that a step will occur, but no certainty. In daily life, one speaks of "cause and effect" relationships as if there is one cause for every effect and as if an effect necessarily follows the presence of a cause. This is too rigid to be useful in epidemiology and especially in carcinogenesis, where the mechanisms are complicated and influenced by numerous external and internal factors. It is not even useful, in this context, to speak of a cause as being either necessary or sufficient, because causes may be interchangeable in the mechanism or may interact.

For example, exposure to either cigarette smoking or asbestos individually is known to result in lung cancer in a roughly predictable probability. Exposure to both increases the risk beyond that of the summed probabilities of either alone, suggesting a substantial interaction. However, most workers who have been exposed to either or both do not develop lung cancer, although they might if they live long enough and are free of other risks to their life. A few unlucky people who neither smoke nor become exposed to environmental carcinogens such as asbestos develop lung cancer regardless, although this is uncommon. Neither asbestos exposure nor cigarette smoking is necessary, sufficient, or predictable in individual cases as a cause of lung cancer, but the association is clear and these factors are truly "causes."

The medical expert needs to review the case with an eye toward many factors in causation. These include:

- Determination of the proximate cause (what was immediately responsible)
- Determination of the underlying causes (what conditions created the situation)
- Liability for the causal situation (who was responsible for allowing it to happen)
- Contributing behavioral factors
- Apportionment among the various causes that are possible
- Preexisting conditions (such as atopy) and personal factors (such as host defense or susceptibility states) that confer susceptibility (a biological condition that makes effects more likely)
- Occupational, environmental justice, and behavioral factors that confer vulnerability (a social condition that makes a person more likely to be exposed or disadvantaged in protecting him- or herself)

Causation is similar to the concept of etiology in clinical medicine but without the implication that there can only be one cause. In clinical medicine, etiology is usually not as important as diagnosis, because in clinical practice, regardless of what caused the condition, the task at hand is to treat the patient. In law and policy, however, the assessment of causation is critical because it establishes liability and responsibility. Causation is even more central than diagnosis in initiating compensation and stimulating prevention. It is not at all unusual for a physician to be able to make a diagnosis without knowing the cause. It is also not always necessary to know the exact diagnosis to assess causation, as long as the pathological process is known. For example, one can know that a worker has nonallergic airways reactivity following an exposure clearly associated with work without determining for certain whether it is occupational asthma associated with irritant exposure, reactive airways dysfunction syndrome, or aggravation of preexisting but subclinical airways reactivity in allergic rhinitis.

The concept of causation has different implications in different disciplines. In epidemiology, the concept of causation assumes that the risk factors bear a "causal" relationship to each other in that they either establish a necessary condition or set into motion a process that results in the outcome. This does not necessarily mean, as in common language, that a cause must be "sufficient" in itself to produce an effect. In toxicology, the concept of causation tends to be more mechanistic, and assumes that there is a chain of biological causation from first exposure to outcome. However, toxicologists are also accustomed to thinking in terms of complex interactions. In OEM, causation is the determination of the most-probable cause of the worker's condition or disability. In workers' compensation, to establish causation means identifying the factor that created the condition and also demonstrating that it arose out of the work setting or conditions.

In law, there are two elements of causation: cause in fact and proximate cause. Cause in fact is the necessary condition, similar to the notion of "underlying cause" on a death certificate. It can be identified by a simple test: would the adverse outcome have been avoided "but for" the presence of the cause? A cause in fact can be necessary but not sufficient. The proximate cause is the particular event or factor that initiated the chain of events leading to injury or damage; it is comparable to the "immediate cause" on a death certificate. In law, especially in adjudication proceedings, a proximate cause may also be a "substantial factor," which contributes to the outcome even if it is not wholly responsible. Thus, in a heavy cigarette smoker who was also exposed to large amounts of asbestos and developed asbestosis, and who subsequently developed lung cancer, the smoking may be a cause in fact, but the asbestos exposure could be a proximate cause and the basis for a judgment. This is because not all or even a majority of cigarette smokers get lung cancer (although they all might if they survived long enough), but the effect of asbestos exposure on a cigarette smoker more than doubles the risk of lung cancer: so most cases would not have arisen but for the asbestos exposure.

A good medical evaluation alone is not enough for causation analysis. Causation analysis must be undertaken methodically on two levels. The individual case must be thoroughly documented and evaluated. Then, the evidence in the individual case must be linked with the broader body of knowledge in science regarding risk, usually derived from epidemiology, taking into account how the individual may differ from or resemble the populations studied.

One systematic approach to causation analysis is the following:

- Confirm the diagnosis and the nature of the injury. Occasionally, a report of the diagnosis will be incorrect.

- Determine the circumstances of exposure. Confirm that there was a plausible route of exposure of sufficient magnitude to place the person at risk.

- Determine other possible exposures that may be causal or significant in the case and their plausibility and likely magnitude. For example, cigarette smoking is by far the most common alternative risk factor in occupational lung-disease cases, so the smoking history is often critical.

- Determine whether the injury is a recognized effect of the exposure. This is relatively easy to do for carcinogens because the International Agency for Research on Cancer is an authoritative body that provides assessment of the evidence for carcinogenicity of chemicals and industrial processes. It is more difficult when the scientific literature is incomplete and may be impossible in a "first case."

- Determine whether the particulars of the individual case are consistent with findings in the scientific literature. This often requires a working knowledge of toxicology because outcomes may differ in human and animal studies.

- Develop a reasonable hypothesis for how such an event might have happened—the simpler, the better. Then test this hypothesis against the facts of the case. Does the theory predict a different fact that can be checked?

Causation may be simple if the disorder is typically associated with a single external cause, such as mesothelioma and asbestos exposure. The challenge in such cases is to demonstrate the opportunity for exposure to an agent that is a known cause, which requires a thorough history. Medical records are usually poor sources of the exposure history because the first person to take the history is rarely trained to obtain a thorough occupational history (see Chapter 15), is not primarily interested in exposure assessment, and is relying on second-hand information from an anxious patient. Subsequent references to the exposure in the medical history often merely copy the first and occasionally distort it, perpetuating errors in the process.

Conditions for which there is a strong or suspected association with occupation on a group basis may be hard to prove on an individual basis. Some workers' compensation systems have schedules of recognized diseases, for which claims qualify more-or-less automatically if there is a history of exposure or if the worker is in an occupation with a demonstrable and accepted risk. However, the association may be disputed in the individual case if there is evidence for another cause, evidence that exposure was not sufficient, or evidence for some other mitigating circumstance. This is called a rebuttable presumption and is an important policy alternative in workers' compensation and legislation. Presumption is discussed later in this chapter.

Identifying a particular cause for the outcome is often difficult. This is illustrated by common occupational lung diseases. The occupational and environmental history certainly narrows down the range of possible exposures and may rule out all but one or a few possibilities, particularly in the case of the pneumoconioses, which never occur without exposure to the causal dust. However, cases of asthma and hypersensitivity pneumonitis are rarely so easy, because the disorders may mimic common nonoccupational and the number of possible exposures triggering the immunologic responses may be large. Toxic inhalation cases are always associated with a discrete event; there may be uncertainty over which particular chemical exposure caused the injury, but the association with the event in question is rarely in dispute. Obstructive airways disease and cancer are exceedingly difficult and often impossible to associate with a particular exposure in the presence of other risk factors, such as cigarette smoking.

In many cases, the OEM physician has available a variety of records to develop an inventory of exposures and possible causes:

- A thorough occupational history
- Employer personnel records
- Industrial hygiene survey records (when available)
- Union records
- Pay stubs, tax records, and income statements that identify particular employers
- Medical records
- Testimony of co-workers
- Past workers' compensation claims

At other times, the medical record and most recent occupation is all that is available. When the information is insufficient to come to a firm conclusion, the expert should say so and then use the best judgment and most reasonable assumptions possible, spelling out in detail at every step what assumptions have been made and the basis for them.

The evaluation of occupational and environmental disease may be assisted by more-advanced diagnostic modalities. Technology has advanced the precision of medical diagnosis, but it does not necessarily help to the same degree in causation assessment and etiological determination. The use of advanced diagnostic tests without guidelines may even bias the system. A claimant who receives sensitive but not specific tests, such as high-resolution computed tomography for fibrotic lung disease, might be more likely to have his or her claims accepted than a claimant whose physician did not use that technology, simply because it looks more convincing to a judge. Likewise, x-rays of the spine that show erosion of the vertebral body and spurring are often accepted as evidence of a structural abnormality for low-back pain alleged to have arisen out of work, yet such lesions are common in people without low-back pain and are not by themselves evidence of an occupational cause. Therefore, diagnostic tests are not always helpful and may sometimes confuse the picture.

The evaluation of occupational disease may appear very conservative to practitioners who are accustomed to applying the latest medical breakthroughs, but there are good reasons for this. Workers' compensation evaluations tend to rely on studies with known and familiar technology. Traditional tests, such as the chest film, have been exhaustively studied in occupational medicine and are well understood; for example, progression of asbestosis on a chest film has a relationship to lung function and cancer risk, but this has not been established for high-resolution computed tomography (HRCT). Insurance carriers may not authorize newer or highly sensitive tests that are not easily interpreted. The history of OEM is littered with nonspecific, unhelpful, or misinterpreted studies: trace element analysis (see Chapter 2), PET (positron emission tomography) scans used for "toxic encephalopathy" (see Chapter 1), serum mold antigens and antibodies, visual contrast sensitivity, and a raft of tests associated with unproven medical theories, such as multiple chemical sensitivity and its progeny. There have also been egregious cases of questionable tests being applied in fitness-for-duty evaluations and periodic health surveillance, where incorrect and invalid results had the potential of costing a worker his or her job or career. This is why the issue of validated testing is so sensitive in health monitoring (see Chapter 5) and OEM ethics (see Chapter 25).

Another peculiarity of causation analysis compared to conventional medical assessment, diagnosis, and management is that treatment records are generally useless. Unless the clinical management of a condition is part of the question being put to the medical expert, as in medical malpractice, nothing that occurred after the disorder appears is of much interest in causation analysis. Treatment records should still be scanned by the expert, however, because every once in a while the later notes reveal a useful fact. Likewise, nursing notes are usually not very informative, except in reporting the patient's state of mind and anxiety, and sometimes introduce or perpetuate errors, especially in matters of diagnostic detail and smoking history. On the other hand, pulmonary function tests incorporate a short smoking history, which may be more accurate than what is found in the history of present illness.

A finding of causation is a reasonable conclusion when a case conforms to risk factors that are described in the scientific literature, and there is a clear consensus that the exposure is associated with the disease outcome. These are the easier cases. The harder cases are those in which the literature is not clear. The first step is to review the literature to determine whether the evidence suggests a causal association. The literature may be clinical, toxicological, or epidemiological. In general, the clinical literature tells the OEM physician that something happened, the toxicological literature tells the physician that something could happen, and the epidemiological literature tells physician that something does happen. None of them can tell the physician what happened in the specific case; that is a matter of inference.

As a practical matter, empirical evidence that can be demonstrated to apply to a given case trumps a mechanistic argument that is based on toxicological principles, which in turn trumps personal opinion based on clinical experience. Toxicological studies may demonstrate that an association between exposure and an outcome in the case exists in animals and may demonstrate a plausible mechanism. The methods, relevance to humans, comparative exposure levels, species, and strain become matters of interpretation.

It is important to know whether the profile of the injured party/worker corresponds to the population the study has investigated. It may matter, for example, that the plaintiff/claimant is younger, has worked longer, does or does not satisfy the expected latency period, or belongs to a particular subgroup in the analysis. An important principle in workers' compensation is to "take the worker(s) as they come," meaning that once they are hired, personal characteristics do not matter. For example, unless there is a policy against hiring people who smoke, an employer cannot argue that an exposure that makes only smokers sick is not work related. Some claimants, by their family history or some acquired condition, may be more susceptible than others to injury. Such persons are known as "thin skull," "eggshell," or "eggshell skull" plaintiffs after an early legal case in which a person sustained a skull fracture after a minor blow. The fact that the victim was more susceptible to a skull fracture than most people did not absolve the person responsible for hitting him on the head from liability and paying damages.

"Aggravational" causation occurs when an exposure makes an existing condition worse or brings out symptoms in a previously silent condition. Exposure to an irritant gas, including passive cigarette smoke, may aggravate reactive airways disorders in an individual with atopy, for example, even if he or she has had no previous asthma. This is not the same as de novo asthma but may be accepted as permanent impairment in some systems if it persists and interferes with the worker's ability to perform his or her usual occupation. Some systems use the term "exacerbation" to refer to a longer-term, often permanent, worsening of symptoms.

"Substantial contribution" is a feature of some legal systems. This doctrine suggests that the condition should be considered to have arisen out of the workplace if the exposure was sufficient to contribute more than trivial risk and would have added enough to the causation of the disorder to tip the balance, all other things being equal. This criterion is particularly common in situations in which strict causation is difficult or impossible to prove or in which the job was particularly hazardous or involved national security and the assumption of personal risk. The Black Lung Benefits Program in the United States is such a system, administered under the Department of Labor (with some supplemental benefits from Medicare).

Some sense of apportionment by cause may be needed to explain the history and presentation of the disorder and to sort out the extent of contribution of work-related factors when the relationship is not simple. In a given case, there may be more than one plausible agent or risk factor responsible for the condition, such as cigarette smoking, exposure to asbestos, and exposure to other chemical carcinogens. Separation of the nonfactors, and attribution of the factors to the correct employer, is an ideal to be sought, but it is rarely feasible in practice. Demonstration of substantial contribution by workplace-associated exposures is usually sufficient to declare the disorder and all associated impairment to be work related. Since 2004, apportionment of cause has been required under workers' compensation law in California. It may be tempting to apportion based on attributable risk, but this is an error. Attribution is an estimate of the contribution of a given cause to disease in a population, based on its role in a proportion of cases; apportionment is an estimate of the contribution in an individual case, where the cause may be all or partial, or may not be a cause at all.

CERTAINTY

Society uses many different criteria for evaluating risk, accepting what is likely to be true, and deciding to act. OEM physicians and others who are well prepared and formally trained know how to evaluate evidence in science and have internalized the "95 percent certainty" principle for statistical significance or a change in baseline condition. However, civil law (and most systems of adjudication) has a different standard for disputes between parties: the balance of probabilities, or "weight of evidence," which translates to greater than 50 percent certainty. When the medical or health expert ventures into the courtroom, therefore, it is like playing a (serious) game with very different rules. By comparison, the standard of certainty for criminal cases, when the accused will be deprived of rights, is "beyond reasonable doubt," a standard even more stringent than 95 percent certainty.

The usual criteria applied in civil litigation and for accepting an association as causal is that the disease in question is "more likely than not" associated with the exposure or act of the defendant. The same standard of "50 percent + 1," or "balance of probabilities," is also the legal criterion for judgment in a civil case, and in a civil case the burden of proof is on the plaintiff. In workers' compensation cases, the benefit of the doubt is given to the claimant. One need only be "50 percent sure" (the exact balance of probabilities, when there is equal weight on both sides of the question) to make a judgment.

Statements of certainty are just that, not statements about relative contribution or apportionment. The expert helps the court to the extent possible to recognize a balance of probabilities where it exists on the basis of evidence. The court is looking for pivotal points, thresholds, or "bright lines" (a term of art meaning a clear distinction) on which to base a decision.

Various jurisdictions use different terminology to express the idea of certainty or a balance of probabilities. All terms are intended to express the idea that one is persuaded, by the weight of evidence, that the evidence for causation by the factor in question is at least as good or marginally better than the evidence for causation by any other factor and by all other factors in combination. These terms should be considered a different vocabulary of expression that is specific to the medicolegal or adjudication setting. For example, many jurisdictions expect the expert to use the phrase "to a reasonable degree of medical certainty" to express confidence in the opinion, as well as recognition that the science and art of medicine have limitations. If so, whether the expert likes it or not, the phrase should be used, because it is actually a signal that the expert understands what he or she is being asked within the context of that system. On the other hand, some terms are universal. For example, where the "50 percent sure" criterion applies, as it usually does, "probable" means yes and "possible" means no, because "possible" means less than 50 percent certainty to most people. No distinction is made between being very sure and being certain; all that is important is that a conclusion based on fact is definite and more likely than not. To be unsure or uncertain is not to support the conclusion. It thus adds little to an expert witness's testimony to go into detail on the witness stand about minor reservations or to express an unlikely alternative opinion as a possibility. When a scientific expert is asked for an expression of certainty, there is a natural tendency to couch the statement in the usual scientific terms, with many qualifiers. This is a mistake. From the legal standpoint it is of no interest, but expressing such reservations may have a psychological effect on the jury or adjudication panel that may confuse the case.

Most adjudication systems give a nominal benefit of the doubt to the claimant in cases where the odds are evenly matched, but these systems zealously guard their right to confer this benefit of the doubt. The expert witness should not assume the prerogative of making this judgment. The role of the expert witness is to outline the framework for a judgment of probable or likely causation clearly and as rigorously as the discipline allows, and then to let the system decide.

Some medical expert witnesses stick to the familiar rules of science and are therefore, by definition, too conservative in their opinions. Others may feel liberated by the looser standard of civil litigation and free to make up theories and opinions that are extrapolated far beyond solid evidence. An example of this is suspect testimony in the wave of litigation over "toxic mold" in the United States today. Litigation has been a spawning ground for so-called "junk science," which has threatened the credibility of experts in general and has probably discouraged many knowledgeable investigators and practitioners from sharing their knowledge when it has been needed.

There is nothing unethical about holding one opinion with respect to the legal interpretation of a set of findings and another with respect to the scientific interpretation. One may legitimately consider a matter to be very likely but not scientifically proven (such as asbestos as a cause of colon cancer). Often, the scientific evidence for an association is strong but not conclusive. In such cases, it is entirely reasonable and responsible for an expert witness to maintain on the witness stand that there is an association on the basis of an interpretation of "the weight of evidence," but to maintain in a scientific forum that the association is not proven, because it has not been proven beyond scientific doubt. The reverse is also true: It is legitimate for an expert witness to believe, as a matter of opinion, that there is not an association but that the evidence against it is not conclusive. (This position, which might apply, for example, to cancer induced by electromagnetic fields, is very common because the doctrine of falsification makes it clear that a negative can never be conclusively proven.) The law is interested primarily in the weight of what evidence exists, and secondarily on how strong the body of evidence is in its entirety. A corollary to this is that the testimony of an ethical expert witness on the stand may not coincide with his or her professional opinion in a scientific setting. (Some sources cite a 1984 decision of the United States Court of Appeals for the District of Columbia—*Ferebee v. Chevron Chemical Co.*, 736 F.2d 1529—in support of this principle; however, this is incorrect. *Ferebee* addressed the sufficiency of evidence supporting an opinion rendered in court and the right of an expert to hold an opinion based on interpretation of the evidence. It did not address consistency or divergence of the same expert's opinions or conclusions based on the same evidence outside of court and in the realm of science. That is a not a matter for courts to decide, anyway.)

Testimony based on the latest findings and just-published studies gives the appearance of being up-to-date and irrefutable. Likewise, a common ploy in cross-examination is to cite a new or obscure study that takes the expert by surprise. (This is called the "gotcha!" strategy.) However, both tactics are actually weak because the latest findings have not had time to be evaluated and integrated into the body of scientific interpretation, which is what really matters, and the most obscure studies never will. Their probative value is therefore limited until they can be examined and, in most cases, confirmed. On the other hand, it is ethical to testify that there is an association on the basis of preliminary evidence while acknowledging that systematic efforts to disprove the hypothesis have not yet been made. It all depends on how the information is used and how the argument is framed. In general, however, an argument that pivots on a very new or very obscure finding is weak. Paradoxically, these findings carry most weight when they are consistent with the body of science, not when they contradict it.

The courts only expect an interpretation based on the best evidence available, not prescience or omniscience. What counts most is the weight of what evidence exists, not how strong the body of evidence is in its entirety. The court cannot wait to make a decision until all the evidence one could want is available.

When an expert concludes that the balance of probabilities, or the weight of evidence, favors the conclusion that a particular hazard caused an injury or disease, the statement only refers to the relationship between the hazard (cause) and the effect. Often the factor in question is the most likely by a plurality, not a majority share. There may be other possibilities and the cause in question may be the most likely among them. That test is whether the likelihood that the outcome was caused by the hazard is the most likely among several possibilities (usually by a wide margin), but not necessarily at a level of 50 percent probability. The expert witness must then explain that the weight of evidence favors the most likely cause against all the other possible causes individually. If the hazard in question is at least equally probable to have been the cause as the combined probability of all other possible causes, then it is already at the balance of probabilities.

Statements of certainty can also be applied to incomplete causes. In this application, they describe how sure one is with respect to whether some factor was a cause at any level. Some adjudication systems find for the claimant if the hazard or action played a role or substantially contributed to the outcome. For example, the managed federal tort systems for railroad workers do not require a conclusion that the hazard caused an illness by itself; it is sufficient if it made a substantial contribution. However, one must still decide whether it is more likely than not that the factor in question contributed anything substantial to the causation of the outcome.

These statements of certainty can be read in one way as descriptions of whether a particular factor was the cause of a particular disorder. This is true only when the assumption is made that there is only one sole and sufficient cause of the outcome. There may be several possible causes, but the argument proceeds on the basis of which cause is more likely to be responsible. This is indeed a common situation, such as in cases disputing whether exposure to a carcinogen was sufficient to cause a cancer or whether there were other causes that could have caused it. Here it is enough to determine that the evidence favors the cause in question being sufficient and more likely than any and all of the other possibilities.

A related issue arises when exposure to a cause is necessary but not sufficient. For example, if a particular exposure raised the risk of a heart attack, but only in persons with high blood pressure, it should be enough to demonstrate that the available evidence shows it to be more likely than not that "but for" the exposure, the person would not have had a heart attack, regardless of the cause of his or her underlying hypertension.

The relative emphasis to be placed on each of these partial roles depends on the case and the weight of available evidence. The more the facts of the case speak for themselves, the less important it is to interpret them and the less work the expert witness must do to establish their validity. As the weight of evidence comes closer to certainty, the burden of interpreting the evidence correspondingly becomes lighter. The expert's role then becomes to explain and present the evidence clearly and accurately.

Judgment remains important in the testimony of the expert witness. Indeed, the expert witness is excluded from the hearsay rule in presenting evidence precisely because he or she is deemed qualified to present an informed opinion based on the collective wisdom of the discipline. However, where judgment is needed, the reasons for making an informed judgment one way or the other should be spelled out. The areas of gray, the reasons for choosing one estimate over another, and the means by which one deals with uncertainty should be made explicit.

Gold (1986) defined three levels of certainty in litigation:

- Burden of proof
- Preponderance of evidence
- Standard of persuasion or belief

The three levels are frequently confused. In particular, the preponderance of evidence and the standard of persuasion are often "collapsed" (in the terminology of Gold) into a single statement of how convincing the evidence may be. It is more useful to think about them separately. Table 23.1 presents the three levels and key descriptors that anchor statements of certainty for each.

Causation—did the exposure cause the damage or not?—is a dichotomy, a true or false proposition. In order to decide, the pertinent facts must be presented, and this burden falls to the plaintiff or claimant. The burden of proof is the responsibility to establish those facts that must be proven if the case is to be resolved. The burden of proof falls to the claimant in an adjudication case and to the plaintiff in tort litigation. In principle, the claimant or the plaintiff is challenging the status quo and must provide the information necessary to establish his or her claim and upset the status quo. This means that the defendant shoulders less of a burden, in theory, because it is only necessary to rebut the claim or assertion, not to establish beyond doubt the absence of culpability or responsibility. In practice, the defendant also usually has substantially greater resources and essential information that the plaintiff lacks. Likewise, in an adjudication proceeding, the insurance carrier or agency receiving the claim normally has much greater access to expertise than the claimant. Such cases therefore often end up with an agency or defendant protecting its position with amassed available evidence on the one hand against an incompletely documented claim of damage on the other. Such claims are often supported by facts of the case that establish the potential for harm but that leave a large degree of uncertainty as to the damage that actually took place in that individual case.

Table 23.1. Standards of Evidence

Strength of Evidence
• Relates to burden of proof
• A statement on the means by which an event occurs and the uncertainty of knowing
• Hierarchy (items above the line are persuasive; items below the line are not)
Empirical evidence
Inferred evidence
<u>Informed opinion</u>
Speculation
Preponderance of Evidence (Frequentist)
• Interpretation of a causal association
• A statement of whether the model suggests an association in fact, taking into account the uncertainty
• Hierarchy (items above the line are persuasive; items below the line are not)
Presumptive
Probable—"more likely than not"
<u>Most probable among causes</u>
Possible
Standard of Persuasion/Belief (Subjectivist)
• Degree of uncertainty associated with a specific conclusion
• Operates for both witness and judge/adjudicator/jury
• Hierarchy (items above the line are persuasive; items below the line are not)
Certain "beyond reasonable doubt"
Probable
<u>"Reasonable medical certainty"</u>
Possible

The burden of proof cannot be described by a statement of certainty, because it is a statement of fact, not supposition. Whether it has been met can be described by a statement about the strength of the evidence. Individual elements of evidence may be compared and assessed for strength and weight. Table 23.1 also presents a hierarchy of the strength of evidence used to discharge the burden of proof; the higher in the hierarchy, the stronger the type of evidence. Informed speculation, permitted in the post-*Frye*, pre-*Daubert* era, is no longer acceptable; it was always the weakest level of evidence. Informed opinion is stronger because the opinion can be based on statements of uncertainty and general principles with more rigor than speculation. However, inferred evidence (drawn from studies that relate to but are not specific to the individual case) and empirical evidence (actual data from pertinent studies) are much stronger.

Whichever the situation, what ultimately matters is the preponderance of evidence when the evidence on both sides is reviewed. If the evidence on both sides is weak but marginally stronger on one side than another, that satisfies the standard of "more likely than not." Adjudicators and judges may be unsure just how important a particular bit of evidence may be, and this may be the deciding factor in the case. If the evidence on the two sides is extensively documented beyond dispute and is in every respect (within reason) equally matched, then a wispy bit of data on one side that has not been effectively refuted may tip the balance. Courts take into account the strength of the evidence, but it is the weight that counts most.

The preponderance of evidence is described by statements of certainty. These statements of probability have been called "frequentist probability" because they refer to the relative frequency of events in a sequence of experiments or, in epidemiology, a time period of risk. The corresponding hierarchy of certainty for the preponderance of evidence is also presented in Table 23.1. Terminology is crucially important here. "Possible" is taken to mean less than probable, therefore less than 50 percent certain and therefore not likely. The word "possible" therefore implies that the evidence does not favor a causal role for the factor involved, even if it admits that there may be an association. A risk factor that increases a person's risk some of the time or only a little for an outcome that is relatively common in daily life cannot be said to be the probable cause, but may be a possible cause among others. This does not establish causation but may carry some weight in certain circumstances. For example, if it can be demonstrated that the preponderance of evidence favors the cause as a contributing factor but not the sole or principal cause, then the possible cause of the condition may become a probable contributing factor. Under some adjudication systems, this may be enough to establish the claim. More generally, however, the most likely exposure among possible causes is the first solid level of certainty likely to be persuasive, and "probable"—more likely than not—is the general standard for certainty. Where an association is well established as the primary and most likely cause in the great majority of cases, it is sometimes still adopted as a "presumption" by law or policy, as described below; that is, the association is assumed to be causal unless demonstrated otherwise through rebuttal.

The standard of persuasion or belief is the degree of confidence imparted to the adjudicator or jury and internalized by them in making their decision. It is a psychological factor for all parties to the case, including the expert witness him- or herself, but it plays a critical role for the judge, jury, or adjudicator. It is a statement about the security of supposition in the face of the unknowable. It reflects the effort required to overcome the subjective uncertainty the adjudicator may feel over the decision and over not knowing what really happened. This statement of certainty has been called "subjectivist" by Gold because it reflects subjective comfort in arriving at the conclusion.

Table 23.1 also presents a hierarchy of certainty for the standard of persuasion. For the adjudicator to believe that it is "possible" that the putative cause resulted in the outcome is not enough. For this reason alone, highly speculative lines of argument and extraneous facts are usually counterproductive. They often convey a sense of weakness of argument that undermines confidence in stronger evidence, and they cloud the perception of adjudicators that there is one clear answer to the problem. A conclusion with "reasonable medical certainty" implies a considered judgment that the relationship is probable but that there is a range of uncertainty around the judgment that may include the possibility that the relationship is not causal. In the absence of definitive evidence, the burden of decision-making placed on the adjudicator is increased. The expert witness, after exercising informed judgment, cannot say for sure, although he or she is inclined on balance to accept the relationship as causal. The adjudicator, with less technical insight, must now apply lay judgment a second time (having first decided whether to accept the expert witness as authoritative), in effect choosing somewhat arbitrarily where he or she will fall within the range of uncertainty implied by the expert witness. "Probable" is not only much stronger, but use of the term implies that the range of uncertainty is much narrower, giving the adjudicator much less room to apply personal judgment (assuming that he or she accepts the expert witness's formulation). Certainty "beyond reasonable doubt" approaches the much higher standard used in criminal cases and is uncommon in these cases.

Gold has pointed out that the frequentist and subjective probabilities are often conflated into a general statement of likelihood. He points out that this confusion distorts the proper analysis of the case in several ways. It devalues the preponderance of evidence because it confuses the notions of weight of evidence and the most convincing evidence, or that evidence most likely to make an impression. It makes it difficult to sort through complicated chains of logic, each step of which is associated with a conditional probability in which the "more likely than not" standard must either apply to each sequential step in the logic (a frequentist approach, relaxing the expected rigor of the testimony) or to an overall summation of the argument (a subjectivist approach, increasing the standard for accepting the testimony). Collapsing also tends to favor certain types of evidence, such as epidemiological studies, that yield clear statements of probabilities and estimates, even though the standard for resolving medical disputes is a conclusion about an individual case, which may be exceptional or for which there may be particular circumstances. It also tends to focus attention on a particular estimate or probability, even though a range or set of values may be more appropriate to the case. Finally, Gold points out that decisions are made on the basis of persuasion—the level of subjectivist probability—not by the other levels of certainty. These are of course critical in arriving at the final level of persuasion, but it is ultimately the confidence in the minds of the adjudicators that decides the case. That depends on the presentation of the case and the expert's explanation of the significance of the evidence.

THE ROLE OF EPIDEMIOLOGY

Epidemiology has become one of the most powerful tools in modern tort litigation and adjudication for occupational and environmental hazards. The epidemiologist is now an essential expert for the resolution of many issues involving health outcomes following exposure to hazards. However, epidemiology is not enough.

Epidemiology is fundamentally a science of generalizations. The basic approach of epidemiology to estimating risk is to measure the experience of a population of individuals with the expectation that, all other things being equal, the overall risk for the group will be a valid estimate for most members of the group. Epidemiology has become increasingly valued in health-related cases precisely because it is a powerful tool for generalization.

However, epidemiology has limitations precisely because it is a science of generalizations. That is its great strength, but also its great weakness. When applied to class actions, generalizations make sense because one is considering patterns in a large population. However, most litigation involves individual plaintiffs, and the individual circumstances of the case must be separately considered. (This is also true in adjudication systems, such as workers' compensation; most legislative acts require that individual consideration be given to each claim.) Thus, epidemiology can inform the expert witness with a description of what happens most of the time or what is most probable, but the interpretation still must be brought to the level of the individual case. This may mean demonstrating that the plaintiff or claimant is similar to a group at demonstrably high risk; or that he or she is different and therefore belongs to a subgroup; or that he or she has unique characteristics, so the risk is not adequately described by summary statistics. This is where a well-prepared, knowledgeable medical expert can play a critical role.

Epidemiological studies have the great advantage of reflecting human experience and the great disadvantage of being generalizations. The science of epidemiology describes patterns in populations, and from this, one infers the most likely history or the most likely future risk in an individual case. However, studies on populations are not the same as predictions for individuals. Individuals may or may not conform to the pattern of characteristics in a population or a relevant subgroup. Individuals have life histories and risk factors that exist in combinations in one person but as frequencies in groups, scattered among individuals in a population. Thus, it is very important to separate three roles of epidemiology as a science in providing evidence for a causal association:

- Observational data that relate the risk factor (putative cause) and effect and provide evidence on a statistical basis from population-based science for causation, even though causation cannot formally be proven by epidemiology
- Frequentist predictions for individuals, based on an estimate derived from the experience of a population from which they were drawn or that they are presumed to resemble
- Population studies that can be used to attribute (but not apportion) cause in a large group, demonstrating that an outcome is associated with a particular occupation, hazard, or exposure
- Descriptive studies that put a problem in context, such as the number of people exposed to the hazard

Causation is an especially elusive concept applied to epidemiology. Human populations are vastly more complex than experimental systems, subject to numerous influences on health, behavior, and social adjustment. Each individual in the population may be subject to numerous other exposures that influence the outcome of interest. Although these are called "confounding" factors, they are often every bit as important in determining the outcome as the risk factor under study; it is a mistake to dismiss them as merely sources of bias. In the presence of numerous "confounding" factors, clear associations demonstrated in epidemiological studies are remarkable observations, with three likely explanations: an association, a statistical chance event, or a bias in the study method. If the latter two "false" outcomes are excluded, the association that remains is not necessarily causal in nature. Often, the Hill criteria (explained in Chapter 2) are applied in such cases and have become popular in courtroom testimony. However, this is incorrect. The Hill criteria are general guidance within the framework of epidemiology and are neither definitive nor grounded in the weight of evidence.

For the epidemiological science to be brought down to the specific case, the science must be understood and then interpreted with knowledge of the circumstances of the specific case. The medical expert contributes most to understanding in going from the broad generalization, which is called "general causation" in American law (does x make y happen?), to an opinion on causation in the particular case (did x make y happen in this individual?), which is called "special causation." This requires an expert who understands the epidemiology and also understands the individual. OEM physicians spend their entire careers doing just this.

Another critical issue is how to apply scientific evidence when the standard is "more likely than not," rather than scientific certainty. In other words, what would epidemiology and biomedical sciences be like if the standard for conclusions (not necessarily individual experiments) were 50 percent rather than 95 percent certainty? What would be the role of the doctrine of "falsification" (the notion that a theory cannot be proven, only disproven) if the standard for accepting a theory were only the weight of evidence rather than a single fact that the theory cannot explain? In effect, this is the issue that confronts the expert in developing a theory of what happened in the individual case, also known as "framing."

Here, epidemiology faces a serious methodological limitation that it has not acknowledged within the discipline. Inference based on conventional "frequentist" statistics are based on an a priori probability: what are the chances of something happening in the future, extrapolated from what happened in the past? An a priori risk is meaningful only before the event has occurred. After the event has occurred, its occurrence is no longer a prediction, and its causes must be sorted out; the risks must be put into the context of an individual risk profile, which requires knowledge of the "posterior" probabilities, or the probability of an association in the past once the even has occurred, however unlikely it may have been going forward. There are some experts who believe that conventional statistics cannot be applied in such cases and that Bayesian statistics are more appropriate, as they are in determining diagnosis in a clinical case. Perhaps because of their complexity, novelty in court, and how difficult they are to explain to nonstatisticians, this is never done in practice. It is at this point that the argument for medical dispute resolution should be based on individual evidence rather than epidemiology alone. Because Bayesian statistics are simply not used, notwithstanding the logic for applying them, epidemiological evidence is always of the conventional "frequentist" variety. (See Chapter 21 for a similar argument applied to workers' compensation.)

The frequentist point of view requires that the epidemiologist place him- or herself in a position in the past, before the event occurred, and to determine whether the probability of the illness or injury was high or low before it occurred. The "bright line" in that construction is whether the risk estimate (relative risk, standardized mortality ratio, or odds ratio) is consistent with a doubling of risk in absolute terms, because a doubling of risk corresponds to the weight of evidence for one individual in the population, all other things being equal. A doubling of risk means both that it is more likely than not that a particular cause or hazard was associated with the outcome in any one case, and also that half the cases are associated with this hazard or cause. It can therefore be applied to the individual or to the characterization of group risks, and therefore it confers eligibility for a "presumption" (the policy that a given case with a given association will automatically be accepted as causal unless there is good reason to think otherwise). For any one case arising out of a group of, say, workers with a risk that is doubled or more (for example, a case of kidney cancer arising in a firefighter), it can be presumed that unless the case had unusual features, the condition was as or more likely than not to have arisen from the cause or hazard. In workers' compensation, presumption is an important way of simplifying procedures and recognizing risk among occupations and workers exposed to particular hazards. In civil litigation, doubling of risk is strong evidence that the association is causal, because it is a relatively strong association and explains the outcome.

The rationale behind making a doubling in risk a criterion for presumption requires some explanation if it is not already obvious. The standard of an exact balance of probabilities means, in this context, that the risk of developing a bad outcome arising from the hazard is equal to the risk of the outcome arising from other causes, or for simplicity, in the general population. In statistical terms, therefore, the attributable risk from the hazard is equal to the expected risk. The balance of probabilities also means at least equal odds, or 1:1, or an odds ratio of 1. A balance of probabilities also means that the overall probability that the condition was due to the exposure or putative causal factor in the population under study is 50 percent, and one half equals the other half. A relative risk of 2 or an SMR of 200 means that the risk due to the exposure is equal to the risk of the general or comparison population. (If the risk of the general population is 1, then a relative risk of 2 can be thought of as 1 plus 1 divided by 1.) This in turn corresponds to an SMR of 200, an odds ratio of 2, or an attributable risk fraction 100 percent of expected. Therefore, if an epidemiological study has a relative risk of 2, then all other things being equal, it is strong evidence for the balance of probabilities and favors the conclusion that there is a causal association by legal standards of civil litigation, although not by the standards of science.

In practice, the criterion of a doubling of risk can be liberally applied, as it should be, given the uncertainties and the wide confidence intervals surrounding most of the available estimates. This criterion still excludes many disorders for which there is a clear association but for which nonoccupational risk factors appear to be much more important in determining risk.

PRESUMPTION

Modern presumption developed as a simplifying doctrine within the workers' compensation system. The concept of presumption makes sense when a disorder is well known—and well documented—to be strongly associated with particular workplace or environmental conditions. A claimant who presents with a particular diagnosis or type of injury in the particular setting that is characteristic for the disorder is presumed to be eligible for compensation and benefits, as long as the conditions are documented.

The justification for presumption is that the disease is either so common within a particular occupation or so rarely found outside certain occupations that any given claimant almost certainly developed the disorder as a result of work-related exposure. The simplest example is mesothelioma, which, in the presence of a work history suggestive of exposure to asbestos, is almost universally accepted as work related. The most controversial presumptions are those for elevations in risk of common disorders. This is the general problem with presumption in the case of most adverse health outcomes relevant to occupations such as firefighting, where lung cancer has been a persistent issue.

In practice, presumption takes one of three forms:

- Scheduled or "prescribed" occupational diseases
- Rebuttable presumptions
- Legislated entitlement programs

Scheduled or prescribed occupational diseases are accepted without any questioning of their association with exposure. Much of the legislation proposed in the middle of the first decade of this century for solving asbestos litigation scheduled asbestos-related diseases. Schedules are also common in countries other than the United States and Canada.

A rebuttable presumption is a policy that a disease will be considered as arising out of work unless there is a reason to dispute (rebut) this conclusion. This is the most common type of presumption in the United States and Canada. The rebuttal is based on the circumstances of the case and the characteristics of the individual worker. The general association between the disorder and occupation is not itself disputed, only the association in the particular case. Although a rebuttable presumption may be contested by the employer, the burden of proof is on the insurance carrier or the employer to demonstrate why the claim should not be accepted. Many rebuttable presumptions are passed as legislation: The states of California and Virginia have enacted rebuttable presumptions for chronic obstructive pulmonary disease or cancer for firefighters, and for myocardial infarction for firefighters and police.

Legislated entitlement programs are presumptions that have been written into law—for example, the Black Lung Benefits Program.

Ideally, rebuttable presumptions should be limited to disorders in which the group risk is at least doubled, such that in every case, the odds are as or more likely than not the result of work-related factors. However, legislated schedules are often based on notions of risk that cannot be documented scientifically or that are historical, but not necessarily current. Once legally established, it is almost impossible to remove such provisions.

Presumption rests on a set of assumptions that are rarely examined in detail. A general presumption of risk rests on the conclusion that any given claim from a particular group (such as workers exposed to lead) for a particular disease (such as lead poisoning) that comes before the adjudication agency is (much) more likely than not to be work related. The claim can be expedited on that assumption. Presumption requires that the individual case match circumstances known to give rise to the condition and that the case is drawn from a specific, defined population known to be at risk. As a practical matter, the probability that the injury came about because of any other cause must be so low that assessing causation is not worth the administrative effort.

This level of certainty may be achieved in two ways:

• Exclusive causation (e.g., pneumoconioses)
• General presumption of risk

Exclusive causation is easy: There are few nonoccupational causes of some diseases (such as silicosis), and the question is only where and when exposure occurred.

General presumption of risk is much more problematic. The analysis of presumptive occupational causation in a disease that is not unique to occupational exposures is a process with multiple steps. First, the association with occupation or, preferably, a specific occupational exposure must be demonstrated. Usually, this is done by means of epidemiological studies, from which a population-specific relative risk (called "population risk") is derived. Finally, the criteria have to be shown to apply in the individual case. Then, rebuttals are formulated and presented or anticipated. These actual hypothetical rebuttals are addressed in the report on file to ensure that other causes have not been overlooked.

Presumption must satisfy the usual compensation standard of proof that the occupational cause must be "more likely than not" responsible for the outcome (giving the benefit of the doubt to the claimant). Therefore, a general presumption of risk requires demonstration that the risk associated with occupation must be at least as great as the risk in the general population. This can be shown if the usual measure of risk in epidemiological studies is at least double the expected risk, making allowances for uncertainty in the estimate. Therefore, a general presumption of risk is only justified if there is a consistent and plausible association with occupation, and the magnitude of risk is at least double that of the general population.

General presumption of risk, on the basis of population estimates, assumes that all members of the population or occupation share in the pooled risk about equally or randomly, and that it is more likely than not, in the individual case, that the cause of the condition is work related. In terms of epidemiology, presumption reflects an attributable risk that is greater than the expected risk in an unexposed or general population. One cannot know for certain that any individual case drawn from the population is due to this exposure, but the odds are enough that it is a reasonable working assumption. A general presumption of risk is not the same as identifying an association, which can be any magnitude. A general presumption of risk implies that the elevated risk is sufficient in magnitude to make it more likely than not that in the individual case the cause of the disorder was related to work. A presumption means that there is not only a relationship, but that it is strong enough and consistent enough to be causal, and that it accounts for more than half of the cases of the disease. Both assume that some association with the exposure or occupation has already been proven to a reasonable standard of scientific or legal proof.

When population risk data are applied to individual cases, there are two questions to be considered in evaluating the association between a putatively work-related condition and occupational exposure: (1) How strong is the evidence for an association? and (2) How strong is the association itself? The Bradford Hill criteria (outlined in Chapter 2) address the former but not the latter. For population risk data to be useful as applied to the individual, however, some indication must be given that the individual risk, inferred from the strength of the association in the population, is at least as great as that from other causes not associated with occupation. This criterion must be satisfied before concluding that an occupational cause is likely to be causal in an individual case. The doubling criterion for epidemiological data does this on a population basis and makes it much easier to argue causation in the individual case. Its value is in evaluating a general presumption that all (or the great majority of) workers in a given occupation are at risk. The specific case must still be evaluated individually. When a general presumption of risk cannot be made, individual assessment of risk should be used to deal with the merits of the case. Some observers believe that in some jurisdictions, such as Texas, risk doubling has been elevated by judicial decision to the exclusive basis for accepting causation in civil litigation. This may be going too far, because epidemiological findings have too much inherent uncertainty, potential for dilution of risk estimates, and potential for bias to be so doctrinaire.

A general presumption of risk is not easily justified or defended for weak associations or when diseases are common in the general population. A more productive approach may be to take the claims on a case-by-case basis, examining individual risk factors and overall risk profile. A general presumption of risk is more easily applied to unusual disorders with high relative risks, particularly when they are unique to or characteristic of certain occupations.

The expert must apply the population risk to the individual case as guidance, not as an accurate estimate of personal risk. A population risk, which conforms to the past experience of the population under study, is only an estimate of the individual risk. Characteristics of the individual—such as age, length of employment, family history, and lifestyle—may substantially modify the individual risk profile. For an individual with few risk factors for the disorder, the population risk may be an overestimate of total risk but an underestimate of the risk due to occupation. Conversely, for an individual with many nonoccupational risk factors for the disorder (or occupational risk factors unrelated to a claim), the population risk may be an underestimate of total risk but an overestimate of the risk that can be attributed to occupation. Rebuttal rests on assessing personal characteristics on a case-by-case basis.

WITNESSCRAFT

There are skills to serving as an expert witness, just as there are skills a physician must master as a clinician. These skills suffer neglect when the expert becomes absorbed in on his or her own presentation skills and value to the case. They flourish when the expert puts ego aside and concentrates on the case.

The responsible expert should be prepared and should know the relevant literature. This does not mean stopping when one finds a passage or evidence supporting a conclusion. This means reading beyond the literature that supports one's position, knowing the arguments on the other side, and being aware of controversies that affect the conclusion.

There is a natural tendency for highly educated people to lapse into the language of their discipline because it is precise, comfortable, and establishes authority. However, it is a destructive tendency that must be resisted in testimony and reports. The expert must cultivate the skill of describing things in common words, explaining complicated things simply, and translating jargon into everyday language. This also means knowing exactly what the jargon means (it can be very embarrassing to have one's definition of a medical term questioned by a knowledgeable lawyer).

The best experts also have a sense of how technical terms are actually used in conversation between experts, as well as how the words would be defined, formally and in common language. For example, the word "neoplasm" is formally defined as a new tissue growth that may be benign or cancerous, but the term is almost never used in that sense outside of pathology textbooks. The specific word "neoplasm" is almost never used between physicians in conversation except as a euphemism for suspected cancer; when that word is used, usually with a pause, it strongly implies that one physician is expressing to the other, if only subliminally, that he or she is worried that a patient's mass is indeed cancerous despite indeterminate tests, and it implies that the physician is trying to figure out how to manage the expectations of the patient in the face of uncertainty.

The expert examines the internal evidence of the case, paying particular attention to anomalies and unexplained facts, which might be the key to alternative explanations. The expert places the case in the context of the literature and external, mostly scientific, evidence, demonstrating how the case fits the profile described by the literature or how the individual case is sufficiently different that the literature does not apply.

The expert will be expected to produce his or her current CV. This should be complete, with explanations entered for all lapses in credentials, periods out of practice, or major career changes, particularly if they are unusual. Unexplained gaps or discontinuities in practice invite scrutiny and challenge at the time of deposition. The expert will need to supply a list of cases in which he or she served as a witness in recent years, indicating which were on the side of the plaintiff and which were for the defense. (The time period varies with the jurisdiction.) If testimony in recent cases has all been on one side or the other, the opposite side will take it as evidence of bias; and if the testimony has been balanced, the opposite side will insinuate that the expert's opinion is for hire. That is how the game is played.

Discovery is the process by which all the records and documentation held by one side are made available to the other. It occurs before trial and is intended to level the playing field so that, as much as possible, the factual evidence can be agreed upon and there will be no surprises. The expert's notes and records are "discoverable" and should also be produced at the time of deposition and trial. These records include marginal notes, personal comments, sticky notes, handwritten outlines, interim and rough drafts, and analyses that may have been preliminary and possibly incorrect at the time. If they show up in a discovery, they will be legitimate subjects for inquiry, and the most embarrassing or inappropriate will certainly be flaunted by the opposing counsel. The result is usually to make something irrelevant to the case into a major issue prejudicial to the expert. Experts should keep their files free of this extraneous material, refrain from making marginal notes, never make rough drafts, and never write on any document that is discoverable.

Bills and invoices should be kept, but in a discoverable file separate from the records of the case. The expert will be asked to disclose his or her rate, and opposing counsel will usually imply that it is too high and that the expert has been bought. An extremely high fee tends to work against the credibility of an expert. However, an extremely low fee raises eyebrows (unless the expert is working "pro bono"— donating his or her time).

The expert must keep a record of key documents, sources, and reference materials on which the expert "relied" in coming to a decision. Most experts base at least part of their opinion on common knowledge in the field. That common knowledge is very likely to be questioned if a specific, relevant textbook passage or authoritative source is not added to the list. Courts are not very tolerant of long lists of standard textbooks or general references: they expect specific articles, chapters, and page numbers. The expert should make copies of all documentation "relied upon," because the lawyer on one side is often required to furnish copies of the relevant textbook pages or articles to the opposing side.

The lawyer will ask for time to "prepare" the expert before trial or deposition. This preparation time is immensely valuable and should not be rushed. The expert is usually focused on a particular technical issue or theory of causation. Because the expert is rarely involved with a case every day for days on end, it is easy to lose track of the sequence of events, names and events that are pivotal in other aspects of the case, and the meaning of the hearing within the overall process (for example, if it is to try the case, to qualify a class action, or to establish admissibility of evidence). The lawyer, however, lives with the case and should, by the time of deposition and trial, have a better knowledge of the facts of the case than the expert. The lawyer will refresh the expert's memory on many forgotten aspects of the case that may come up. The lawyer will want to hear, one last time, what the expert plans to say and how he or she will say it. This is also a time when the lawyer will impress upon the expert the particular legal burden of proof in the case and terminology that has special meaning in that jurisdiction.

Depositions are pretrial question sessions in which lawyers examine and cross-examine experts and other witnesses on the record. They will be available to the judge and the evidence provided in deposition may be used later in trial. The purpose of the expert's deposition is to discover the expert's argument, command of the evidence, and theory of the case before the trial. It is an important step in the case, but only rarely is testimony given in deposition later discussed at the trial itself, and then only when it is flagrantly contradictory or when it appears that new testimony is being introduced at the trial that was not covered in discovery and deposition. Deposition testimony is often important in signaling to the opposing side the strength of the case and motivating them to settle.

There is a predictable pattern to questioning on the stand and in depositions. Counsel for the side that has called the expert will usually start first, and one of the first items covered will be the qualifications of the expert. The expert should show neither arrogance nor defensiveness; no matter how much emphasis the attorney places on them, qualifications are only to set the stage and justify why the expert has been called. Opposing counsel, starting cross-examination, will almost always start off with a pleasant and cordial manner and then turn aggressive and even hostile, often feigning outrage over some contentious point; one should always expect it. The expert should answer the question and refrain from giving a seminar on the topic. This is a situation in which less is often more, and a long-winded answer carries a risk of raising secondary issues, distracting from the pivotal issues, or creating misunderstandings that do not help the court. This is no time to deliver a sermon. The expert should not volunteer information. A good lawyer will already know the answer to every question he or she will ask and will adapt and change tactics in the event of an unanticipated response, leaving the expert one step behind. Experts who try to outsmart the lawyer often end up confusing and outsmarting themselves. "Trick" questions are perfectly acceptable in the courtroom, and the expert who cannot handle them, unpack their various parts, and explain the answers on the levels required probably should not be on the stand. The expert should take his or her time, answer thoughtfully, and stop when the question is answered without going further and introducing new and confusing elements into the discussion. If the deposition is being recorded on video, however, overlong pauses may seem like equivocation.

The trial is similar to the deposition in format, but it is a very different experience. All eyes will be on the witness. In the courtroom, unlike in a deposition, hesitation in giving answers gives the impression of insecurity and sometimes falsehood. The expert is bound to stick to what has been covered in the deposition and cannot introduce entirely new lines of argument or a new and undiscovered pivotal fact. At trial, it is never entirely clear whether the jury, or for that matter the judge, has actually understood the testimony. In general, juries seem to understand more than they let on, and trying to "read" a jury is hard enough for a lawyer and pointless for an expert.

Aids to testimony are distracting and should be kept to a minimum unless they make a major difference in understanding. Models, graphics, PowerPoint presentations, and other aids interrupt the flow of testimony and are often interpreted too literally by jury members, who may get hung up on a detail and miss the bigger picture. They are most useful in showing anatomical relationships, spatial relationships, and details of key pieces of evidence. They should be used by the lawyer, not the witness.

Lawyers are at least as smart as experts, and many of them are much smarter. Experts should never assume that they are smarter than the lawyer. One should not try to play intellectual games in his or her testimony, nor should one try to engage in one-upmanship or try to anticipate where a lawyer's line of questioning is going.

It is an accepted tactic for the opposing counsel to attack the qualifications, credibility, honesty, motivation, and competence of the expert. These attacks can be stinging but should not be confused with personally motivated attacks. Their only purpose is to impugn the evidence, and one easy but intellectually bankrupt way to do this is to show that the expert is undisciplined and untrustworthy. Baiting the expert in order to cause him or her to become angry or defensive is a sign that the opposing counsel has run out of steam and is frustrated in its efforts to counter the evidence. It is a desperation maneuver, especially at trial, because the lawyer risks appearing abusive to the jury. It is essential that the expert react not by losing control, but by remaining professional and therefore credible throughout the personal attack. It should be viewed as a backhanded compliment to the preparation of the case. It is not about the expert.

It is also important to realize that the counsel representing the side the expert is assisting is motivated to win the case, not to make the expert look good. The lawyer has a strategy and knows, or should know, how he or she plans to use the expert. The expert should have no strategy, because the case is not about him or her.

New experts are often concerned about what they should wear and how they will appear on the stand. This is a very minor part of being an expert witness. An expert does not have time to establish his or her persona and the depth of his or her understanding of the field in the short time available on the stand. As a result, much depends on first impressions. The expert should therefore look the part of a responsible and meticulous physician: professional, well-groomed, conservative in dress, confident but not arrogant, and careful in manner and use of words. Beyond that, the expert should look as neutral as possible, because anything that draws attention to the expert distracts from the case itself.

In preparation to do this kind of work, the OEM physician should have "errors and omissions" professional liability insurance, which goes beyond clinical practice. It is important to maintain a clinical practice at all times, because current engagement in providing patient care is important in establishing the expert's qualifications and credibility. Mixing plaintiff and defense work is helpful in establishing credibility, and argues that the expert is responsible and takes cases on their merits. Whether to advertise and list with commercial directories is a personal choice, but many experienced experts prefer not to do so, because it creates the appearance that they are "hired guns."

EVIDENCE-BASED MEDICAL DISPUTE RESOLUTION

Medical knowledge has many uses outside of medicine. When operating outside the medical profession, the physician must consciously accept that medical norms do not necessarily apply.

Extension of biomedical research into commercial applications in the pharmaceutical and biotechnology industries is an obvious example. In these settings, the principles of business and engineering run the show, not those of the physician or biomedical investigator. Medical knowledge is also useful to resolve conflicts arising from injury, regulation to prevent future risk, and public policy. When this occurs in the context of the resolution of legal disputes, the physician plays the role of expert, applying medical knowledge to a practical problem that is outside the context of medical practice or biomedical research and that is not governed by the rules of medical practice or research. In court, the judge runs the show, not the physician serving as a medical expert witness. The expert defers to the logic of the legal system.

On a practical level, the legal system lacks the capacity to evaluate the validity of knowledge as evidence and relies heavily on expert opinion. There are no broad, socially agreed-upon rules for the application of medical knowledge, public-health knowledge, or for that matter any scientific knowledge except in the rules of evidence and decisions of the law. This is particularly evident in tort litigation, when liability for causing injury is under consideration, and often rests on theories of disease etiology and the circumstances surrounding exposure to a hazard.

A similar problem once existed for the clinical practice of medicine. Over the last twenty years, an approach called "critical appraisal" has established norms for the acceptance of evidence in clinical practice that are now almost universally accepted. Critical appraisal is a systematic approach to evaluating the evidence based on clinical epidemiology; evidence-based medicine is the practice of medicine justified by valid studies correctly interpreted.

Is it possible to develop a framework for applying the knowledge of health and medicine that is similar to the concept of critical appraisal? How can the evaluation of medical knowledge be adapted to the rules of the dominant framework of dispute resolution in our society: the law? Is it possible to develop an evidence-based approach to the expert's work, which one might call "evidence-based medical dispute resolution"?

Thirty years ago, a movement toward evidence-based medicine revolutionized clinical practice. Critical appraisal of the medical literature and the reliance upon evidence-based principles by managed-care organizations and utilization-review organizations led to the adoption of evidence-based medicine as the dominant mode of clinical practice today. The concept of critical appraisal and evidence-based medicine was not embodied in legislation or enforced as governmental or judicial policy. This movement advanced for many years through education in medical schools, debate, and consensus until it was ready to be institutionalized in practice. It became the accepted norm because it met a need, satisfied a rising demand, and made sense to all participants. Evidence-based medicine did not end controversy in medical practice, but it confined the scope to the scientific issues and rooted controversy in evidence rather than unsubstantiated opinion.

The current state of affairs in the courts is not unlike the situation in medicine at the time clinical epidemiology was "invented." The "practice" of medical expert witnesses is not standardized or governed by a consistent set of principles. Each expert witness is essentially autonomous. An expert witness cannot link, at present, to a community of other experts who have a consistent view of how to approach a problem or interpretation. Medical practitioners thirty years ago were similarly autonomous. That all changed for medical practitioners as a result of increasing external demands for consistency and persuasion.

It should be possible to develop a similar framework for the evaluation of scientific evidence in legal settings. It will not be possible—or even desirable—to distill a set of rigid rules for dealing with scientific evidence in legal settings. However, if the broad outlines of reasonable interpretation can be agreed upon, all parties will have advanced much further and can concentrate on the factors of the individual case. There is a need for evidence-based medical dispute resolution.

There is no formula or easy set of rules that can be derived for the universal application of this approach to scientific evidence. What would evidence-based medical dispute resolution consist of? A rational approach to evaluating evidence in the health sciences requires both a capacity to generalize, usually on the basis of a population, and a capacity to individualize to the specific case. If the mechanism is known, the explanation enhances the credibility and therefore the persuasiveness of the conclusion. This approach should be useful in the development of a specific case and in guiding the development of the administrative systems in which it is used. Ideally, it should contain these elements:

- Epidemiology and the interpretation of population data
- Individualization of the evidence to the specific case, using methods of clinical medicine, toxicology, and (in the future) genetics
- Statistical treatment that does not necessarily rely on conventional assumptions designed for scientific studies
- An understanding of science that takes into account the social nature of the scientific enterprise, as shown in contemporary studies in the history and philosophy of science
- Adaptability to a variety of applications, including public policy, statutory adjudication systems, and tort litigation

RESOURCES

Gold S. Causation in toxic torts: burdens of proof, standards of persuasion, and statistical evidence. *Yale Law J.* Dec 1986;96:376–402.

Guidotti TL, Rose SG, eds. *Science on the Witness Stand: Evaluating Scientific Evidence in Law, Adjudication and Policy.* Beverly Farms, MA: OEM Health Information; 2001.

Jasanoff S. *Science at the Bar: Law, Science and Technology in America.* Cambridge, MA: Harvard University Press, Twentieth Century Fund; 1995.

Meufeld PJ, Colman N. When science takes the witness stand. *Sci Am.* 1990;262(5):46–53.

Muscat JE, Huncharek MS. Causation and disease: biomedical science in toxic tort litigation. *J Occup Med.* 1989;31(12):997–1002. [This paper explains the importance of a doubling of risk and why it is equivalent to the "balance of probabilities."]

NOTEWORTHY READINGS

Black B. Evolving legal standards for the admissibility of scientific evidence. *Science.* 1988;239:1508–1512.

Black B, Lilienfeld DE. Epidemiologic proof in toxic tort litigation. *Fordham Law Rev.* 1984;52:732–785.

Brent R. Medical, social, and legal implications of treating nausea and vomiting of pregnancy. *Am J Obstet Gynecol.* 2002;186(suppl 5):S262–S266. [A particularistic discussion of the *Daubert* case.]

Cohen FL. The expert witness in legal perspective. *J Legal Med.* 2004;25(2): 185–209.

Goss PJ, Worthington DL, Stallard MJ, Price JM. Clearing away the junk: court-appointed experts, scientifically-marginal evidence, and the silicone breast implant litigation. *Food Drug Law J.* 2001;56(2):2727–240.

Guidelines for the physician expert witness. American College of Physicians. *Ann Intern Med.* 1990;113(10):789.

Guidotti TL. Evidence-based medical dispute resolution in workers' compensation. *Occup Med.* 1998;13(2):289–302.

Guidotti TL. Evidence-based medical dispute resolution. In: Demeter S, Andersson GBJ. *Disability Evaluation.* 2nd ed. Chicago: American Medical Association; 2003:86–94.

Guthell TG, Hauser M, White MS, Spruiell G, Strasburger LH. "The whole truth" versus "the admissible truth": an ethics dilemma for expert witnesses. *J Am Acad Psychiatry Law.* 2003;31(4):428–431.

Hollingsworth JG, Lasker EG. The case against differential diagnosis: *Daubert*, medical causation testimony, and the scientific method. *J Health Law.* 2004;37(1):85–111.

Kulich RJ, Driscoll J, Prescott JC Jr, et al. The *Daubert* standard, a primer for pain specialists. *Pain Med.* 2003;4(1):75–80.

Meyer C, ed. *Expert Witnessing: Explaining and Understanding Science.* Boca Raton, FL: CRC Press; 1999.

Price JM, Rosenberg ES. The war against junk science: the use of expert panels in complex medical-legal scientific litigation. *Biomaterials.* 1998;19(16): 1425–1432.

Price JM, Rosenberg ES. The silicone gel breast implant controversy: the rise of expert panels and the fall of junk science. *J R Soc Med.* 2000;93(1):31–34.

Reference Manual on Scientific Evidence. 2nd ed. Washington, DC: Federal Judicial Center; 2000. [Use current edition.]

Science, Technology and the Law. Science and Technology Policy Forum. New York: New York Academy of Sciences, Science in Society Policy Report; 1998

24 REGULATORY AGENCIES

This chapter provides an overview of the principal regulatory agencies in the United States and a brief description of the much less complicated but province-specific regulatory framework in Canada. The regulatory frameworks for specific hazards, workplaces, special occupations, and environmental risk are discussed where these respective issues are covered elsewhere in the book.

The occupational and environmental medicine (OEM) physician should know the missions of these agencies as they pertain to both environmental risks and occupational health protection. However, this chapter is for general orientation only. Specific guidance from legal counsel or another authoritative and competent legal source should be sought for any question of law or for any question regarding jurisdiction of these agencies, particularly as it may apply to a particular issue. Do not rely on this or any other text or general reference book for legal guidance.

ENVIRONMENTAL PROTECTION AGENCY

The National Environmental Protection Act (NEPA) of 1970 created the Environmental Protection Agency (EPA), which soon became the largest and arguably most powerful regulatory agency in the United States government. Almost all significant environmental health protection and some occupational health functions fall within the purview of the EPA. NEPA gave EPA wide authority for environmental protection, including:

- Standards and enforcement for water quality and emissions (pollution release)
- Standards and enforcement for air quality and emissions
- Standards and enforcement for land disposal and hazardous materials
- Standards and enforcement for radiation and radioactive substances in the general environment, other than nuclear waste
- Standards and enforcement for solid-waste disposal
- Standards and enforcement for asbestos in school buildings
- Standards and enforcement for large-scale ecosystem disturbance such as stratospheric ozone depletion and climate change
- Standards, enforcement, and prioritization for abandoned hazardous waste sites, and management responsibility for abandoned sites of high priority
- Standards for pesticide residues in food
- Guidelines for indoor air quality and safe housing
- Protection of ecosystems and adverse effects within its mandate that affect endangered species (the Department of the Interior is the lead agency for this, however)
- Protection of oceans and wetlands
- Planning for and response to oil spills
- Registration and regulation of pesticides
- Occupational health protection for pesticide workers
- Occupational health protection for hazardous materials (hazmat) workers

- Registration and regulation of toxic substances
- Enforcement of standards and regulations under the applicable legislation
- Grant-making authority for environmental-protection infrastructure
- Research on environmental problems, both intramural (conducted by scientists within the agency) and extramural (funded by grants and contracts)
- Environmental monitoring and dissemination of information
- Reviewing and ability to deny approval of Environmental Impact Assessments, a comprehensive review of the environmental implications of any federally supported project
- Reviewing and ability to approve state implementation plans for air and water pollution control
- Promotion of energy efficiency consistent with the Energy Policy Act of 2005 by using its authority to stimulate use of renewable energy, mandate fuel efficiency and blending, and prevent greenhouse gas emission
- Management of the implementation by the United States of treaties and international conventions related to environmental protection
- Programs in support of environmental justice, children's environmental health, emergency planning, and community right to know

The EPA also has oversight authority over state, territorial, and tribal departments of environmental protection. With few exceptions, EPA does not directly regulate utilities, such as water distribution companies, because these are normally supervised directly by the state department of environmental protection. EPA does not handle local environmental issues that fall under state or municipal jurisdiction, such as landfills, although it sets standards and guidelines.

The EPA plays only a supporting role in many important environmental issues that are primarily handled by other federal departments. It is only peripherally involved in the following:

- Noise (local government agencies; EPA once did regulate ambient noise, but no longer)
- Protection of habitat (Department of Interior)
- Endangered species (U.S. Fish and Wildlife Service)
- Nuclear waste (Department of Energy, Office of Civilian Radioactive Waste Management)
- Wetlands management (U.S. Army Corps of Engineers)
- Indoor air quality (Consumer Product Safety Commission for building materials and mobile homes, local public-health agencies for safe housing)
- Traffic-related dust and noise (local government agencies)
- Emerging infections (Unless waterborne, EPA is not usually the lead agency for infectious agents; the Centers for Disease Control and Prevention provide this role.)

The EPA is organized by problem sector and by region. There are ten federal regions, each with a regional administrator and an organization chart similar to the federal EPA's, but proportioned to local issues and including some offices specific for problems, such as protection of the Chesapeake Bay in EPA Region 3 (based in Philadelphia and covering Maryland, Virginia, Delaware, Pennsylvania, and West Virginia). Aside from the staff functions and administrative offices, there are assistant administrators, who each manage several "offices" devoted to major divisions of the environmental mandate. The administrative divisions on the level of the assistant administrators include:

- Air and Radiation
- Enforcement and Compliance

- Environmental Information
- International Affairs
- Prevention, Pesticides, and Toxic Substances (which is mostly concerned with individual or categorical pollutants, and with administration of the Toxic Substances Control Act and pesticide registration)
- Research and Development (including major laboratory complexes in North Carolina, Cincinnati, Las Vegas, and elsewhere)
- Solid Waste and Emergency Response (which is unified by hazardous materials and mainly deals with toxic materials and covers Superfund, brownfields, underground storage tanks, and emergency management, including hazmat).

The EPA is one of the few remaining major regulatory agencies that retains intramural research facilities for work useful in setting and validating standards. This is counter to trend: OSHA is advised in this regard by the National Institute for Occupational Safety and Health; the Nuclear Regulatory Commission by the Department of Energy. However, this legislative trend appears to be reversing because the Food and Drug Administration, faced with a need for much better scientific grounding for its regulatory activities, has massively expanded its internal research infrastructure in recent years.

History

The history of EPA is perhaps best understood through the history of its legislative authority. The U.S. Environmental Protection Agency (EPA) came into being in 1970, the same year as OSHA, after the passage of the National Environmental Protection Act of 1970. A number of environmentally related agencies were detached from various federal agencies and consolidated to create the new EPA, which had the great advantage of bringing enforcement, state grants for environmental protection, standards setting, mission-oriented research, and training and education under a unified management structure. EPA also combined the authority to protect living species and to conserve ecosystems (mostly a domain of the Department of the Interior) with the authority to protect human health.

The EPA quickly established itself as one of the most powerful agencies in the federal bureaucracy. One reason for the influence EPA has exercised has been the intensity of public concern over environmental issues. The year NEPA was passed, 1970, was also the year of the first Earth Day commemoration (April 22, annually) and the crest of the popular environmental movement that started in the 1960s. Another reason was the considerable legal authority vested in the new agency; it had the power to obtain convictions resulting in jail terms and to block expenditures for huge public projects. However, an often underappreciated source of its influence was its large budget; this derived for the most part from the EPA's role in funding water projects, which in the early history of the agency made up a disproportionately large share of the federal budget for environmental protection and a significant source of funding for public works at the state level.

In 1970 Congress passed the Clean Air Act, which, with the Federal Water Pollution Control Act (which was amended in 1972), gave EPA huge and centralized authority over the two major worlds of pollution control of the day. The Federal Pesticide Control Act (1972) gave EPA authority over individual toxic chemicals, as well as media pollution, and the authority to ban DDT in 1972; this came in addition to the EPA's responsibility for administering the Federal Insecticide, Fungicide, and Rodenticide Act (1947). This authority kept growing with the Toxic Substances Control Act and the Resource Conservation and Recovery Act, which dealt with hazardous materials, both in 1976.

The Clean Water Act, also passed in 1970, gave EPA a mandate to act as a public-health agency that other environmental protection agencies, at the state level and in other countries, have usually lacked. This authority permitted one of the great public-health achievements of the time: the ban on lead in gasoline, which began in 1973 as a gradual phaseout to 1986.

In 1979 EPA introduced a major regulatory innovation known as the "Bubble Policy," which allowed local sources of air pollution to determine for themselves how they would manage their pollution, as long as their total emissions (within the "bubble") were in compliance. This innovation gave the agency recognition for regulatory flexibility and enhanced its authority over regulated sources of pollution. It also freed EPA from the need to prescribe specific control measures, which would have been very unpopular and would have constrained technology. Perhaps more important in the short term, however, the Bubble Policy allowed industry to make progress quickly by controlling emissions where it was easiest to do so. This created an early win for the agency and the expectation of further progress as technology improved. That same year, EPA ordered and sued to obtain cleanup at Love Canal, a highly visible toxic-waste disposal site in Niagara Falls, New York, a strategy that served as a model for managing hazardous waste sites.

On the other hand, EPA did not hesitate to ban chemicals outright, as it had DDT, and in 1978 the agency banned fluorocarbons in aerosol products as a measure to protect the stratospheric ozone layer and then banned PCBs in 1979.

In 1980 the agency had its authority expanded even further—and its budget increased by billions—by the passage of the Comprehensive Environmental Response, Compensation, and Liability Act (CERCLA), which created the Superfund for the remediation of hazardous waste disposal sites. Superfund faced its first challenge in 1981 in funding cleanup of the Valley of the Drums, an abandoned site for chemical waste dumping near Louisville, Kentucky.

In the mid-1980s, during the Reagan administration, the agency was criticized for pliant leadership and allegations of political favoritism. The founding administrator, William D. Ruckelshaus, was brought back and reappointed to bring credibility back to the agency; he brought in a new policy of transparency called the "Fishbowl Policy."

During the 1980s, Superfund, because of its magnitude and complexity, had increasingly come to dominate the agenda of the EPA. By the 1990s, the slow pace of cleanup of abandoned, illegal, or unclaimed hazardous waste sites under the Superfund program was widely seen as an embarrassment to the agency. However, there was progress on many other issues, notably air toxics, radon, watershed protection, prohibition of ocean dumping, and large-scale ecosystem health issues such as stratospheric ozone depletion, with EPA being the competent agency in the United States for the Montreal Protocol. In 1989 the Exxon Valdez tanker collision in Alaska and management of the resulting oil spill thrust the spotlight back on the EPA's responsibilities for ecosystem protection.

The 1990s were marked by further progress on a variety of fronts, especially once EPA faced less constraint from a more-sympathetic Clinton administration. The United Nations Earth Summit in 1992 had set a global agenda for sustainability as well as the traditional environmental missions of conservation and pollution prevention. EPA had the power and the mandate to advance the agenda in the United States, with congressional support, from the local level, with restrictions against passive cigarette smoke, to the planetary level, with bans on chlorofluorocarbons to protect the stratospheric ozone layer. New initiatives were seen in remediating "brownfields," industrial sites requiring cleanup for other land uses, which restored contaminated urban sites to productive use and allowed "in-filling" of the urban landscape for better regional planning and management of density.

The public-health mission inherent in the EPA's health-based standards was broadened, expanded, and elevated to an agency-wide priority with the creation of the Office of Children's Health Protection in 1997. Children's environmental health protection became a highly effective policy for crosscutting programs and public education. It was also politically neutral and unassailable, and therefore served for many years as a means of achieving bipartisan and community support for environmental protection initiatives, despite a polarized political environment.

The EPA also launched a variety of initiatives collectively referred to as "right to know," which expanded the information resources available to citizens and advocacy groups and brought transparency to environmental monitoring. As in the case of children's environmental health, this was politically neutral because it made information more accessible to all citizens, whatever their purpose.

During the administration of George W. Bush, EPA was widely perceived as taking a big step backward and becoming less effective. A case in point was the decision not to revise the regulation for permissible levels of arsenic in drinking water, despite new evidence suggesting a higher risk of toxicity than previously believed. Another was the diminishing number of enforcement actions taken by the agency compared to previous years. However, the agency generally maintained forward progress until the last years of the administration, when it was caught in a series of policy maneuvers that were more directly aimed at halting or reversing measures for environmental protection. One was an initiative and proposed legislation that would have amended the Clean Air Act in a bill called the "Clear Skies Act," which was perceived as weakening air pollution regulation; reducing control of emissions from power plants; and, toward the end, permitting unacceptable emissions and long-range transport of mercury. This initiative stalled in Congress in 2005. The low point for the agency in the 2000s, however, was probably when EPA Administrator Christie Todd Whitman, a former governor of Connecticut, reassured residents about the health risk of inhaled dust during rescue efforts at the site of the World Trade Center after the September 11, 2001, terrorist attacks. Within a short time, she was contradicted by studies suggesting significant respiratory effects. Administrators, of course, are dependent on their staff and expert advice, but in this instance there was also concern over the degree to which the White House may have influenced her remarks at the time, injecting politics into a scientific and health issue.

The environmental laws and regulations administered by EPA are too numerous to describe in this chapter, but some major acts are described in Chapter 12.

The direct role of EPA in occupational health is relatively narrow, but considerable in its sectors. EPA has regulatory authority over the application of pesticides, and as a consequence, its standards and enforcement procedures are critically important in agriculture. (Pesticide manufacturing comes under OSHA.) EPA also establishes procedures and monitoring programs for workers involved in cleaning up hazardous waste sites.

OCCUPATIONAL SAFETY AND HEALTH ADMINISTRATION

The Occupational Safety and Health Act of 1970 (OSH Act) established the Occupational Safety and Health Administration (OSHA) in the United States and its power to set and enforce federal standards for worksite safety and health. The 1970 OSH Act was passed to ensure employees legal protection against occupational injury and disease: "To assure so far as possible every working man and woman in the Nation safe and healthful working conditions and to preserve our human resources."

OSHA sets occupational-health exposure standards; requires safe work practices and specifically mandates some for serious hazards; requires maintenance of a log of injuries at the worksite (the "OSHA 300" log); requires training and communication regarding hazards; petitions courts on behalf of workers in case of imminent danger; inspects workplaces (although it is required to give advance notice of routine visits); and approves state programs. There are hundreds of standards covering machine guarding, materials handling, toxic chemicals, noise, radiation, exits, walking and working surfaces, sanitation, fire prevention, welding, staging and shoring, scaffolding, operation and design of machinery, and other hazards. If no specific standard is set for a workplace, there is a "General Duty Clause" in the OSH Act that states, "Employers are required to maintain a workplace free from recognized hazards." Temporary emergency standards can be set until permanent ones are established to protect workers when new hazards are introduced in the workplace.

History of the OSH Act and OSHA

Unlike the Environmental Protection Agency, which was created from the consolidation of several preexisting agencies, OSHA was newly created under its legislation. OSHA is also much smaller and narrower in its mission, and therefore more vulnerable to political challenges. OSHA is easiest to understand through an appreciation of its history.

Passage of the OSH Act was the result of a long and concerted effort on the part of organized labor. During the 1960s, there was growing concern about dangerous working conditions, and organized labor was at a high point of influence. OSHA was a response to this concern and, in practice, an extension of the oversight relationship already exercised by the federal government over its contractors. The states had been responsible for worker health and safety prior to 1970 by default. The OSH Act allowed individual states to develop their own state OSHA equivalents, as long as enforcement procedures and standards were at least as stringent as those of OSHA. Thus, the adoption of OSHA was more incremental than a break with the past.

The single most important part of the act is probably what is known as the "General Duty Clause," part of which reads: "[Each employer] shall furnish to each of his employees employment and a place of employment which are free from recognized hazards that are causing or are likely to cause death or serious physical harm to his employees." In theory, therefore, the act provides a strong mandate for worker protection and includes an implied expectation that hazards will be studied in order to be recognized. However, read another way, the General Duty Clause applies to hazards that cause "death or serious harm" and so may be viewed as intended to apply only to life threatening or potentially disabling risks. At the same time, the original act did not explicitly declare the right of a worker to refuse an assignment that may result in serious injury or death and not be punished for such refusal. That had to come later by regulation, almost as an afterthought, and as a Supreme Court ruling in 1980 (*Whirlpool v. Marshall*). This ambiguity pervades the act and its subsequent history.

Unlike the National Environmental Policy Act, which was passed the year before and created the Environmental Protection Agency, the OSH Act did not create a single, strong agency with enforcement powers, extramural funding capacity, and standards based on mission-oriented research. It created a group of individually weak organizations with divided responsibilities:

- OSHA, the enforcement agency, was embedded in the Department of Labor, rather than the department responsible for health (at the time, the Department of Health, Education, and Welfare), in order to align it with other labor standards.
- The National Institute of Occupational Safety and Health—a relatively small agency now absorbed into the Centers for Disease Control and Prevention—had a mission of research and training, and was given the mandate to propose new standards, most of which have not been adopted by OSHA.
- The Occupational Health and Safety Review Commission is the appeals body for OSHA citations.

Occupational health and safety standards then in existence had been written by industry associations and professional organizations; they were intended to be voluntary guidelines for management. They became mandatory for federal contractors under the Walsh-Healey Public Contracts Act of 1936, which, among many other provisions, required covered private companies providing services and products to the federal government to adhere to safety and sanitation standards. The OSH Act adopted by reference the Walsh-Healey standards, which consisted of relevant guidelines defining unsafe, unsanitary, and dangerous working conditions, and elevated them to the status of federal regulations for industry as a whole and created an enforcement agency to ensure compliance. By then, many of the standards and guidelines were already dated, however, and coverage of workplace hazards was not complete. For this reason, the initial set of OSHA standards also included then-current voluntary guidelines that represented a "national consensus" in 1970, namely those of the American Conference of Governmental Industrial Hygienists (ACGIH) and the American National Standards Institute (ANSI). The body of health standards that governs occupational health and safety in the United States is therefore more than forty years old, for the most part, and some provisions may be seventy years old.

Two mechanisms were adopted by OSHA for enforcing chemical safety. One was the Permissible Exposure Level (PEL), a limit on exposure to chemicals that is primarily based on the assumption that level of exposure (such as concentration in air) and duration of exposure can be treated as a product or a cumulative toxicity model in the form of an eight-hour, time-weighted average for the approximately 600 chemicals so regulated. Though approximately true for some chemical hazards, this is not so for many; but the ease of applying this toxicological simplification, the relatively low risk of toxicity at current levels, and the precedent and body of recommended standards of organizations such as the American Conference of Governmental Industrial Hygienists made this approach attractive and fairly robust. (Ceiling levels and Short-Term Exposure Levels—for chemical exposures in which peak exposures are more significant—were supplemental to the PEL approach.) The other approach was the bundled or comprehensive standard, which laid out in one package exposure limits, mandated surveillance, required personal protection, and special issues such as medical removal, as exemplified by standards on asbestos, arsenic, and lead. These three particular standards demonstrate a number of complications because of differences between the general industry standards and the construction standards for asbestos and especially lead; the calculation of allowable exposure for longer work shifts for arsenic and lead; and the medical removal provisions and criteria for return to work for lead, which differ slightly between the general industry and construction standards.

Notwithstanding the long history and general acceptance of the major part of its body of standards, OSHA was immediately ridiculed as being standards obsessed and lampooned in jokes and cartoons, which very effectively undermined its image and mission. Throughout this early period, OSHA emphasized voluntary compliance over stringent legal enforcement, but even so, the organization gained a reputation for heavy-handed enforcement and had to contend with numerous efforts to legislate exemptions to its jurisdictions. OSHA did exempt employers with ten employees or less from record-keeping requirements as a measure of "regulatory relief" and introduced a consultation service in 1975 designed to help employers, especially in small enterprises, achieve compliance with standards. A brief but apparently baseless scandal erupted during the Nixon administration in 1974 over whether OSHA enforcement was politically manipulated.

By then, the late 1970s, OSHA was getting a rather late start on new standards setting, which was intended to be a major role of the new agency. However, in the latter half of the decade, this became the priority. A watershed event in standards setting was the standard for benzene, which was the subject of a 1980 Supreme Court ruling that required documentation of the significance of a health problem and effectively introduced quantitative risk assessment into occupational health standards setting.

Among other initiatives, OSHA started the New Directions program (now called Susan Harwood grants) in 1978, providing small financial awards to support training employers and workers in occupational health and safety. OSHA also maintains a network of training centers to provide technical education for compliance officers and interested health and safety professionals in the private sector.

Under the Reagan administration, OSHA was a favorite target for allegations of regulatory abuse, but it scored a major victory when the cotton-dust standard was upheld by the Supreme Court, which held that cost-benefit analysis was not an acceptable basis for a health and safety standard. During the first half of the 1980s, OSHA was caught up in the deregulation effort of the time, which diminished its authority again, a process not helped by a series of messy and highly visible regulatory issues that were interpreted as either withdrawal from a commitment to worker protection or professional incompetence.

In order to be seen as responsive to employer's concerns, OSHA introduced the so-called "regulatory relief" package in the 1980s— a series of policy changes to reduce the perceived burden of federal regulation of industry. Rather than concentrating on eliminating hazards from the workplace, this policy emphasizes increasing use of protective gear such as respirators and earplugs. OSHA had allowed only temporary reliance on respirators and similar personal protective devices, which is seldom as effective as engineering controls. A more positive development was the Voluntary Protection Program, which enlisted employers as partners in cooperation for occupational health protection and helped OSHA's troubled relations with the employer sector. Outside of OSHA, however, many saw this and later partnership programs, such as the Alliance Program initiated during the George W. Bush administration, as effort recognition programs that did little to improve enforcement where it was actually lacking. In 2004 a report by the General Accounting Office questioned the effectiveness of such programs.

In 1991 the agency promulgated the Bloodborne Pathogen Standard in response to rising rates of occupational infection from hepatitis B and the risk of HIV among health care workers. This move was unique in having been directed by Congress in a rider to legislation. The standard appears to have been one of its most successful, paving the way for universal precautions and later amendments for the prevention of needlestick injuries (and the Needlestick Safety Act of 2000) and precipitating a major and sustained decline in transmission.

During the Clinton administration, OSHA's emphasis shifted to assistance in compliance with regulatory standards, building on the consultation program that provided technical assistance to employers who asked for it. Skepticism on the part of employers and reluctance to have attention drawn to their issues, even with the intent to avoid enforcement activities, reduced participation in this program.

In 2000, after years of preparation, OSHA faced its most severe test when it promulgated the standard on ergonomics, a well-documented regulation for the prevention of musculoskeletal disorders. (The ergonomics standard did combine low-back pain and repetitive strain injuries, which have different characteristics, into one regulation, which in retrospect may have been a mistake.) It was ferociously opposed by employer groups led by the United States Chamber of

Commerce, and despite a favorable review of the underlying science by the National Academy of Sciences, it was ultimately repealed by Congress in what was viewed as a stinging rebuke.

OSHA remained a weakened agency for the duration of the Bush administration. Its regulatory initiatives came primarily in the form of voluntary compliance and cooperative programs for voluntary adherence to guidelines, which largely vitiated the role of the agency in enforcing mandatory compliance with regulations. An example of this weakness was the manner in which OSHA, which had the responsibility to ensure the safety of workers so as not to compound the tragedy, was marginalized in the immediate aftermath of the September 11, 2001, terrorist attacks on the World Trade Center in New York, where its role was largely restricted to handing out respiratory protection on-site for rescuers who could be persuaded to use it. Later, it played almost no role in the investigation of the assault using anthrax, although almost all of the victims were exposed in the course of their work duties.

By the close of the Bush administration, OSHA seemed to be struggling mightily with two seemingly straightforward issues. The first was the appropriate hazard standard to be promulgated for prevention of a newly recognized serious lung disease (colloquially called "popcorn lung") caused by diacetyl and seen in commercial popcorn operations. The second was enforcement of regulations dealing with the imminent hazard presented by combustible dusts, specifically with respect to explosion hazards in the sugar and grain industries, for which there has been an applicable standard since 1987. Although enforcement of a major action arising from a fatal explosion in a sugar factory resulted in a large and highly publicized fine to the employer, what seemed to be an obvious and intolerable hazard appeared to be mired in confusion as OSHA discovered that seventeen different standards could apply. The issue was met with a National Special Emphasis Program rather than the emergency standard that was recommended by the Chemical Safety Board.

Under the Obama administration, new as of the time of writing (2009), OSHA is likely to have much more support in both Congress and the executive branch. OSHA has many more options open to it than in the past, among them the development of generic and class standards, adoption of recommended exposure limits (RELs) proposed by NIOSH, a return to process safety management as a key regulatory tool, a closer alignment with public-health agencies, the introduction of innovations and simplified approaches such as control banding, harmonization of occupational health standards with the European Union (where the process has continued to advance), and greater engagement with training and education.

OSHA has made several efforts to deal with the inertia of regulation by adopting generic or comprehensive standards for categories of exposure (one unsuccessful effort would have provided a template for regulation of carcinogens) and for policies that broadly support regulation—most notably the 1983 Hazard Communication Standard (also called "Right to Know"), which had the effect of raising worker awareness and capacity for self-protection.

OSHA also initiated an awards program for exemplary employers called the Safety and Health Achievement Recognition Program (SHARP), which involves a voluntary inspection.

Enforcement

Standards are enforced through inspections. Once a job hazard is encountered, it should be brought to the attention of the employer. If no action is taken, an employee may contact the OSHA area office, where the employee will be able to file a complaint in writing. All complaints are evaluated, and priority is assigned by the perceived severity of the hazard. On the basis of this, OSHA staff members decide whether to conduct an inspection. OSHA policy has been to inspect all potential serious violations within three working days.

The first priority for inspections is imminent hazard, when there is an immediate risk and action must be taken quickly to prevent the potential for death or serious injury. When there is evidence for this, the compliance officer normally requests voluntary abatement by the employer, and if it is refused, the officer seeks a court injunction against the employer to suspend operations until an inspection can be completed. The second priority is the investigation of fatalities or catastrophic events resulting in three or more employees hospitalized. These must be reported to OSHA by the employer within eight hours. The third priority is to respond to formal complaints from employees or other interested parties. Programmed or routine inspections come last and are prioritized by the safety record of the employer and the industry, or by the presence of potential hazards of concern.

Inspections for enforcement purposes are surprise visits; employers are not notified in advance unless there is a fatality reported, a clear reason why the inspection would require it, or an imminent hazard that should be corrected before an inspection is possible. There is an initial meeting with management (a workers' representative may be present) called the "opening conference," followed by meetings with responsible managers and employees, and a visit to the location of the suspected violation. Following the inspection, there is another meeting with management called the "closing conference," at which preliminary findings are discussed. OSHA then issues a report in the form of citations, which are outlined in a letter citing the specific violations and a date by which the hazard must be abated or the violation corrected. A fine may also be assessed. There may be follow-up inspections to determine whether a hazard has been abated.

The employer has the right to dispute the citations but must do so within fifteen days. The first level of appeal for citations by OSHA compliance officers is through the OSHA area director to the Occupational Health and Safety Review Commission, which uses a system of administrative judges with a final level of review by the commission itself. The counterpart appeals system for state OSHA plans is generally similar but involves state review boards.

Should a violation be found, fines are determined by how serious a risk the violation presents to workers. There are categories of violation:

- "Other-than-serious" violations
- Serious violations

- Willful violations
- Repeated violations
- "Failure to abate" a prior violation

Citations on grounds of imminent danger are very rare; when they are made, the shop is closed down immediately until the danger is corrected. Serious violations are those that have substantial probability of causing death or physical harm. If management shows "good faith" in trying to keep things safe, there is a reduction in the penalty and a further reduction for small businesses. Additional fines can be added for various reasons, such as failure to post notice of the violation within the required time period (three days) until it is abated. Additional fines and possible criminal sanctions are levied for falsifying or concealing records and reports, or for assaulting or interfering with a compliance officer.

Various factors are weighed before citations and fines are issued, such as the size of an employer's business, the seriousness of the violation, the apparent good faith of the employer, and any record of prior violations. After all these factors are taken into consideration, penalties are frequently minimal. Because it often costs considerably more to correct a hazard than to pay OSHA fines, abatement dates may be missed or ignored by employers. An employer may be assessed a civil penalty of not more than $1,000 for each day during which a violation continues past an abatement date. Extensions beyond the abatement date are common. During this time, employees may continue to be exposed to the hazard.

On the other hand, there is no limit on the dollar amount of a fine. In 1987 federal OSHA imposed a fine of $1.6 million on Chrysler Corporation's Newark, Delaware, plant for multiple violations. In 2005 the biggest fine in OSHA history, $2.78 million, was levied on Cintas, a laundry company in Tulsa where a worker was dragged to his death in a dryer and multiple willful violations were discovered. This is very unusual, however, and such cases are widely interpreted as efforts by OSHA to show visible strength.

Under Section 11(c) of the OSH Act, an employer is prohibited from firing or discriminating against any employee "because of the exercise by such employee on behalf of himself or others of any right afforded by this act." Specifically included in this section are the rights to file a safety and health complaint, to institute a proceeding under the OSH Act, and to testify at any hearings. Despite Section 11(c), however, many workers fear that their employer will nonetheless find grounds to discipline or even fire them on other grounds or on pretexts if they exercise their rights. Unfortunately, this appears to happen often enough to confirm such fears. Once an employee is singled out as a "troublemaker" by management, it is easy to accumulate real or imagined complaints that may lead to termination, ostensibly on other grounds.

State OSHA Programs

The enabling legislation for federal OSHA assumed that most states would eventually assume partial responsibility for occupational health and safety under broad federal supervision. Most were slow to do so. At the time of writing (2009), there are now twenty-six state programs, of which three cover only public employers. State regulations, as permitted under the OSH Act, are to be at least as strict as the federal law and may be even stricter in setting standards and enforcement policies. Much depends on financial resources available, however.

The story of the state agency in California is illustrative. California had been considered at the forefront of worker protection, largely due to the progressive administration in the state department. In 1987 the California state OSHA (CalOSHA) was rescinded by the governor from the budget and dissolved, although the state contribution to the agency represented only an $8 million expenditure per year. Fifty percent of CalOSHA's budget came from the federal government, and fifty percent came from the State Department of Industrial Relations. As budget cuts on the federal level reduced the federal contribution, maintenance of the state agency had become increasingly more difficult. After the governor's decision, California was covered by an office of federal OSHA that included many former CalOSHA employees. In an initiative referendum in 1988, voters restored CalOSHA, but by then many of the staff had changed careers or left their jobs at what was briefly the California office of federal OSHA in search of stabler careers. The net effect was a considerable weakening of the agency that became CalOSHA again in1991. CalOSHA was reestablished and restaffed and went on to regain its clout and to become an assertive regulatory agency again. However, its close call with oblivion underscores just how fragile state OSHA programs may become.

The Legacy of OSHA at Forty Years

How one views OSHA depends on who one sees as the victim in the enforcement of occupational health protection. Worker advocates see workers as the victims, with companies inflicting suffering on them through unhealthful working conditions and time pressures. This does not necessarily mean that workers are solidly in support of OSHA as the advocate of their best interests, however. Workers do not always see OSHA or other issues from a "worker" point of view. They hold their own political opinions and often view it as an example of regulatory excess, depending on their views. Employers and managers, on the other hand, show more consistency in their opinions against "government regulations." Their advocates typically see the employer as the victim, with OSHA, the workers, unions, and government in general inflicting excessive and unnecessary regulation, which causes delays, frustration, and increased costs. Intrusion into the production process is not easily accepted by the business manager or owner who expects to control that process.

OSHA has been widely seen as too weak on enforcement. What OSHA has accomplished generally, however, is the ever-greater and more-sophisticated appreciation of the problems of workplace health and safety. Nothing has been as important as the message that has come from the existence of OSHA: change the workplace, not the worker.

Until the passage of the OSH Act, personnel or industrial relations managers rarely had more than the most rudimentary safety and health training. Few industrial relations and personnel courses or texts contained more than a mention of theories of accident causation. Hazard control was delegated to maintenance or engineering departments. Top management was little involved in hazard controls. Supervisors in these departments were directly responsible to line management, whose major concern was production and not the improvement of working conditions. The safety director rarely had much influence or support from top management unless a major accident occurred. Many companies regarded accidents from a cost standpoint and retitled their safety and health director as the "loss control" supervisor. The old approach tended to consider safety issues only after an accident or illness had occurred. Then, attention was often focused on laying blame, especially on the worker who was seen as carelessly committing an unsafe act, rather than on correcting for human limitations in performance in an intrinsically unsafe environment. It may be said that attitudes toward safety on the part of management lag at least a generation behind the knowledge base of safety science (see Chapter 6), and by much more in some sectors. (Shipyards and hospitals are particularly slow in this regard.)

Today the situation is far from ideal, but it is much improved, as it should be after forty years. A vigorous effort has been made to clean up the workplace. A keystone of this effort has been the direct training of workers to recognize hazards, to participate in their control, to have the means to control them, to monitor hazards in the workplace, and to know and to exercise rights under the law.

MINE SAFETY AND HEALTH ADMINISTRATION

The Mine Safety and Health Administration (MSHA) is an agency within the Department of Labor. MSHA separated from OSHA in 1978 and took with it responsibility for occupational health and safety regulation in mines, including underground and surface mines and quarries. MSHA administers the Federal Mine Safety and Health Act of 1977. However, it had a much longer antecedent history prior to union with OSHA in 1970, and for most of its statutory life, it was part of the Bureau of Mines of the Department of the Interior, a status that ended with the OSH Act of 1970.

MSHA inspects underground mines four times a year and surface mines twice a year to assess occupational hazards. MSHA also has responsibility for approving respirators, the principal personal protective equipment for respiratory hazards.

In 1978 the research functions attached to MSHA's predecessor agencies were moved over to the National Institute for Occupational Safety and Health (NIOSH). In addition to supporting the certification of personal respiratory protection, which is the one MSHA responsibility that affects general industry, NIOSH conducts surveys for coal workers' pneumoconiosis through a medical surveillance program to assess progress in eliminating pneumoconioses.

Mining has always been among the most dangerous industries in the United States, as it is elsewhere. The history of coal mining in particular is inextricably entwined with occupational health and safety as well as society's understanding of occupational health risks over several generations (see Chapter 25). Mining presents many specialized hazards—mostly associated with underground mining—which was the major reason MSHA was removed from OSHA and restored as a separate agency. These specialized problems include dust exposure; tunneling and sinking shafts, and preventing their collapse; roof support and preventing roof collapse, roof falls (rocks detaching and falling from overhead), and outbreaks (rocks separating from the sides); pockets of explosive gas (methane, sometimes with hydrogen sulfide); explosive dust; diesel exhaust; safety and reentry during intentional explosions; ventilation; lighting; electrical hazards; fire (and generation of carbon monoxide); flooding; and mine rescue, which is a highly specialized field of emergency management. Underground mines are, of course, confined spaces and present many problems of access and egress; it is easy to get trapped during a mine accident. Surface mines, on the other hand, are usually more like large construction sites in their hazard profile.

Dust exposure is a particular and characteristic hazard, including silica in both underground coal and "hard rock" (noncoal, further divided into "metallic" and "nonmetallic" in the industry) mines that require excavation and drilling through rock, and coal dust in coal mines; pneumoconioses, especially silicosis and coal workers' pneumoconiosis, are therefore the signature occupational diseases in the mining industry. Historically, the high priority of respiratory hazards in mining has led to MSHA, rather than OSHA, becoming the leading agency in certifying respiratory protection equipment, although NIOSH conducts research on standards and testing for respiratory personal protection equipment.

The federal effort to regulate safety in mines began in 1891, with an act that set minimum ventilation requirements and addressed child labor, establishing a minimum age of twelve. The largest fatal industrial incident in U.S. history occurred in a coal mine in Monongah, West Virginia, in December 1907, when 392 men and boys working in the Fairmont Coal Company died in an underground explosion. Later in the month, another mine explosion in Dary, Pennsylvania, killed 239 workers. It was followed two years later by a mine fire in Cherry, Illinois, that killed another 300 miners. These mining disasters killed mostly immigrants from Italy and Hungary, not native-born Americans, and so had less impact on public opinion than they otherwise might have had, but the magnitude and frequency of the disasters still motivated Congress to pass legislation establishing the Bureau of Mines in the Department of the Interior, which was the predecessor to MSHA.

The Bureau had the responsibility of encouraging the exploitation of mineral resources and supporting the critically important extraction industries, as well as regulating safety. Its safety authority was limited to research and education. However, during the 1920s and 1930s mining fatalities and injuries increased, demonstrating that this weak approach was not working. The Bureau did not acquire the power to inspect mines until 1941, at which time a code of regulations was also adopted by Congress, largely through the influence of the United Mine Workers and its president, John L. Lewis. The Federal Coal Mine Safety Act of 1952 strengthened the agency in the coal sector, where occupational injuries were particularly common, severe, and often affected more than one worker in one incident; but the act did not give the Bureau the power to levy fines for noncompliance with regulations, leaving enforcement possible only through civil litigation. In 1966 these provisions, which in the 1952 act applied only to certain coal mines, were extended to all coal mines and to non-coal mines as well, but with still-weak enforcement measures. Meanwhile, sporadic mine disasters continued to plague the industry and mining communities, where the burden of health effects was also being felt in the form of coal workers' pneumoconiosis (colloquially called "black lung" and other respiratory diseases). In 1968 another mine explosion, this time in Farmington, West Virginia, very close to the Fairmont site, killed seventy-eight miners and abruptly drew attention to the extreme risk of coal mining. In 1969, the year before the OSH Act, the Coal Mine Safety and Health Act of 1969 was passed partly in response to the Farmington incident; the act required regular inspection of surface and underground coal mines based on risk, and it increased enforcement powers, including the authority to levy fines and to lay criminal charges.

In 1973 the Department of the Interior created the Mine Enforcement and Safety Administration (MESA) in order to separate occupational health and safety regulation in mines from the Bureau's larger mandate to support the extractive mineral industries. The Federal Mine Safety and Health Act of 1977 amended the 1969 coal act; brought together regulation of coal and non-coal mines; shifted MESA into the Department of Labor, as a sister agency to OSHA; and transformed it into MSHA, with greater enforcement powers. The act also created a Federal Mine Safety and Health Review Commission, parallel to the Occupational Health and Safety Review Commission, for appeals of MSHA citations and actions.

The 1980s and 1990s were characterized by a number of contentious enforcement cases, some of which involved allegations of fraud in monitoring dust levels and most of which reinforced the traditional stance of mine owners and operators as a sector among the most resistant to regulation in American industry. Mining is driven by commodities prices, which are highly volatile. The revenue generated by a mine, coal or non-coal, peaks when the price is high, but this generally does not last long. (The early 2000s, with the expansion of industry and the rapid development of China, have been an exception, and in the current economic climate as of this writing, prices have plummeted.) Mine owners are motivated to take profits in the short term while they can and otherwise to keep costs at a minimum in order to keep the operation sustainable when commodity prices are low. This economic motivation is often put forward as a reason for the resistance of mine owners and operators to changes in work practices and regulation.

During the George W. Bush administration, MSHA, like OSHA, emphasized partnership and voluntary programs with employers. Over the 2000s (as documented in a story in the *New York Times,* March 2, 2006), MSHA levied generally fewer citations for much smaller amounts and did not collect a large fraction of these fines.

During MSHA's three decades, it has generally been considered disappointing in its performance. Whether from resource constraints, lack of political will, or a few highly publicized incidents of irregularities, MSHA has been widely perceived as excessively deferential to the industry and weak in enforcement. Since the creation of MSHA, fatalities and serious mine injuries have declined overall, but beginning in 2005, another series of disasters began—Sago (WV), Alma (WV), Darby (KY), Crandall Canyon (UT)—reversing the trend and raising questions regarding the adequacy of regulation and whether MSHA had acted on prior indications of deficiencies in mine safety. In 2007 NIOSH reported that the incidence of coal workers' pneumoconiosis, which had been falling, was rising again, in younger coal miners.

CONSUMER PRODUCT SAFETY COMMISSION

The Consumer Product Safety Commission (CPSC) is responsible for protecting the consumer, who may be in the role of a worker or a private citizen, from hazards associated with consumer products, including but not limited to durable goods (such as appliances), building materials, mobile homes, tools, household (but not industrial) chemicals, and toys, which have been of particular interest and concern in its history. CPSC does not regulate food or medicine, medical devices, or cosmetics (Food and Drug Administration); pesticides (Environmental Protection Agency); automobiles and other vehicles (National Highway Traffic Safety Administration, Department of Transportation); boats (U.S. Coast Guard); alcohol, tobacco, or firearms (the latter three are regulated by the Bureau of Alcohol, Tobacco, and Firearms, which for historical reasons of collecting taxes is part of the Department of the Treasury).

CPSC's main activities include the following functions:

- Issuing and enforcing mandatory standards
- Developing voluntary standards with industry representatives
- Ordering the recall of products identified as hazardous
- Ordering the repair of products identified as hazardous
- Consumer education
- Market surveillance to identify hazardous products in commerce
- Surveillance of imported products at ports of entry
- Surveillance of injuries related to consumer products through a reporting system based in 100 hospital emergency rooms (the National Electronic Injury Surveillance System)
- Surveillance of deaths related to consumer products
- Liaison with foreign governments to harmonize and raise safety standards (especially in manufacturing and distribution processes)

CPSC can replace a voluntary standard with a mandatory standard only after determining that the voluntary standard is inadequate or is unlikely to be complied with. CPSC's most visible actions are product recalls. These may occur on an expedited basis with cooperation of the manufacturer or distributor through the "Fast Track" program, or more conventionally through legal action.

CPSC was created in 1972 when Congress passed the Consumer Product Safety Act, which directed the new agency to "protect the public against unreasonable risks of injury associated with consumer products." This act was amended by the Consumer Product Safety Improvement Act of 2008. CPSC also administers six other federal laws:

- Children's Gasoline Burn Prevention Act of 2008 (portable gasoline containers)
- Federal Hazardous Substances Act of 1960 as amended several times (household and consumer products)
- Poison Prevention Packaging Act of 1970 (child-resistant packaging)
- Pool and Spa Safety Act of 2007 (preventing suction-caused entrapment and drowning of children in draining pools)
- Refrigerator Safety Act of 1956 (requiring that the door can be opened from the inside to prevent confinement and suffocation)

The Federal Hazardous Substances Act has been a particularly important source of regulatory authority and has been used to ban carbon tetrachloride, potentially dangerous aerial fireworks, strong liquid drain cleaners, and products containing cyanide and asbestos. It also mandates labeling for consumer products containing hazardous chemicals.

Although a freestanding federal agency, it is relatively small compared to other regulatory agencies (420 employees to manage 15,000 categories of consumer products). Its administration is divided into functional units, of which the operational (as opposed to support) offices are Compliance and Field Operations, Hazard Identification and Reduction, and International Programs and Intergovernmental Affairs.

CPSC has established itself as a leading innovator among federal agencies, creating a single portal ("one-stop shop") for managing recalls by all federal agencies with the authority to order them, an Early Warning System to identify and disseminate information on new products and emerging safety issues, a National Injury Information Clearinghouse, and electronic systems to transmit information on product recalls to media and participating Web sites electronically. The agency's generally proactive approach has served it particularly well in recent years during a period of challenges involving the risk of imported toys contaminated with lead, use during natural disasters of portable generators (which when used indoors create a serious risk of carbon monoxide toxicity), and toy magnets (which, when more than one is swallowed, can attract one another and pinch the bowel, causing necrosis and bowel infarction or intussusception).

OTHER U.S. FEDERAL AGENCIES

In the United States, workers in sectors that are outside the mainstream of general industry or defined by special hazards are often regulated by agencies other than OSHA. This is primarily to ensure access to relevant technical expertise but also, as in the case of aviation and the military, to ensure that there is not a conflict between worker protection and carrying out sensitive duties.

The Department of Transportation (DOT) requires regular fitness-to-work evaluations for drivers, pilots, and seamen. Also, branches of DOT require drug testing for these transportation workers and pipeline operatives. This is discussed in Chapter 12.

Within DOT, the Federal Aviation Administration (FAA) has regulatory authority over the occupational health and safety of aircraft-maintenance and flight personnel. The FAA is responsible for occupational health protection of flight personnel in civil aviation (mostly pilots and flight attendants) during periods of operation, which are defined strictly as when the first member of the crew arrives and the last departs, whether the airplane is in flight; on the ground, either in motion or holding; or whether engines are running or off. At other times, and at all times for the maintenance and ground crews, occupational health is the responsibility of OSHA. FAA has promulgated regulations regarding health and safety in airplane cockpits, including lighting, seat-belt use, ventilation, and smoke evacuation, but not noise, which has been controversial. FAA regulations are most visible in terms of evaluating pilots' fitness for duty, discussed in Chapter 18.

The Department of Defense (DOD) has a very large responsibility for occupational health and safety, covering the protection of active-duty personnel (including those with combat status) as well as civilian employees. The military maintains numerous facilities for the maintenance, development, and production of weaponry, support equipment, and vehicles. A military base may function more as a location for industrial-scale technical activity than for deployment and training. The same exposures common in industry generally are common in the military, and many military activities also involve potential exposures that are unusual or exotic, such as torpedo fuel (nitrate compounds that cause vasodilation and hypotension if absorbed), particles from jet aircraft brakes (beryllium alloys), and classified agents of warfare. Each branch of service maintains occupational health and safety units and supervises workplace safety in facilities under its direct control. In the past, DOD resisted being placed under the authority of other federal agencies and did not accept OSHA standards as binding. This impasse was resolved in the late 1970s by executive order, and in the 1980s DOD developed a strong intramural occupational health and safety program consistent with OSHA regulations.

The nuclear industry is another sector that has been carved out for special management of occupational health protection, a legacy of the Atomic Energy Act of 1954. The Department of Energy (DOE) is the federal agency responsible for occupational health and safety related to the nuclear industry's radiation hazards and for DOE national laboratories and test facilities. The Nuclear Regulatory Commission (NRC), which licenses nuclear plants and nuclear medicine in health care, is responsible for establishing exposure standards for ionizing radiation, chemical hazards that arise from radioactive materials (for example, uranium, which is nephrotoxic), and plant conditions that may affect radiation safety. The NRC also sets exposure standards for the diagnostic and therapeutic use of radionuclides in nuclear medicine. OSHA has authority over other occupational health hazards, such as chemical exposures. In practice, the agencies take a team approach. The Department of Transportation manages regulations on transport of radioactive materials; EPA regulates ambient exposure in the environment; and the Food and Drug Administration manages food irradiation and pharmaceuticals. This is a complicated area, and specific guidance should be sought if an issue involving radiation falls within the responsibility of an OEM physician.

The Department of Agriculture has programs to promote farm safety and health. It also regulates laboratory-animal housing and management. Because laboratory-animal handlers have a high rate of occupational injuries and allergies, this is a significant responsibility with implications for worker health protection.

CANADIAN REGULATORY FRAMEWORK

Environmental Health

Under the Canadian constitution (devolved from the British North America Act), environmental regulation and conservation is a provincial responsibility, as is health. The role of the federal government is therefore circumscribed.

The lead federal department (ministry) for environmental issues is Environment Canada. Federal responsibility is primary in issues involving inshore or offshore fisheries (a responsibility shared with the Department of Fisheries and Oceans), aboriginal lands, waters, national parks, and a few issues that are defined as being of "national concern," such as management of toxic substances, migration of contaminants through the ecosystem, protection of endangered species, management of Canada's engagement in international treaties and conventions, and so forth. Federal action on the environment otherwise is generally undertaken in partnership or collectively with provincial and territorial agencies, which vary in their capacity but are generally consistent in environmental regulation. Environment Canada also has responsibility for research, monitoring, and prediction of weather, climate, and environmental trends, making it Canada's lead agency in matters of climate change.

Provinces (of which there are ten) and territories (of which there are three) have ministries of environmental protection, which are responsible for environmental standards, monitoring emissions, local habitat and ecosystem conservation, environmental assessment, inspections, and enforcement. OEM physicians who practice in Canada or who have responsibility for Canadian operations are advised to find out about local regulations and environmental regulation in the relevant province or territory.

Canada operates primarily by a system of guidelines that represent targets for attainment rather than mandated standards, although mandated standards may also be adopted by the provinces. Guidelines for standards setting are negotiated by a federal-provincial working group and are implemented as emissions standards at the provincial level. These include the Canadian Drinking Water Guidelines and similar guidelines for recreational water use and air quality. Remediation standards for contaminated sites (including hazardous-waste disposal sites and brownfields) are governed by a set of consensus guidelines negotiated directly by provincial ministers responsible for environmental protection: the Canadian Council of Ministers of the Environment.

Occupational Health and Safety

Government services in occupational health vary widely across Canada because those services are primarily a provincial (or territorial) responsibility. Each of the ten provinces and three territorial governments as well as the federal government (primarily on behalf of its own employees) has its own occupational health and safety agency, freestanding in Quebec but attached to departments of labor in other jurisdictions, for a total of fourteen jurisdictions. In British Columbia, uniquely, occupational health and safety is joined with the Workers' Compensation Board. These agencies are responsible for administering the individual occupational health and safety acts relevant to their jurisdictions, conducting inspections and investigations, surveilling occupational injuries and illnesses, recommending standards, and supporting training or research. Most acts cover only nonagricultural workers. They vary somewhat in services, coverage, and enforcement policy. There is some uniform legislation for some occupational health and safety functions, primarily the hazard communication and "right-to-know" through the Workplace Hazardous Materials Information System, which covers labeling, worker education, and access to material-safety data sheets.

The federal government is responsible for occupational health and safety for federal employees and employees of Crown corporations and employees in industries that operate across provincial boundaries (including banks, transportation, telecommunications, and grain elevators), which together cover 10 percent of the Canadian workforce. The federal government is also involved when a role exists for it in facilitating voluntary and cooperative efforts. For example, the federal government sponsors the Canadian Centre for Occupational Health and Safety, a Crown corporation (government-owned, nonprofit company) that primarily disseminates information on occupational hazards but has no legal authority in issues of standards-setting enforcement or national policy.

Separate from the agencies (except in British Columbia) are the workers' compensation boards, which are Crown corporations that serve the dual functions of claims processors and insurance carriers (rather than allowing multiple private insurance companies). In general, there is little interaction between the occupational health agencies and the workers' compensation boards, with the latter focused on claims, rehabilitation services, and insurance services, except for exchanging statistical information. In a few cases, efforts have been made to innovate, such as Alberta's "window of opportunity program," which provided a financial incentive for employers in selected industries that improved their performance in the short term.

The OEM physician with responsibility for operations in Canada should become familiar with the provincial and federal legislation and regulations affecting the industry.

General

In Canada, reimbursement for health care services to physicians is a responsibility of provincial governments through their provincial health-insurance plans, with federal contribution from transfer payments and regulation. The system functions as a government-administered health insurance company paying physicians on a fee-for-service basis. (Hospitals are funded through direct annual allocations.) Remuneration for occupational physicians for services not directly related to the treatment of patients must be from third parties.

Government-based provincial health plans, whether the provincial health plans or workers' compensation, do not usually reimburse physicians for work done related to occupational health protection or occupational health services related to work capacity, such as pre-placement or periodic health surveillance programs. These costs are the responsibility of the employers. In Ontario, government, labor, and industry have supported a network of occupational medicine clinics: the Occupational Health Clinics for Ontario Workers. In Quebec, some occupational health services are provided by departments of the "community health centres," a network of service facilities supported by the government and usually attached to regional hospitals.

MULTILATERAL AGENCIES

Several important agencies in North America represent shared responsibilities and governance over environmental issues. These agencies do not have direct regulatory authority, but they are influential in actions taken by the national regulatory agencies.

Because they are official bodies and quasi-regulatory in their functions, they are included in this chapter.

The International Joint Commission (IJC) is a binational organization governed by appointed commissioners from the United States and Canada. Since the Boundary Waters Treaty of 1909 was ratified by the parties, the IJC has had the responsibility of overseeing and proposing nonbinding recommendations for environmental issues that straddle the U.S.-Canada border. Historically, most of its work has been directed at preventing pollution, conserving resources, or mitigating degradation of watershed for bodies of water, such as the St. Lawrence River and the Great Lakes. There are standing bodies, or "boards," for the major rivers and lakes. The Great Lakes Water Agreement of 1978 has dominated the agenda of the IJC in recent years, and the organization has been very active in monitoring water quality, studying the interaction of air deposition and bodies of water, and relating the ecosystem to human health. Although primarily concerned with water issues, one of the IJC's first important health issues involved air (involving a smelter in Trail, British Columbia, in 1910) and much of its most recent activities include monitoring and advising on transboundary issues involving air pollution, particularly through its International Air Quality Advisory Board. The IJC can only take up issues that are referred to it by both national governments and has only advisory powers; but its recommendations have been influential, and it has had an active program of community education and has supported research and education relevant to ecosystem and human health, including sponsoring a task force of health professionals.

The U.S.-Mexico Border Health Commission is an advisory body created in 2000 by international agreement; it consists of state health officers (four American and six Mexican states) or their delegates and appointed representatives. It is concerned with environmental health issues within 100 kilometers on either side of the international border. To date, it has dealt with tuberculosis, lead in traditional pottery, and air pollution from a power plant, among other issues. It acts mostly as a forum and through advocacy, coordination, setting achievable objectives, and public education. The commission has close ties with the El Paso regional office of the Pan American Health Organization and the Association of State and Territorial Health Officers, the organization representing state health officers in the United States.

The Commission for Environmental Cooperation of North America (CEC) is a trilateral organization established in 1993 by the North American Agreement on Environmental Cooperation, a side agreement of the North American Free Trade Act. The CEC monitors environmental issues in the three member countries (the United States, Canada, and Mexico), particularly with respect to trade and the impact of international trade on resources, environmental quality, and potential conflicts. It receives and investigates submissions from the public on issues but has no enforcement or regulatory authority.

RESOURCES

Information from and on regulatory agencies is abundant on the Web and in both professional and nontechnical publications. However, much information and opinion tends to be ephemeral, issue specific, and often partisan. Regulations also change and agencies evolve in response to politics and social demands. Readers are advised to do their own Internet searches on any significant issue to ensure currency and accuracy, and not to rely on books for anything other than historical guidance.

Bassett WEH, ed. *Clay's Handbook of Environmental Health*. London: Taylor & Francis; 2002.

Collin RW. *The Environmental Protection Agency: Cleaning Up America's Act*. Westport, CT: Greenwood; 2005.

Fletcher SR, Copeland C, Luther L, McCarthy JE, Reisch M, eds. *Environmental Laws: Summaries of Major Statutes Administered by the Environmental Protection Agency*. Haupauge, NY: Nova; 2008.

Silverstein M. Getting home safe and sound: the Occupational Health and Safety Administration at 38. *Am J Public Health*. 2008;98(3):416–423.

NOTEWORTHY READINGS

Bingham E. On the need for reform of the OSH Act. *Am J Ind Med*. 1992;21:891–893.

Cheit RE. *Setting Safety Standards: Regulation in the Public and Private Sectors*. Berkeley: University of California Press; 1990.

Doniger DD. *The Law and Policy of Toxic Substances Control: A Case Study of Vinyl Chloride*. Baltimore: The Johns Hopkins University Press / Resources for the Future; 1978.

Lofgren DJ. *Dangerous Premises: An Insider's View of OSH Enforcement*. Ithaca, NY: ILR Press / Cornell University Press; 1989.

McCaffrey DP. *OSHA and the Politics of Health Regulation*. New York: Plenum Press; 1982.

Smith RS. *The Occupational Health and Safety Act: Its Goals and Its Achievements*. Washington, DC: American Enterprise Institute for Public Policy Research; 1976.

25 SOCIETY, CRITICAL SCIENCE, AND ETHICS

Occupational and environmental medicine (OEM) is unique in medicine in many respects, among them its dual emphasis on the individual patient, worker, or community resident and the population, workforce, or community. Because of this concern for protecting the health of people both as individuals and in communities, occupational medicine is rightly called "public health for the employed population," and environmental medicine is rightly considered to stand at the interface between medicine and public health.

OEM is also unique in that it is driven by changes in demography, the economy, and technology more than medical science. Occupational medicine practice scarcely changes with the introduction of a new antibiotic or anti-inflammatory agent, but it changes profoundly as the workforce ages, as employment patterns change, and when a new chemical hazard is introduced into the workplace. Occupational medicine is characterized by an innate conservatism scientifically because the biomedical science on which it relies must be validated and well accepted; its epidemiologically derived knowledge base requires rigor; and its procedures must be legally and ethically defensible after experience in practice. Environmental medicine is more responsive than occupational medicine to advances in biomedical science because of the rapid advances of bioindicator technology, molecular epidemiology (a term that is falling from favor), and toxicogenomics, which examines gene expression and gene-toxicant interactions.

Coming from their different histories and traditions, the merging medical fields of occupational medicine and environmental medicine are harmonizing their different relationships to the community and different orientations toward social issues. As the fields continue to knit together, their common alignment will come from the notion of OEM as a medical field or specialty that bridges to public health and serves defined populations, whether in the form of a workforce or a broader community. For the time being, however, the two poles of OEM are best discussed separately, after a brief introduction to the concept of "critical science," which applies to both sides of the field.

OEM AS "CRITICAL SCIENCE"

Another concept of OEM is that it is one of several scientific or medical fields that document and seek to correct problems of technology and society.

The economic success of technology and applied science has had mixed social blessings. OEM, like the environmental sciences and risk assessment, is at a deep level a critique of the technology and society of the day. Such a critique is not in automatic opposition to progress. Rather, it is a means of correcting the errors of technology and of economic growth before they threaten to impede progress and to undermine human values. To see how this works—and how it has come to define a new form, or "mode," of science—requires an understanding of why science and technology are not the same thing, and a realization that science can legitimately study and critique the effects of technology and the economy.

Basic science and applied science are the two commonly accepted "modes" of scientific research, the latter being associated with technology. Scientists and academics talk about the difference between basic science and applied science, but the public rarely follows the distinction, considering science and technology to be two sides of the same coin. To decision makers, it often sounds like the distinction is merely a justification for grant funding for basic research. However, the differences between the two are important outside of academic debate because they have different functions altogether.

Basic science pieces together a worldview in part by documenting the unexpected, which expands society's vision beyond narrow applications and documents the unpredictable. This is the mode of science that fills in the uncharged white spaces of the metaphorical map, the mode on which society falls back when confronted with the unexpected and from which come so many fortuitous observations and unanticipated applications, as well as an understanding of mechanisms. It is basic science that pieces together a world picture. Basic science cannot have a ready answer for every question as it arises, but such answers may come closer when investigators have been allowed to extend their investigations into areas that appeared improbable for application before the question arose.

Applied science and problem-oriented technology, on the other hand, are mission oriented and involve problem solving. They create value and innovation. However, they are by their nature poorly equipped to anticipate problems because they are goal oriented and therefore one-sidedly searching for the predictable.

The emergence of a third mode was the result of a new way of thinking. The idea emerged in the 1970s that a systematic evaluation, using the tools of basic science, of the negative risks of technology could create a new mode, which was named "critical science" by its principal theoretician, Dr. Jerry Ravetz, of the University of Leeds (United Kingdom). He described it as a new approach that critically evaluates and analyzes the impact of technological developments within the context of the real world (not the engineer's world of simplifying assumptions), and which draws primarily on basic science and collaborative critical research to predict, document, and correct physical and human problems of technological origin.

The concept of a "critical science" describes much of the role that OEM at its best plays in society. For its more inquisitive practitioners,

OEM is very much in the mode of a critical science. It addresses issues of occupational health and of environmental health risk as they arise from changes in technology and the economy. The objective is to identify and then to correct these problems for the good of humanity and the sustainability of society. The whole point of a critical science is to identify and correct social problems, particularly those that arise from technology. As such, it is profoundly in support of progress and change, because it seeks to remove obstacles to progress, to prevent adverse and unintended consequences, and to correct what has gone wrong.

Occupational medicine, at one pole of OEM, is a critical science because it seeks to identify, document, and correct the problems of the workplace, which arise from technology, work organization, and economic development. Environmental medicine, at the other pole, is a critical science because it seeks to identify, document, and correct the environmental problems caused by human activity, which reflect changing technology (which introduces new hazards while also correcting others), failure to use technology (for example, to provide clean water in the developing world), and economic change. Environmental medicine is also closely aligned with ecology and environmental sciences, the disciplines Ravetz first cited as examples of critical science. Like its sister critical sciences, OEM, as a whole or at its two poles, uses the methods of basic science and research to investigate practical problems, and it depends on basic science to identify previously unsuspected or undocumented problems. Applied science and technology build on the insights and mechanistic studies of basic science, but they do not do very well at anticipating unintended consequences. Disciplines such as epidemiology and toxicology identify and evaluate problems, and that is, of course, the first necessary step in their correction.

The notion of OEM as critical science is not unlike Rudolph Virchow's admonition that:

Medicine is a social science, and politics is nothing else but medicine on a large scale. Medicine, as a social science, as the science of human beings, has the obligation to point out problems and to attempt their theoretical solution: the politician, the practical anthropologist, must find the means for their actual solution.

This idea, which neatly embraces OEM, applies equally well to public health. At its best, OEM is in the same tradition with Virchow's social medicine in treating health as a human right—a means of achieving full expression in one's personal life and social role—and an end result of the struggle for fairness, freedom, and material security. It cannot solve every problem, of course. It is embedded in a social, economic, and management system that has a responsibility to be responsive on a larger scale and to change when necessary.

Both poles of OEM will be discussed separately—environmental medicine first because it fits more obviously within Ravetz's definition.

Environmental Medicine as a Critical Science

Health professionals in North America are often deeply concerned with the environment in their personal lives, and some physicians have been prominent as activists. The environmental movement in North America often speaks in terms of health, and health is a driving concern for the public in shaping the response to environmental problems. However, the term "environmental health" has a different meaning in the health professions, including public health and OEM, than in the environmental movement. Health professionals perceive "environmental health" as pertaining to environmental determinants of human health. To environmentalists, and to many members of the public, "environmental health" is as likely to mean "the health of the environment." Some have dubbed the latter "ecosystem health." The public generally sees human and ecosystem health as mixed together and both fundamentally related to social justice and fairness.

Public health professionals and environmentalists often find themselves frustrated in communication with one another. The concept of environmental determinants of health as expressed by the public health professional may appear very limiting and even self-serving to an environmentalist accustomed to the big picture of "the environment," or of ecosystem stability. On the other hand, the concept of ecosystem health or health in a holistic sense, as used by environmentalists, may appear to be vague, indirect, and unprofessional to a health professional accustomed to thinking of specific exposures, calculable risks, and specific disorders.

This difference in understanding becomes most contentious when health issues are presented as evidence of environmental degradation on the basis of evidence that may not meet the rigorous standards of epidemiology. If one takes the environmental movement, especially its more radical elements, literally on a technical level as an alternative interpretation of exposure to toxic and physical hazards, it sometimes appears to bend the science and, at the extreme, to be antiscientific and even irrational. The discrepancy between the approach of scientists, environmental health professionals, and OEM physicians, on the one hand, and environmental advocates and activists on the other is not unlike the difference in standards of certainty described in Chapter 23 for scientific and for medicolegal issues. Environmentalists are using a standard often described as the "precautionary principle," which for this purpose can be described as requiring action to protect against risk if there is any evidence of an environmental hazard—even if there is scientific doubt about the evidence—because the consequences are considered to be unacceptable. (There are other definitions of the precautionary principle.) This scenario is played out over and over again in issues such as the risk of cancer from common herbicides used on lawns and parks, the risks of electromagnetic fields, and popular assumptions regarding the risk of getting certain diseases, usually those with unknown causes, such as multiple sclerosis, autism, and sarcoidosis. At its best, the precautionary principle leads to continuous improvement, such as green technology, without the need to justify every step along the way. In public health and OEM, however, it often leads to priorities that are questionable in public health practice—such as emphasizing the putative risk resulting from disinfection byproducts in water over control of waterborne infectious-disease risk—and wrong public health decisions—such as discouraging breastfeeding because of the putative risk resulting from PCB residues when breast milk is known to have unequivocal benefits to infants.

There is also a tendency among naive environmentalists to use health concerns as a rhetorical device to raise awareness of a skeptical public to an issue that is considered to be critical to the environmental agenda. Environmentalists may perceive themselves to be sounding the alarm on important health issues that illustrate the link between the environment and human health, and therefore called upon to motivate people to political or social action. To health professionals, however, attributing health problems to environmental causes without rigorous evidence sounds alarmist, and the science often seems suspect. It is also threatening to the hard-won and fragile credibility that public health professionals and OEM physicians always seek to protect.

For all these reasons, health professionals are often inclined to disassociate themselves from environmentalists, at least as professionals, for fear of losing public trust. Environmentalists, who usually are primarily concerned with getting action on what they consider to be the big issues, may therefore see their health professional colleagues as hair-splitting, timid careerists who shy away from the root causes of health problems, which in their view lie in the perverse relationship between human society and the environment.

What is the most appropriate role for physicians in environmental issues? Obviously, well-trained and focused physician investigators will continue to make substantial scientific contributions to the field. A relatively small number of highly motivated physician activists will also continue to make contributions in public awareness and on specific issues. An individual physician may feel an ethical obligation to speak out on environmental issues, but for most there is a limit to their comfort level. Physicians are generally most comfortable playing a personal role in environmental issues when there is a practical objective to be achieved that is related to a health problem they know, when there is a clear health connection supported by evidence, and when a clear distinction is made between the professional role of clinician and the personal role of citizen. They generally show a preference for incremental rather than radical change and a preference for advocacy over activism.

Physicians' awareness of new hazards and the process of disease as well as the influence that physicians have from the profession's high public acceptance and esteem give physicians a special role. That role suggests several opportunities for action, depending on the physician's training and commitment:

- Work within organizations, such as companies and government, to correct and prevent environmental problems
- Document through research the health effects of environmental degradation
- Endorse, support, and advocate for an effort to improve human health by moving toward environmental sustainability
- Work within the health sector to ensure that it is environmentally responsible in its operations and facilities
- Act responsibly by example, both as an individual practitioner and employer
- Work with organizations outside the health sector to help them understand issues of the environment and health
- Work within medical organizations locally, nationally, and on an international level to help them understand issues of the environment and health and to take responsible policy positions

Physicians need to take account of their standing and of the respect that they receive from local communities, and to use this respect responsibly to act as advocates for ecosystem health and human health. The first obligation of the physician who becomes active in environmental issues must be to prepare him- or herself—as thoroughly as possible for a new medical practice—to learn enough about environmental sciences and health issues to speak responsibly and knowledgeably.

On the other hand, organized medicine may also speak collectively for the individual physician. What are the appropriate roles of the profession as a whole and of "mainstream" medical organizations?

Assuming that physicians are confident that the organization demonstrates sound judgment, it is reasonable to present a collective voice for physicians that is cautious, authoritative, and concerned but also effective. Certain organizations, such as the International Society of Doctors for the Environment, the Canadian Association of Physicians for the Environment, and the International Physicians for Prevention of Nuclear War and their affiliates (Physicians for Social Responsibility in the United States, and Physicians for Global Survival in Canada), will play a role in the vanguard of medical participation in these issues.

Occupational Medicine as a Critical Science

Just as environmental medicine fits Ravetz's description of a critical science for environmental issues, the other pole of OEM, occupational medicine, is dedicated to preventing, identifying, and correcting problems and unintended consequences in the workplace, as well as to improving conditions of working life. This extends to using the workplace and the employment relationship as a platform to enhance the health of workers and to contribute to the community. Occupational medicine is a critical science for working life, and is not limited to hazards on the job. However, it is in the realm of workplace hazards that the function of occupational medicine as a critical science is most obvious.

For any form of occupational health protection to be effective, the employer and the worker need to know what is going on. That is the crucial role of occupational medicine as a critical science. A fundamental issue in occupational health in general is who controls the workplace and whether employers have an obligation to share governance of issues such as health and safety with the workers they employ. In the United States, it is the employer who controls the workplace and the working environment and who must therefore bear full responsibility for occupational health protection. This creates a tension between the employer's prerogatives and ownership and the right of workers to be protected or to be given the means to protect themselves. This tension is irresoluble in a country—the United States—that defines itself in terms of entrepreneurship, private ownership, and creative destruction. However, the more informed, educated, trained, and involved workers are, the more likely OHS is to be effectively monitored and managed. That is why worker participation features so prominently in the ethics of occupational medicine (discussed below). But without knowledge about workplace hazards and information from the particular workplace, neither employer nor worker can take effective action. This is the role of occupational medicine as a critical science.

The Imperfect Emerging Economy

New hazards will continue to emerge as technology develops and exposure patterns change in the workplace. Europe, Japan, North America, and some parts of the middle-income, developing world have moved into a largely "postindustrial" society. Services in this new economy are as highly valued and important as manufactured products. Among the features of this postindustrial society is an emphasis on information as a commodity and automation of much manufacturing, which comes to resemble agriculture in that it produces at high volume but with a small workforce. Much production is outsourced overseas, currently mainly to China, and then, by China as well as North America, to other countries with lower wage levels. There is a potential for new or rediscovered occupational hazards with each new industry, whether it be high-technology electronics; advanced materials such as composites, ceramics, or biotechnology; or the shift work and stress that accompany a global trading network, requiring split-second decision-making and devastating consequences for error.

The old hazards that result in predictable injury and disease, with their burden of disability and insecurity, do not disappear, however. They go overseas to affect workers in other countries where the work is outsourced. They persist in low-margin industries that are difficult to outsource, such as construction. They hide in the informal sector or in industries with a history of abusive practices, often disproportionately harming immigrants and other vulnerable populations. They are perpetuated by ignorance or lack of awareness in small enterprises that lack the means to improve conditions or do not see the point. As the economy changes, it gets harder to find occupational hazards, but not because they have disappeared. They become less visible and affect workers who are least able to protect themselves and earn the lowest wages.

Workers who are vulnerable and are not provided with the occupational health protection they need are called "underserved workers." Underserved workers are most often thought of as well-defined groups, such as recent immigrants, disadvantaged minorities, illiterate workers, and the economic underclass. However, it may be more useful to think of underserved workers as an underclass workforce defined by broad social issues. These issues include the concentration of dirty and dangerous work by class, geography, and sector as well as ethnicity, migration status, and income level, into poorly documented, less accessible corners of society largely hidden from the majority population and the media, often in marginal industries where employment is unstable.

Occupational health problems are relatively invisible already because they are spread through many industries and many workplaces. Occupational health has not coalesced into a social issue that people get excited about. Occupational health issues are perceived, wrongly, by the public as the concern of a special interest, such as organized labor, or a narrow problem in a particular industry or employer. The deaths or illnesses tend to occur one at a time, or in small clusters. They tend to occur quietly and are obscured by the bureaucracy and statistical categorization of agencies like workers' compensation boards and occupational health and safety regulatory agencies, necessary as those statistics may be.

It is a fundamental tenet of occupational medicine that old hazards always reappear in new technologies. For example, in the manufacture of semiconductors and other electronic components, gallium arsenide is a very important constituent. There were cases of arsenic intoxication among semiconductor workers when the industry began, and a great deal of denial and disbelief at first that such a "clean" industry could cause this problem. However, arsenic is a very old hazard, well known and well studied, and its risks and measures to control exposure were understood long before the semiconductor industry was invented. However, the people who pioneered the manufacture of electronic components were not thinking in terms of the mining and smelting industry. For them, this was a bright, new, unique technology starting from the beginning. Truly, old hazards never quite go away; they just reappear in a new technology.

North American society seems to have entered a twilight zone in occupational health and safety. The European Union has taken the lead in occupational health protection. The United States and Canada are passing from an era in which there were certain clear ideas of what the major issues were—and these issues had strong evidence of commitment from government and public policy—into a new and ill-defined place, an uncharted territory through which both countries are still feeling their way.

The problems of greatest concern have changed over the last two decades, although it is difficult to be sure how much of the change is a real difference in changing impact on society and how much is a change in perception. Asthma and reactive airways, solvent-induced neurological problems, repetitive-strain injuries, soft-tissue injuries, passive smoking, injury control, and violence emerged as the growth areas of interest. Soft-tissue injuries, particularly in the context of repetitive-strain injury, have been primarily perceived as an issue in ergonomics rather than medicine. The old, characteristic diseases of occupational medicine, such as silicosis and noise-induced hearing loss, seem not to inspire any great interest anymore because of the (false) assumption that they have disappeared.

For historical reasons, so much of the American social insurance system is tied to employment (health insurance, pension benefits, disability, unemployment insurance) that managing these issues far outweighs managing work-related hazards as a practical problem, from the employer's point of view. General health issues, such as health insurance, disability management, wellness, and managed care, now command much more attention from employers and government than occupational health and workers' compensation. There is little interest and less reward in going looking for occupational health problems in obscure places or unpopular corners of the economy. In the new economy, occupational safety could fall to an even lower priority because of the perception, incorrect as it is, that the injury problem is solved.

Occupational medicine is the medical arm of occupational health, which in turn is part of the broad field of occupational health and safety. The mission and fortunes of OEM are therefore linked to the priority given to occupational health and to the attention paid by management and by society to occupational health and safety (OHS) in general. In recent years, just before the time of this writing (2009), OHS went through a long period of marginalization and neglect, especially on the federal level. This was justified at the time on the questionable grounds that injury rates were falling and that industry was overregulated. The former was hard to be sure of, given changes in the way that injuries were counted during the period, and the latter was certainly arguable. In such a policy and management environment, it was hard to sustain interest and momentum for health protection at the level of individual employers, especially for small enterprises. OEM physicians had to adapt in many ways, but they mostly maintained their positions and continued to do well, if not flourish.

Hazard control interventions are intended to keep something bad from happening, and it is always more difficult to document that bad events have not happened than it is to show that positive changes have occurred. Control of workplace hazards is difficult to sustain as an enthusiastic interest of management, but once the controls are in place they are difficult to change. Safety measures, to prevent incidents of trauma, are usually easier for management to comprehend and to evaluate than health protection. Safety, although it can be very sophisticated as a field, tends to be less technically complicated in practice because the measures required to control safety hazards are relatively straightforward by comparison to health protection. Safety science is more a problem of behavioral engineering than technical engineering. At the heart of sound safety practice is the difficult problem of motivating and sustaining behavior.

OEM physicians must be aware of trends in OHS in general, and their implications for the field and for practice. Interest in health, as opposed to injury, runs in cycles, just as does interest in occupational medicine. There is a seesaw in management interest between safety and health. At intervals, the seesaw tilts rather sharply toward safety, usually following highly publicized incidents, especially those involving fatalities. Concern over cancer, hazardous chemicals, and other, more subtle effects usually tips the balance back the other way, but does so more slowly, bringing health back as a major management concern over time. It is important for the OEM physician to realize this dynamic, because it is often reflected in management perceptions, proposed reorganizations, and cooperation between safety and health professionals. Safety departments in major companies are often more or less autonomous and generally resist being incorporated in the same administrative unit with medicine and occupational health. The emphasis seesaws between safety and health; however, it is ultimately pointless for there to be a pendulum swinging between safety and health. Protecting workers is a common goal and a shared professional commitment between the two fields.

A positive change in the workplace has been that OHS is increasingly considered standard operating procedure. This is critical: if health and safety are not built into line responsibility, they simply will not be a priority. It is not appropriate to make the health or safety professional "responsible" for health protection: it has to be a commitment of the organization followed through with policies, procedures, and work practice. For this to work, in turn, occupational health has to be part of performance evaluation. Supervisors need to know that they can be fired for failure to perform diligently in health and safety issues. Today, performance review policies generally are more accurately characterized as likely to deny a promotion to a supervisor who fails miserably in occupational health and safety, but such a failure hardly ever leads to a supervisor's termination unless a worker is killed or seriously injured.

Occupational health and safety professionals in industry are always afraid of losing resources. In the 1980s and 1990s, many corporate medical directors in large companies resisted the introduction of health promotion programs, because they were concerned that hazard control would get short shrift. Others adopted health promotion, incorporated it into their departments, and were able to keep their focus during the ensuing popularity and then plateau of enthusiasm for worksite health promotion.

Periodically, management and social fads distort priorities in health protection and affect the mission of occupational health and safety, including OEM. These come and go, and like all management fads, they capture the imagination of managers who are looking for a new, simple solution. An illustration of the general principle was the movement called "quality of working life" (QWL), or "conditions of work," which built up a substantial following in the 1970s. QWL emphasized the conditions of work and personal control over the working environment. It took a very general approach, assuming that the major determinants of a worker's sense of well-being have to do with the immediate social and physical environment of the work-place and the amount of control the worker has over personal comfort and work pace. QWL advocates were frequently shortsighted in assuming that the principal occupational health hazards had been controlled already. Some QWL advocates, who by and large were isolated from the realities of work outside of offices, even went so far as to say that occupational health was no longer pertinent to the modern world, because industry was no longer as hazardous as it was during the Industrial Revolution. In effect, QWL advocates were substituting for substantive hazard control what they believed to be the nonspecific and probably nonexistent "Hawthorne effect" (see Chapter 13) of enhanced worker productivity and satisfaction stimulated by management attention. QWL, if done well, may have provided the worker with greater control over the working environment. It is more likely that it served little purpose other than the manipulation of the working environment to achieve management objectives. There was also a considerable commercial potential in selling management on aesthetic changes that improve office and plant decor. Both worksite health promotion and quality of working life were aggressively marketed, but occupational health was not.

At the time, QWL was seen as reflecting good and enlightened management. On the other hand, occupational health implies a need to solve problems that perhaps should not be present in the first place. No supervisor or manager wants to admit that the workplace for which they are responsible is hazardous. No supervisor or manager wants to believe that a worker was injured due to a preventable hazard in the workplace that they overlooked or allowed to exist. It is much easier for managers to deny the problem, to turn to a quick fix, to provide incentives for underreporting injuries, or to assign responsibility to someone else without giving them real authority. It takes courage and professional commitment to accept that a workplace is hazardous and to take steps for occupational health protection. That is why occupational health services that work well and that have the backing of employers are uncommon and to be commended. It is also why the management tools that focus attention on occupational health and safety—such as written policies, worker and management training, performance evaluation of supervisors that includes safety performance, and audits—are critical to sustaining an OHS effort overall and maintaining support for the OEM physician.

Occupational health is often at a disadvantage for management attention and priority for allocation of money and resources. There is a very real danger that when the heat is off, occupational health services will be rolled back and replaced by the more popular and less expensive health promotion and QWL measures. Control of workplace hazards is difficult to sustain as an enthusiastic interest of management, but once the controls are in place it is possible to show management the ongoing benefits. Hazard control requires resources and sustained commitment; it requires constant vigilance; and it is usually not perceived as exciting or responsive to the workers' psychic needs in the way that both health promotion and quality of working life are. In the end, however, it is the heart and soul of occupational health and safety and of OEM.

HISTORICAL PERSPECTIVE

The history of occupational health illustrates the importance of OEM and the historical contributions of science in a critical role, documenting the problems of technology.

Western society moved through several distinct phases along the technological path to modernity. Europe and its North American colonies started out as agrarian societies, but England and Scotland soon developed urban centers that depended on technology rather than trade alone. Britain was first to enter a very difficult, technologically driven Industrial Revolution. Some parts of the world are only now entering theirs and are having similar difficulties, although history never repeats itself exactly.

North Americans, having prospered and become as much a fountain of innovation as was Britain (and France) in the past, now live in a very different technological age than the one that began with the Industrial Revolution. North American society has moved into a phase beyond the Industrial Revolution in which it is trying to solve the lingering abuses of an earlier technological age and at the same time to move on to another, qualitatively different and more egalitarian era of more sophisticated technology and organizational management. A natural concomitant of this progress has been an aversion to risk. Each generation became more affluent and acquired the technological means and the purchasing power to insulate itself, or at least a majority of the population, from risks to a greater and greater degree—first the risk of starvation, then poverty and privation, then discomfort and inconvenience, and now risks that would have been tolerable or even acceptable to this generation's parents. Societies become more risk averse as they grow more affluent, age in their demographics, and mature socially. North American society is now in the enviable position of being able to worry about small risks of cancer and about reproductive hazards, which would have been inconceivable to this generation's grandparents.

However, the aversion to risk is selective. It focuses on hazards that are visible (usually through the media), associated with dread outcomes, and affect the middle class, but it largely ignores the persistent hazards of the workplace and problems such as contaminated water, which is still the major environmental hazard worldwide (see Chapter 7). The social aversion to risk was not enough to motivate measures to prevent global climate change, the greatest environmental risk of all, despite years of warnings. The gains of the last century may not be held. The economy is again restructuring and is, at the time of this writing, in deep trouble worldwide. It has been said that the now-passing generation of "baby boomers" may be the first in North America to have expectations of a life less affluent than their parents.

Until the present generation, Western society has tended to equate the progress of technology—with its promise of more and more engineering and organizational breakthroughs—with progress in terms of better lifestyle and better individual opportunity economically. (In another era, this was the ideology of the party known as the "Whigs.") It would be a mistake to think that progress is uniform, however, and naive to think that technological progress necessarily brings a better life for all. The early Industrial Revolution caused enormous dislocation in the fabric of British society at the time. It emptied the English and Scottish countryside of people and impoverished half the United Kingdom. It caused severe urban impaction, to a degree never seen before, and caused epidemics and plagues of injuries and illness of historic proportions, exceeding even the contemporary developing world, where the situation is bad enough. This led to a profound cynicism regarding technology's role in society, perhaps best expressed in the 1936 silent movie *Modern Times* starring Charlie Chaplin. This film focused on what technology seemed to be doing to the individual during the Great Depression, which represented a failure of progress. The world had created technology, it seemed, and now that technology had not only failed but was creating its own negative effect on the world.

Coal Mining as a Mirror

There is no industry in which these issues are clearer than coal mining, not because it was necessarily typical but because it showed all of these problems so vividly and was so closely linked to technological change as the dominant energy source. The fabric of society in coal-mining communities was very thin and very much dominated by the hard work of mining coal. The social effects of living in a one-company town were limiting. When the pay is good (or better than the alternatives) and family is rooted to the place, workers accept the risk because they have to. The miner who went down into the mines in the 1880s had little protection in the way of safety: there were no hardhats, and light was available only from an oil-fired lantern that gave off a very dim light (and caused "miner's nystagmus," a now-forgotten occupational disease). The work was hard and hazardous. It was not unusual in coal-mining communities of the late nineteenth century and early twentieth century for a woman to be widowed three or four times in her lifetime, one husband after another dying in mine-related accidents.

It was standard practice in those days for canaries to be brought down in the mines by miners as an early detection device for toxic gas (carbon monoxide or hydrogen sulfide). If the canary dropped dead off its perch, the foreman knew that the mine was unsafe and the miners would evacuate it. Today, the term "canaries" is used in occupational health to indicate those workers who become ill first, because they are often the first indication of a problem in that particular workplace. The canary became an important metaphor in the English language and one of the few metaphors drawn from occupational health that is regularly heard in common speech.

Technological progress sometimes results in occupational disease. Technological progress does not necessarily mean progress in the health and working environments. For example, the prevalence of "black lung," or "coal-worker pneumoconiosis," and "silicosis" in coal miners increases the higher the respirable dust level. In the 1880s, holes were drilled in coal seams using fairly primitive equipment. Less dust was generated, and those miners tended not to get "black lung" as often as those in later years. Of course, mining was very primitive and dangerous anyway, because of other hazards. The introduction of more effective equipment brought ever more serious safety hazards, including unprotected open gears and belt drives, which required people to be sitting next to operating machinery. A drilling machine, substituting for the hand drills of the early eighteenth century, operated at a much higher speed. The dust that was generated was much greater in concentration and much finer in size than the dust the manual drill could have produced. The effect of this was "black lung." Today, there are many practical methods to keep dust levels down, and the drill bit is kept wet.

Child labor was also extremely common in those days. A child about seven or eight years old might have lived underground for most of his life. He might get up in the morning and go down to the depths of the mine around 5:30 a.m. and spend his entire day doing various jobs or pulling small carts removing coal from the mine. By the time he finished for the day and went topside, he may have gone without seeing daylight for days on end. Another job performed by young boys in England and America was to pick pieces of slate out of the coal as it came by on a conveyor belt. For girls, the same story was repeated in the textile mills. As children grew older they could do heavier jobs, move away from home, and live in dormitories. This was done for ten hours a day with a half-day on Saturday. They went to church on Sunday. The life of adults was not much better in those days.

Mining today is vastly different than in those days, and although it is much safer than it was, it is still dangerous. Underground mining still takes its place among the most hazardous occupations, as evidenced in modern China and other developing countries. Early on, however, progress brought its own problems, and improving technology introduced new and different hazards. Hazards without effective controls place workers at risk. If the controls are not used they may as well not have been invented. But if hazards are identified and controlled by means of effective protective measures, both the employer and the worker benefit from technological progress and society moves forward. The environmental costs of coal mining—from water pollution to mountaintop removal—also serve as a demonstration that occupational and environmental health are linked, often in indirect ways.

The history of coal mining is ancient and may seem passé today, but there are lessons in it for all time.

ATTITUDES TOWARD OCCUPATIONAL MEDICINE

OEM and OHS, so rich in science, history, and social relevance, has never truly broken through to receive appropriate recognition as a discipline and remains marginalized, although much progress has been made (see Chapter 1). This problem is also shared by public health and preventive medicine in general. One might think that occupational health would escape the trap because of its demonstrable usefulness and well-documented cost-effectiveness. The conventional explanation is that OEM has failed to make its case and that those in the field are ineffective at communicating its value. However, there is another explanation: occupational health has been marginalized not because it has failed but because people want it to fail and consider it, at some level, immoral!

The explanation is based on arguments made by George Lakoff in his 1996 book *Moral Politics: What Conservatives Know That Liberals Don't*, which discusses assumptions and cognitive frameworks in which political concepts are judged. Lakoff's contribution is to observe that attitudes toward private matters and public issues alike are conditioned by two belief systems in North American society, which he calls the "Strict Father" and the "Nurturing Parent." Lakoff suggests that this reality is more complicated than labels of "liberal" and "conservative," representing two opposed, highly structured, deep, and contradictory sets of attitudes modeled on experience with the family. The two views of the world may be held on different issues by the same person and different views may be applied to different issues.

The Strict Father emphasizes character above all and considers it to be an attribute, rather than a behavior, with separate and evaluable components of virtue, discipline, resourcefulness, responsibility, and enterprise. The Strict Father values focus and clarity in goals. The worthy person must demonstrate that self-restraint, self-discipline, and self-reliance come from within. The Strict Father has a duty to protect only when children are immature, but once the children are grown, he has a duty to be strict with them. "Character building" is a responsibility of the Strict Father. Character building is a process that fosters self-discipline and self-control. Rewards that are not earned are immoral. To deny a child the opportunity to take risks and to suffer the consequences is immoral. It denies the child the opportunity to grow and become self-reliant. Value is placed in single-mindedly achieving an objective, one goal at a time, because this demonstrates perspicacity and character. The Strict Father paradoxically values, at the same time and to the same degree, both heritage (and the validation that comes from precedent) and the freedom to take risks and to innovate. The defining freedom for the Strict Father is not the freedom to move in any direction of one's choosing but the freedom to take a risk that will result in personal advancement. Risk, in this paradigm, is evidence of character, in that one puts oneself on the line for progress and personal gain. The Strict Father bases his moral framework on a model of family life and morality that is reflected in the nuclear family and in child rearing. It places the burden of responsibility squarely on the individual, in return for which the individual has liberal (small *l*, in the classical sense of individualism) freedoms and opportunities without many obligations to others, except for the primary responsibility, which is to allow his or her children (or dependents) the same opportunity to build character. The Strict Father also places heavy emphasis on tradition, loyalty, and preservation of the social order.

The Nurturing Parent treats personality and achievement as learned and mutable in response to society, not as inherent or forged by uniquely personal experience. Good character will arise in an environment of social responsibility, human rights, diversity, dignity, health and safety, and freedom of expression and action. Interdependence is the reality in this view, and recognition of interdependence defines character. The expression of that good character is empathy for others, a desire to help others, communitarian action, and the healthy recognition that in order to take care of others, it is important to take care of oneself. Self-reliance and the nurturing of others are inseparable in a healthy personality. The Nurturing Parent considers complete independence from others to be an illusion. Protection is a form of caring, and it is reasonable for people to protect the weakest among them when the hazards are beyond one's control. Although personal advancement may be a good thing, it should not take place at the expense of the common good, nor should any member of society be so arrogant as to believe that one's own efforts in isolation, without the social framework, could have accomplished anything worthwhile.

It may seem that there could be no more divergent systems and that between them they cover all possible political and social ground, but really these paradigms are two extremes of one dimension and far from exhausting all possibilities. The two paradigms actually have much in common. Both are based on the idea that the family is a proper model for society and that the education of a child is the proper model for social relationships. The goal of this developmental model in both cases is an independent, self-directed adult capable of playing a constructive role in the community. They do not describe the relationship of adults to one another very well, because they are based on child-rearing models. Both paradigms abhor neglect of responsibility and assume that behavior reflects moral values. Both place great emphasis on the *meaning* of behavior, interpreting actions, beliefs, and rhetoric as consistent or inconsistent with their value systems, whatever the issue and however great the stakes riding on the issue. Both paradigms are profoundly concerned with character as an inherent quality that determines how a person will act under all conditions, which does not allow the idea that behavior in context reflects a specific set of conditions.

Lakoff uses his powerful analysis to demonstrate how these paradigms can explain almost every contradiction in, specifically, American political life. The implications are obvious for certain key issues where moral or "wedge" issues are involved, particularly those with a moral dimension, such as abortion rights and gun control.

Lakoff extends his analysis to perceptions of work and the value of labor. He observes that under the Strict Father paradigm, employment is not an equal relationship. The work relationship reflects the moral order: the employer is in a legitimate authority position, and work is associated with risk and personal advancement and is subject to the same meaning with respect to character and self-discipline as any other aspect of life. Work is a service to the employer, and pay is the reward for obedience in providing this service as instructed, at a fluctuating price set by the market in relation to the demand for the worker's skill. Workers are therefore expected to be obedient and to welcome the opportunity to prove themselves, demonstrate character, and advance themselves. A high, even brutal, level of competition is welcome and builds character. On the other hand, the Nurturing Parent considers that work should be a social relationship of equals, in which labor is exchanged for fair compensation based on the value added by the labor, and that the workplace should support individual aspirations and provide opportunities for growth in a secure environment.

There is much of value to occupational health in Lakoff's analysis. It explains why attitudes toward occupational health and safety, and toward individual injured workers, often reflect a seemingly irrational hostility and resistance on one extreme and empty rhetoric on the other.

Occupational health protection is difficult to fit into the paradigm of the Strict Father. Hazards are inevitable to the Strict Father, and to face them squarely and to take risks is a sign of character. If the risk does not pay off and there is an injury, it is unfortunate, but such is life. The injured worker should receive treatment, fair indemnification by a strict standard that does not foster dependence, and then be prepared to move on, accepting that the market value of his or her labor has diminished. The privilege of returning to work must be earned by effort and loyalty. Indemnification for permanent disability is suspect and destructive to the moral order because it is a reward unearned by effort.

The Nurturing Parent, on the other hand, sees risk taking in the workplace as corruption. In this view, risk is assumed by the worker primarily for the benefit of the employer. Hazard, which is always preventable, is imposed on the worker, and for the worker to accept unsafe conditions is a sign of servility; the right to refuse dangerous work is therefore fundamental to a free society. If an injury occurs and it is serious, it is a tragedy that may affect many lives—those of the worker and his or her family—and the employer should make the worker whole through indemnification, admitting responsibility, and demonstrating concern. Temporary, partial, or total disability is a loss of opportunity to live one's life and diminishes the injured worker's ability to function fully in society. Permanent impairment is a state of need, deserving of compassion. People in need should be helped for the duration of their need. The injured worker or the disabled applicant has a right to equal access to work, after a fair test of ability to do the job with accommodation if necessary.

From these widely divergent points of view come differences of opinion on what to do in the workplace. Safety measures beyond the most obvious may be seen by the Strict Father as evasion of self-discipline on the part of the worker and, on the other hand, as the responsibility of the employer by the Nurturing Parent. Regulation, in the form of occupational health standards, may be seen by the Strict Father as interference with an enterprise that is an engine for social betterment and an expression of moral behavior; the same regulation may be seen by the Nurturing Parent as a necessary but entirely insufficient bureaucratic evil that treats symptoms rather than causes. Enforcement of occupational health standards may be seen by the Strict Father as harassment and an immoral compromise in the opportunity to take risks, whereas the Nurturing Parent may see such enforcement as a failed exercise that is never adequate, equitable, or comprehensive. Government-sponsored programs that support employers' assumption of "internal responsibility" or "partnerships" (in which employers police themselves, such as OSHA's Alliance program described in Chapter 24) may be seen by the Strict Father as government interference in the workplace, but at least as an admission that employers should be allowed to govern themselves; such programs may be seen by the Nurturing Parent as an untrustworthy, immoral collusion between government and industry in an effort to avoid enforcement. To the Strict Father, regulatory agencies are stupid, but to the Nurturing Parent they are corrupt because they do not go far enough. Regulatory policies either promote moral hazard by removing the need for self-discipline, as seen by the Strict Father, or they are tainted by compromise, as seen by the Nurturing Parent.

These attitudes intensify when workers' compensation is considered. Workers' compensation is generally a minor cost of doing business, but claims often provoke ferocious resistance on the part of some employers, often out of proportion to their exposure to financial loss, and this resistance is met by outrage on the part of workers' advocates. To a Strict Father, workers' compensation benefits are a nonproductive social expenditure that undermines discipline and the social order. To the Nurturing Parent, such benefits are an insufficient social support system and a means by which employers evade responsibility. Workers' compensation satisfies neither.

In Lakoff's analysis, issues related to occupational health and workers' compensation, almost uniquely, generate negative interpretations on both sides. Neither side likes occupational health and both consider the field marginal at best and immoral at worst.

Is there a way forward? Perhaps there is, but only if the paradigms are challenged.

Both paradigms are predicated on the same basic idea: that the work relationship reflects the nuclear family. This is nonsense. Workers are not children and employers are not parents. Neither the workforce, the firm, nor the nation is a family. Occupational health is a matter between (mostly) adults with shared interests in health, economic productivity, and security. It can be dealt with apart from these metaphors of family, with an emphasis on prevention, benefit, and human rights. Occupational health and safety—and by extension

OEM—is a normal part of working life, neither a favor to servants nor a trophy for organized labor. It is a branch of public health and a part of daily life, ideally carried into the community in a seamless regard for safety and health.

ETHICS IN OCCUPATIONAL MEDICINE

Ethics is the normative, or prescriptive, study of behavior that arises from social interaction. It is a way of guiding behavior by deriving a set of rules that govern duty and appropriate action that would be considered good or right. When an ethical principle is violated, the reaction is expected to be proportionate to the magnitude of the infraction, and it is accepted that in a diverse society ethical principles may vary and may require periodic re-evaluation.

Morality, on the other hand, is the law handed down by a higher authority, in religious tradition a deity. In secular society, Immanuel Kant proposed that the whole of humanity, acting in its own collective interest, serves to create morality instead of a deity. Moral laws are not negotiable, because they come as an indivisible whole. The moral system must be accepted or rejected in its entirety. The system is received from an absolute authority, so the elements of the system are presumed to be immutable. The moral system may rest on an initial premise, such as the existence of God, such that its elements all flow from this assumption or belief, and it may be structured to be internally consistent. Such moral systems are fragile, resting on deductive logic, and their parts are inseparable. Sometimes moral systems conflict with social needs and freedoms, but that does not reduce their power. In fact, a tension between social freedoms and a moral system may reinforce the moral system, as believers discipline themselves in the exercise of what they believe to be their imperiled faith. When morality is violated, the response is disproportionate, because violation of one moral law threatens the integrity of the structure as a whole and so cannot be permitted.

Laws are human inventions that are part of a code of behavior more concrete than ethics, incorporating both natural laws of inadmissible behavior and rules for the settlement of conflicts that could, in a different context or society, be resolved differently by honest arbitrators (see Chapter 23). Ethics is, in a sense, the test of the goodness of a law. The law is one means to determine what society as a whole believes is appropriate behavior under certain conditions but it is also full of compromises, balances, and adjustments to the exigencies of the "real world." This section only provides general guidance on issues of ethics and touches briefly on law. Whenever legal issues are or might be involved, the reader is always advised to seek a legal opinion from an expert qualified or knowledgeable about current law in the jurisdiction involved.

Ethics, at least in the tradition of Western philosophy, derives from two traditions: deontology and relativism. Each handles issues of competing ethical duties differently.

Ethical principles that flow from morals, religious interpretation, revelation, the instructions or commandments of the deity, Kant's categorical imperative (a secular view of what must be done), or a collective cultural agreement on what is right and just (such as Confucianism) are called deontological. They tend to be absolute (such as "thou shalt not kill") and therefore subject to fine parsing and reinterpretation when applied to complicated events in the real world (". . . except in self-defense?"). This inevitably leads to a large body of theology or philosophical interpretation (such as the Talmud, the fatwas of Islamic scholars, or commentaries on the Bible in Christian tradition) and to competing schools of thought. Traditional medical ethics are deontological and are based on the following four principles:

- There should be respect for the autonomy of the individual ("autonomy").
- Physicians should do no harm ("non-malfeasance").
- Physicians should strive to do good ("beneficence").
- All individuals have equal rights and responsibilities ("distributive justice").

From these principles flow subsidiary ethical rules such as truthfulness, privacy, confidentiality, and fidelity.

Relativism, which is sometimes used in a pejorative sense, holds that ethical principles are meaningful only in relation to one another and to the facts of the situation. It accepts that there may be conflicting obligations and conflicts between legitimate but competing rights and responsibilities, forcing often uncomfortable decisions. Hard choices must often be made. Within relativism there are other paths, such as consequential ethics (taking into consideration the consequences and effects of applying the ethical principle) and utilitarianism ("the greatest good for the greatest number," associated with the philosopher Jeremy Bentham).

In general, medicine has favored deontological ethics, but increasingly the deontological approach is proving inadequate. Physicians experience being caught between competing interests, constraints on how they can practice, limits on their ability to advocate for their patients, and ambiguous ethical dilemmas, regardless of their practice. Because occupational medicine places the physician in a direct relationship with parties other than the individual patient, potential conflicts of interest and competing ethical obligations often occur, and ethical issues may grow quite complex in OEM. Relativistic ethics is the only clear way to resolve these issues, but the nature and priority of competing obligations and rights must be clear. Occupational medicine has had many years to grapple with this problem. Medicine as a whole, at least in North America, is really just waking up to the reality that ethical duties often require balance.

In occupational medicine, much depends on the role of each of the agents or parties in the relationship. In occupational medicine, distinct agents can be identified by role:

- The service provider, who is the OEM physician or his or her designate. The service being provided may be a service of assessment and treatment, assuming responsibility for care, or of evaluation and recommendation without assuming responsibility for care.

- The client, who receives the service. This is usually the worker, who may or may not be a patient, in the sense of having a health problem, and there may or may not be a physician-patient relationship.

- The customer, who buys and in a sense "owns" the service. This is usually the employer (or a unit within a large employer) or the workers' compensation carrier.

- Stakeholders, who may have a legitimate interest in the provision of care or the identification of the case. These may include regulatory bodies, appeals tribunals, suppliers who are concerned with use of their products (for example, chemical manufacturers and distributors involved in Responsible Care®), voluntary organizations, the injured worker's personal physician, and others, including family members of an injured worker. Some of these stakeholders have a right to confidential information, outlined in law, and others do not.

In addition, the worker who is being provided care by the occupational physician may fill different roles, some of them at the same time. A worker who is well and who may be undergoing a periodic health surveillance program is not generally regarded as a patient—that term is usually reserved for someone receiving individualized medical services for a condition. A worker who has been injured or made ill is often called an "injured worker" (this term is regularly used in workers' compensation circles) rather than a patient. A worker, whether injured or not, may be employed, self-employed, or unemployed (because "worker" describes as much the intent to work as employment). If employed, the worker is also an employee, which implies that the worker is bound by contractual obligations and policies that may influence his or her care (such as selection of the initial treating physician).

These are not distinctions without a difference. These distinctions matter. In the past, some occupational physicians believed that their true client was their customer, the employer, and that they did not owe the worker disclosure or even consideration. They identified with management and saw no conflict in ethics, because they did not see themselves as having a physician-patient relationship with the worker; they considered the company to be their "patient." No right-thinking occupational physician should think that way anymore. Clients have rights that should not conflict with customers' rights if the system is working.

The physician should put the interests of the patient or injured worker first, but not at the expense of truthfulness or the potential to do significant harm. The corollary rights of the other parties must be respected and balanced, though the heaviest weight should favor the patient or injured worker. In case of conflicts, it is best to make the balance clear to each party and to document the situation in writing. This is so common that it can usually best be done on forms and confirmed by obtaining a signature to document that the worker was informed.

Occupational medicine practice and the bounds of ethics absolutely require clarity on when a physician-patient relationship exists and on making it clear to the worker when it does not. When the worker is being assessed and treated by the physician, a physician-patient relationship exists. When a medical evaluation is conducted solely for the purpose of a third party—such as a fitness-for-duty evaluation, disability evaluation, an independent medical evaluation, or periodic health surveillance—a patient-physician relationship does not normally exist, and if it does not, this has to be made clear to the worker. In situations where the client is not a patient, this should be made clear to the parties involved, and there is still an obligation for fairness, protection of confidentiality, and non-malfeasance (in the sense that the physician should not intentionally do harm but still has a duty to be truthful in reporting his or her findings).

In cases where the worker is also a patient of the physician in another context, such as serving as his or her personal physician, it is difficult and sometimes untenable to separate these roles. Understandably, there is also a trust issue and enough examples and stories of abuse for workers to generally prefer to seek the opinion of their own physicians in matters such as disability evaluation or fitness to return to work. Some physicians assume that their role is to advocate for their patients' wishes, which may or may not be justified, rather than maintain arm's-length objectivity, as required by the occupational health or workers' compensation system. In so doing, they put themselves in an untenable situation, and their opinions may not carry much weight. That is why it is much better for occupational health services to be provided by qualified (and of course ethical) physicians who do not have an ongoing relationship with the worker in personal health matters. However, this is not possible in many situations, such as when there is limited access to qualified physicians. As in so much else in occupational medicine, this problem often needs to be managed on a case-by-case basis.

Some ethical issues are almost unique to occupational medicine, such as the appropriate management of periodic health surveillance and fitness-for-duty evaluations and disclosure of information. Others are common to the practice of medicine as a whole and are separate problems only as they must conform to the occupational health system, such as confidentiality of medical records. The majority of ethical problems that are of particular concern to the occupational physician are those that pertain to the behavior of the physician as confidant of the worker and as agent of the employer.

The physician who is seeing a patient on behalf of an employer or insurance carrier has an obligation to report to those parties such information as is directly pertinent to the employee's work capacity or work-related disorder and no more. The employee cannot enjoin the physician from conveying such information, nor can the employee enjoin the physician to fail to notify the appropriate government agency of a work-related injury or illness, as these are legal responsibilities of the physician. The employee has an absolute right to know the nature, name, and probable cause of a disorder that is found, and the physician has an absolute duty to inform the patient-employee of these findings and of what information will be conveyed to third parties. Under workers' compensation rules, however, the employee may not necessarily be free to select any physician to treat a disorder beyond the first encounter with the expectation that unauthorized fees will be paid. When circumstances arise in which these rights and responsibilities create a conflict, something is wrong. The physician must then analyze the situation to determine who is out of line and stand firm in an unambiguous position, regardless of personal interest and sympathies.

Confidentiality of medical records is a major issue in occupational medicine, as it is in medicine in general. The general rule applies that the physical medical record is the property of who owns the file or the platform in which it is recorded, but that the information it contains belongs to the person who created it and is at all times available to the worker or patient. This leads to conflict when supervisors or human-resources managers attempt to access an employee's record. They are not entitled to do so. Disputed workers' compensation cases and litigation are subject to law, and the record must be supplied. At that point, control is often lost by the occupational health service. However, the OEM physician should always treat the record as confidential, just like any other medical record, securing it and limiting access to qualified health professionals. Although it is not clear that HIPAA (the American law governing handling of medical information) necessarily applies to occupational health or workers' compensation records, the OEM physician should not put it to the test and should have no reason to try; one should follow the same procedures as for medical records in general medicine.

Occupational health records are normally retained in the United States for at least thirty years (up to forty in some OSHA standards, such as for lead and arsenic) and for the duration of employment, as required by OSHA. (Employees who work for less than one year are not subject to this requirement as long as their records are given to them on separation.) As a matter of ethics, the records should be kept securely under the control of the OEM physician or the occupational health service during that time, or they may be transferred with the worker's consent to another party, including the worker's personal physician. Some state agencies and OSHA will also receive and store records when an employer goes out of business, but normally the record becomes the property of the business that takes over ownership.

Codes of Ethics

Codes of ethics for occupational medicine and for occupational health professionals in general emphasize seven basic themes:

- An obligation on the part of the employer and responsible occupational health professionals to provide a safe and healthy workplace environment for the worker
- An obligation on the part of occupational health professionals to maintain professional competence
- An obligation on the part of occupational health professionals to report problems and advise on solutions
- An obligation on the part of occupational health professionals and employers to maintain the confidentiality of the worker's medical records
- An obligation on the part of occupational health professionals to avoid conflicts of interest
- An obligation on the part of occupational health professionals and employers to avoid discrimination, intended or otherwise
- An obligation on the part of occupational health professionals and employers to maintain ethical standards

Obviously, it is much easier to apply and enforce these ethical standards on occupational health professionals than on employers.

The world standard in ethics for occupational health is the International Code of Ethics for Occupational Health Professionals of the International Commission on Occupational Health (http://www .icohweb.org/core_docs/code_ethics_eng.pdf). The most recent revision at the time of this writing was approved in 2002 and is available in eight languages. The International Commission on

Occupational Health (ICOH) code has been widely adopted by other organizations (including the Association of Occupational and Environmental Clinics) and has been adopted as the legal standard of practice in Italy and Argentina. The American College of Occupational and Environmental Medicine was revising but had not completed its code of ethics at the time of this writing (2009). The Occupational and Environmental Medical Association of Canada has a short, streamlined code adopted in 1989—adapted from the Canadian Medical Association and the Ontario Medical Association—that is compatible with the ICOH code. The ICOH code will therefore be the basis for further discussion in this section.

The ICOH code covers all occupational health professionals, reflecting a shared set of values. This is also important in practical terms because of the confusion and the potential for exploitation that would result if different occupational health professions (physicians, nurses, hygienists, psychologists, ergonomists, and so forth) followed different rules on, for example, confidentiality. The ICOH code therefore applies to any professional who works in the domain of occupational health and overlays the standard of practice and ethics for the profession or discipline. In the case of medicine, the ICOH code guides the physician within the domain of OEM practice, but neither replaces nor subordinates medical ethics in general.

Principles of the ICOH code are laid out in a lengthy introduction, omitted here. Key provisions include the following:

- The highest goal of occupational health practice is protection and prevention.
- A safe and healthy workplace is the responsibility of the employer.
- The workplace should be changed; healthy working conditions should be provided; and work should be adapted to, rather than exclude, the worker.

- "Occupational health professionals should assist workers in obtaining and maintaining employment notwithstanding their health deficiencies or their handicap." This reflects the emerging view that disability is a condition, not a characteristic, and that the way to manage it is to remove barriers to full participation of the worker to the extent feasible, and that a worker's individual needs should be considered.

- Occupational health professionals are defined by their role, not by credentials or formal titles. This role comes with responsibility for workers' health, which, once assumed, requires the practitioner to protect and promote workers' health and commitment to a safe and healthy workplace.

- Discrimination is not acceptable.

- Occupational health professionals should be independent, free to give advice, adequately provided with resources, and allowed to practice according to the highest professional standards. (This provision implies but does not spell out a duty on the part of the occupational health professional not to practice at all if it cannot be done right.)

- Recognition that protection of workers' health is primary, but that there are balances between, for example, protection of employment and protection of health (for example, when a worker has a condition that might present a threat to him- or herself or others but does not wish for it to be disclosed) and conflicts between individual and collective interests (in the same example, between an obligation to the worker and the obligation to prevent harm to other workers on the job).

- Recognition that much of occupational health practice is governed by law and regulation, and that there are also various International Labour Organization conventions and recommendations that are binding in countries that have ratified them. (Several of them require worker representation in occupational health services, which is not the norm in the United States.)

Basic Principles

Following the introduction, the text begins with a set of three basic principles:

- *The purpose of occupational health is to serve the health and social well-being of the workers individually and collectively. Occupational health practice must be performed according to the highest professional standards and ethical principles. Occupational health professionals must contribute to environmental and community health.*

  This is a strong, cohesive statement, not a string of platitudes. The first principle requires high, not merely adequate, standards of practice, but recognizes a potential balance between the interests of the individual worker and the collective interest of fellow workers where they may conflict; this is different from the almost exclusively individual-patient-centered focus of conventional medical ethics. It lays the groundwork for the doctrine of balance among the interests of the parties in occupational health without considering such balance to be an ethical compromise.

- *The duties of occupational health professionals include protecting the life and health of the worker, respecting human dignity and promoting the highest ethical principles in occupational health policies and programmes. Integrity in professional conduct, impartiality and the protection of the confidentiality of health data and of the privacy of workers are part of these duties.*

  Again, this may appear obvious, but it lays a foundation. The OEM physician (in this case) is being admonished to behave according to the highest standards of (in this case) medical practice and not to consider occupational health to be an area in which one can let down one's guard or compromise on behavior.

- *Occupational health professionals are experts who must enjoy full pro-fessional independence in the execution of their functions. They must acquire and maintain the competence necessary for their duties and require conditions which allow them to carry out their tasks according to good practice and professional ethics.*

This principle puts the occupational health professional, in this case the OEM physician, on notice that it is one's own responsibility to determine whether his or her work is adequate, competent, and sufficiently well supported to be effective. The purpose of this principle is not to force any OEM physician to quit if he or she does not get all the support he or she wants. It is intended to require occupational health professionals to be careful about their relationships to ensure that their work is undertaken honestly and that they can follow their best judgment, rather than management dictates. Otherwise one ends up being merely a tool or mouthpiece, or a name to demonstrate compliance with local requirements, with no real authority. The principle also requires that occupational health professionals, in this case the physician, be diligent in preparing to practice in this field, so that, for example, a physician who markets his or her practice to employers in order to get occupational injury cases without learning anything about the workplace, work capacity, workers' compensation, or other important aspects of OEM would be considered an unethical practitioner.

Duties and Obligations

The body of the ICOH code then commences with a section on the duties and obligations of occupational health professionals.

1. *The primary aim of occupational health practice is to safeguard and promote the health of workers, to promote a safe and healthy working environment, to protect the working capacity of workers and their access to employment. In pursuing this aim, occupational health professionals must use validated methods of risk evaluation, propose effective preventive measures and follow up their implementation. The occupational health professionals must provide competent and*

honest advice to the employers on fulfilling their responsibility in the field of occupational safety and health as well as to the workers on the protection and promotion of their health in relation to work. The occupational health professionals should maintain direct contact with safety and health committees, where they exist.

This passage is straightforward. It should be noted that for employers of significant size, the ICOH code expects there to be joint (worker-management) health and safety committees or other mechanisms for the review, evaluation, and correction of workplace hazards and the assessment of safety performance, injuries, and incidents. American OEM physicians may have difficulty with this provision because such committees are uncommon in the United States (except where they have been written into a collective-bargaining agreement), but they are required by law in Canada. Employers may be reluctant to allow OEM physicians who work under contract to participate regularly in these internal company meetings. The OEM physician should at least ask to be on the distribution list for the minutes of the meetings, read them carefully, and follow up on any topic of medical concern.

2. *Occupational health professionals must continuously strive to be familiar with the work and working environment as well as to develop their competence and to remain well informed in scientific and technical knowledge, occupational hazards and the most efficient means to eliminate or to minimize the relevant risks. As the emphasis must be on primary prevention defined in terms of policies, design, choice of clean technologies, engineering control measures and adapting work organizations and workplaces to workers, occupational health professionals must regularly and routinely, whenever possible, visit the workplaces and consult the workers and the management on the work that is performed.*

This provision has become increasingly difficult for OEM physicians who work in the community and not as part of a corporate medical department or in a plant facility. It requires that an effort be made to see the actual workplace and to talk to workers, both outside and inside the clinic, in order to better understand the realities of the workplace. This requires management cooperation, and the lack of such cooperation may be a sign that management will not provide the support and acceptance that the OEM physician needs to do his or her job. In some cases, it may be possible to visit similar workplaces elsewhere to gain a general understanding of hazards and jobs, but the heart of this provision is that the OEM physician should be familiar with the specific workplaces where the workers under his or her care are employed.

3. *The occupational health professional must advise management and the workers on factors at work which may affect workers' health. The risk assessment of occupational hazards must lead to the establishment of an occupational safety and health policy and of a programme of prevention adapted to the needs of undertakings [enterprises] and workplaces. The occupational health professionals must propose such a policy and programme on the basis of scientific and technical knowledge currently available as well as of their knowledge of the work organization and environment. Occupational health professionals must ensure that they possess the required skill or secure the necessary expertise in order to provide advice on programmes of prevention which should include, as appropriate, measures for monitoring and management of occupational safety and health hazards and, in case of failure, for minimizing consequences.*

The major thrust of this provision is that occupational health practice is not a solo affair to be assigned to the occupational health professional. It is management's responsibility and should be governed by a policy, as are other aspects of business and corporate responsibility. The employer needs to have a well-defined and explicit policy, and there needs to be a systematic program for carrying out that policy. If the employer does not have such a policy (a serious mistake, for many reasons, that can lead to big trouble for an organization), the OEM physician (or other occupational health professional) should propose one, and it should be sound in principle and appropriate to the workers' needs. A policy might include a statement on the company's commitment to prevent injury and illness; a statement committing the company to meet or exceed compliance with all applicable regulations and laws; safe work practices (confined spaces, lock-out procedures, working alone or in isolation, and special needs of the industry); hazard evaluation and management (hazard communication and training); occupational hygiene surveys and monitoring; plant inspection; fire and security procedures; management accountability; first aid and access to medical care; early and safe return to work; training; incident investigation; reporting incidents and injuries; drug testing and substance abuse in safety-sensitive jobs; fitness for duty and work capacity (for example, compliance with the Americans with Disabilities Act); and training, at all levels, including drills. However, it is not enough to write the policy and hand it over to management, which may then put it on the shelf unread and unused. Management must be engaged in its development and must "own" it for it to be an effective document.

4. *Special consideration should be given to the rapid application of simple preventive measures which are technically sound and easily implemented. Further evaluation must check whether these measures are effective or if a more complete solution must be sought. When doubts exist about the severity of an occupational hazard, prudent precautionary action must be considered immediately and taken as appropriate. When there are uncertainties or differing opinions concerning nature of the hazards or the risks involved, occupational health professionals must be transparent in their assessment with respect to all concerned, avoid ambiguity in communicating their opinion and consult other professionals as necessary.*

It may not be obvious why this provision is included, but there is often a tendency in occupational health to wait for the perfect solution instead of controlling the hazard quickly and expeditiously. This provision also calls on the OEM physician, in this case, to respect that there may be differing opinions regarding risk, but to be clear in his or her assessment and to consult other professionals, most often occupational hygienists, rather than guessing. This provision reinforces the emphasis throughout the document on prevention and on prompt action.

5. *In the case of refusal or of unwillingness to take adequate steps to remove an undue risk or to remedy a situation which presents evidence of danger to health or safety, the occupational health professionals must make, as rapidly as possible, their concern clear, in writing, to the appropriate senior management executive, stressing the need for taking into account scientific knowledge and for applying relevant health protection standards, including exposure limits, and recalling the obligation of the employer to apply laws and regulations and to protect the health of workers in their employment. The workers concerned and their representatives in the enterprise should be informed and the competent authority [government regulatory body] should be contacted, whenever necessary.*

This provision requires the OEM physician, in this case, to speak up and not let control of potentially serious hazards drop due to lack of management interest or action. However, it is also clear that the threshold for pushing the issue this far is an exceptional and substantial risk. Minor injury does not rise to this standard.

6. *Occupational health professionals must contribute to the information for workers on occupational hazards to which they may be exposed in an objective and understandable manner which does not conceal any fact and emphasizes the preventive measures. The occupational health professionals must cooperate with the employer, the workers and their representatives to ensure adequate information and training on health and safety to the management personnel and workers. Occupational health professionals must provide appropriate information to the*

employers, workers and their representatives about the level of scientific certainty or uncertainty of known and suspected occupational hazards at the workplace.

This provision requires transparency and effectiveness in risk communication on the part of the OEM physician.

7. *Occupational health professionals are obliged not to reveal industrial or commercial secrets of which they may become aware in the exercise of their activities. However, they must not withhold information which is necessary to protect the safety and health of workers or of the community. When needed, the occupational health professionals must consult the competent authority in charge of supervising the implementation of the relevant legislation.*

This provision acknowledges the legitimacy of trade secrets but holds the OEM physician, in this case, to a higher duty committed to health protection. Even so, it requires that local laws and regulations be consulted.

8. *The occupational health objectives, methods and procedures of health surveillance must be clearly defined with priority given to adaptation of workplaces to workers who must receive information in this respect. The relevance and validity of these methods and procedures must be assessed. The surveillance must be carried out with the informed consent of the workers. The potentially positive and negative consequences of participation in screening and health surveillance programmes should be discussed as part of the consent process. The health surveillance must be performed by an occupational health professional approved by the competent authority.*

This provision is not clearly written. Periodic health surveillance to screen for health effects has been more controversial in many countries (including Canada) than in the United States. Sometimes tests have been used that had little value or were even medically contraindicated (such as low-back x-rays). (See Chapter 5.) This provision requires that the methods of surveillance be evidence based. It also requires that participation be voluntary and based on informed consent such that a worker can opt out, for example if a worker is concerned that his or her job might be at risk if he or she is found to have an adverse health effect, or if the worker just does not want to know. This provision would not apply to mandated surveillance, such as that required by OSHA standards, or drug surveillance for workers covered under the regulations of the U.S. Department of Transportation. If there is a legitimate need for health surveillance and it is not covered by a regulation, the procedure and the rationale for it should be documented thoroughly in a policy, and permission to carry out the surveillance should be included in the work contract. As always, seek the advice of legal counsel.

9. *The results of examinations carried out within the framework of health surveillance must be explained to the worker concerned. The determination of fitness for a given job, when required, must be based on a good knowledge of the job demands and of the work-site and on the assessment of the health of the worker. The workers must be informed of the opportunity to challenge the conclusions concerning their fitness in relation to work that they feel contrary to their interest. An appeals procedure must be established in this respect.*

In much of the world, fitness-for-duty evaluations are considered part of surveillance, hence the inclusion of both in this provision. This provision requires the OEM physician to disclose to the worker the results of surveillance testing and to explain their significance. The major part of it, however, outlines the approach to work capacity and fitness for duty (as presented in Chapter 18), and requires that the worker have some mechanism for appeal. In North America, medical conclusions on fitness for duty for new hires or return to work are not normally subject to appeal, although decisions based on those conclusions, being management decisions, can be challenged on legal grounds, as under the Americans with Disabilities Act. This provision requires an appeals mechanism, and fairness and transparency would dictate that the conclusion be reviewed by a physician not involved in the first evaluation.

10. *The results of the examinations prescribed by national laws or regulations must only be conveyed to management in terms of fitness for the envisaged work or of limitations necessary from a medical point of view in the assignment of tasks or in the exposure to occupational hazards, with the emphasis put on proposals to adapt the tasks and working conditions to the abilities of the worker. General information on work fitness or in relation to health or the potential of probable health effects of work hazards, may be provided with the informed consent of the worker concerned, in so far as this is necessary to guarantee the protection of the worker's health.*

This provision is set in the context of pre-placement and periodic health evaluations required by law or regulation in many countries. However, its requirements also apply in North America, where practices differ. As required under the Americans with Disabilities Act (ADA) and Canadian law, the employer is not normally entitled to the diagnosis or any specific information on the medical condition of an employee or even details of the disability (although under ADA the employer may ask about the nature of the disability if the disability is obvious), except a conclusion regarding fitness for duty (expressed as "fit," "unfit," or "fit with accommodation/modification") and the accommodations or modifications required in the event of a disability. (This provision would also apply to certification of illness as grounds for absence by any physician; the "doctor's note" should not mention diagnosis.) Exceptions arise when disclosure of otherwise confidential medical information is required by law or regulation (as in workers' compensation claims), with informed consent, when disclosure would be in the worker's own interest (for example, if the worker became seriously ill at work), and when disclosure would be necessary for the public interest (for example, if the worker had a highly communicable disease). The first two are unequivocal, but the latter two are relative and place the OEM physician in a difficult position of balancing interests. The standard for disclosure without the protection of law or consent would be very high: serious injury or risk to life.

11. *Where the health condition of the worker and the nature of the tasks performed are such as to be likely to endanger the safety of others, the worker must be clearly informed of the situation. In the case of a particularly hazardous situation, the management and, if so required by national regulations, the competent authority must also be informed of the measures necessary to safeguard other persons. In his advice, the occupational health professional must try to reconcile employment of the worker concerned with the safety or health of others that may be endangered.*

This provision acknowledges that the worker's right to employment must be balanced against the potential hazard to others if the worker's duties would endanger others. For the protection of others, "safety-sensitive" workers are held to a higher standard of fitness and reliability, and it is this standard that justifies more frequent periodic health surveillance and mandatory drug testing. However, the emphasis in this provision is on making the worker him- or herself aware of the risk to others, which gives the worker a chance voluntarily to request a change in duties. The provision sets a higher threshold for notifying management and government regulatory agencies; the situation must exceed the usual degree of risk in any workplace.

As in many ethical questions, there is also a legal dimension to this, which, insofar as it represents a social consensus on what is right, informs the ethical argument. In the United States, the decision in a highly influential 1976 California case, Tarasoff v. Regents of the University of California (551 P.2d 334), established a "duty to warn" for health care providers, which overrides confidentiality of medical records when there is a serious risk to others. Many states have laws requiring physicians to disclose information germane to public safety, such as a medical condition that would interfere with safe driving, and others protect the physician who discloses against the will of the patient in such cases but do not require it. However, case law is thin. Canadian law and consensus on ethics accept the principle that confidentiality of medical information is not absolute and that public safety may override it, but this consensus sets a high standard, such as a risk of serious injury or death that is imminent and concrete, not distant or theoretical. Thus it would appear that at least in North America society has decided that confidentiality should be protected to the extent possible, but not at all costs, and that serious injury and death are unacceptable costs.

The ethical principle is that neither the confidentiality of medical information nor the duty to warn of possible risk is absolute. They must be weighed, and the only sure balance favoring disclosure is when the consequences of failure to disclose information are unacceptably high to society. To the maximum extent possible, the OEM physician should avoid such situations, such as by persuading the worker to disclose the information voluntarily (and documenting the effort); by making a judgment of "unfit" for duty; or by seeking guidance through regulation, contract language, and strong employer policies.

12. *Biological tests and other investigations must be chosen for their validity and relevance for protection of the health of the worker concerned, with due regard to their sensitivity, their specificity and their predictive value. Occupational health professionals must not use screening tests or investigations which are not reliable or which do not have a sufficient predictive value in relation to the requirements of the work assignment. Where a choice is possible and appropriate, preference must always be given to non-invasive methods and to examinations, which do not involve any danger to the health of the worker concerned. An invasive investigation or an examination which involves a risk to the health of the worker concerned may only be advised after an evaluation of the benefits to the worker and the risks involved. Such an investigation is subject to the worker's informed consent and must be performed according*

to the highest professional standards. It cannot be justified for insurance purposes or in relation to insurance claims.

Biological tests, in this context, mean clinical, laboratory, bio-monitoring, or personal sampling tests (such as biological exposure indices). To be acceptable, they must conform to the characteristics of a well-performing test as outlined in Chapter 5, particularly with respect to predictive value. The provision discourages or prohibits tests that have not been scientifically validated (such as visual contrast sensitivity as a test for toxicity), that do not have well-defined outcomes (such as neurocognitive testing), that are not demonstrably related to work exposures or capacity (such as pelvic examinations for female employees), and that have poor predictive value (such as color vision tests as an initial screen for solvent toxicity). The provision also prohibits tests that carry an unacceptable risk (such as low-back x-rays) or inconvenience the worker (such as 24-hour urine collections). Every so often, someone invents a new test and tries to use it for screening workers without waiting for appropriate validation and acceptance by the scientific community. (A real, recent example was a proposal to test urine for asbestos fibers, which made no medical sense.) As a practical matter, this means that only time-tested, reliable, and well-validated tests should even be considered for screening, periodic health surveillance, and fitness-for-duty evaluations. Otherwise, the risk of discrimination because of false positives or negatives is too high.

Genetic testing is particularly sensitive. In addition to providing inappropriate information on individual susceptibility and health risk to employers, genetic testing can be used unfairly to exclude workers from a workplace with a hazard, even though the focus should be on controlling the hazard.

13. *When engaging in health education, health promotion, health screening and public health programmes, occupational health professionals must seek the participation of both employers and workers in their design and*

in their implementation. They must also protect the confidentiality of personal health data of the workers, and prevent their misuse.

This short provision is particularly important because it insists on the involvement of workers in the means for their protection. It treats occupational health and health promotion as a matter of equity, in which workers have the right to a say in how their health and interests will be protected, without denying that primary responsibility always rests with the employer.

The ICOH code has provided occupational health and safety professionals around the world with consistent guidance for appropriate behavior and has established a global standard of practice. It cannot solve every conceivable dilemma, but if its principles are followed diligently and documented, the OEM physician will be on firm ground.

THE WAY FORWARD FOR OCCUPATIONAL HEALTH AND SAFETY

Occupational health and safety (OHS) is like a cork in a sea of economic activity, bobbing up and down as the waves pass under it, never completely sinking but carrying little weight, and always at the mercy of forces much larger than its pull on gravity. As the U.S., Canadian, and world economies pass through a wrenching transition, it is time to consider where occupational health and safety may be headed and how the forces at play just now, at the time of writing (2009), are shaping it. The future of OHS will define, to a large extent, the future of OEM.

Occupational health and safety has been seen in many different ways in its long history. The field has passed through eras in which it has been perceived to be primarily an issue of public health, of production efficiency, of labor-management relations, of corporate responsibility, of loss containment, of liability control, and now of human-resources management. What is needed now is a new conceptualization that strips occupational health and safety of its accreted social and political agendas and returns it to a practical field in public health and medicine. This does not mean backing off from a commitment to workers' health protection as a human right. It does mean that this right should be served by a professional system that is stable, objective, and separate from political agendas. (The system should not be neutral, however, because it exists to protect workers.)

Society as a whole has never placed a high priority on safe workplaces as a public health goal or value, preferring to deal with issues of productivity and loss control and to avoid the human rights dimension of occupational health protection. Occupational health and safety is generally perceived as something to be managed, like warranties on equipment or maintenance on a plant. Occupational health and safety functions are perceived as an expense of production, to be kept under control but not likely to yield a return on investment (although they can!). Identification and control of highly specific occupational hazards may not hold much appeal in terms of benefit and cost in the new economy, especially because so many employers are persuaded that the major industrial hazards, such as asbestos, belong to the past. Occupational health services are easily lost in the shuffle in health care policy and management. That is why reform of occupational health and workers' compensation should not be folded into the mainstream of health care reform; there, it will always be an afterthought.

New Challenges

A major challenge to OHS professionals is to create an attitudinal change in the workplace. OHS is considered in industry and by most workers to be an add-on responsibility, not a normal part of doing business. For OHS professionals to achieve their potential, occupational health and safety must be an integral part of the mainstream.

It is instructive to compare interest in the environment with interest in occupational health and safety. The two are clearly related in some people's minds but are very distinct to others. Environmental quality is clearly an issue of public concern; occupational health and safety is perceived by the public as a much narrower issue, of concern only to selected groups of workers and special interests. Environmental quality is always highly visible; occupational health and safety is recognized only in times of crisis or in dramatic cases. Environmental quality is an end in itself and a desirable enhancement of the quality of life; occupational health and safety is a means to an end, because it facilitates productivity and removes obstacles to efficient operation. Small wonder that the quality of the environment is a powerful shaping issue in our society, but the quality of the working environment goes through cycles of neglect and rediscovery.

Since about 2000, the United States has entered a new and rather regressive phase in occupational health and safety. The emphasis today in industry, government, and organized labor is "back to basics"—a renewed emphasis on the essentials, dispensing with more-sophisticated approaches. There is a feeling that occupational health and safety may have become too complicated and technical, and that the basic commitment may need to be reviewed. The result has been a turning inward to reexamine basic issues, rather than reaching outward for new ideas and initiatives. It is an odd phase of rediscovery because it fails to build on what has gone before.

As a result of the election of 2008, there have been fundamental changes in political leadership in the United States that have raised interest in occupational health and safety and environmental protection. However, the onset of the global recession has left government, major corporations, labor, and public opinion with a sense of confusion. The forward momentum expected in occupational health and safety may be over before it started. On the other hand, environmental protection remains high on the national agenda, and emerging green technology makes it easier to align environmental priorities with fiscal incentives and economic reconstruction.

In the economy that emerges from the current recession, occupational health and safety will probably become a production and sustainability issue for some industries, mostly those on the economic margins, and a health services management issue for most. Employers are likely to give higher priority to issues that affect more workers, that affect the workers in higher-value-added jobs, and that involve greater monetary losses or potential productivity gains. These are the issues that relate to low-risk workplaces, such as ergonomic hazards and psychogenic stress—issues that increasingly dominate the occupational health and safety agenda. Occupational hazards of a physical and chemical nature are likely to get worse, or they will at least continue to present management problems in manufacturing sectors that are already under intense economic pressure, as well as in small enterprises that are least able to manage them well.

Occupational health and safety professionals in the new economy may have to learn, as a business proposition, to deal with occupational health primarily through issues embedded in productivity, personal health insurance, disability management, adjudication processes, and wellness. In order to keep employers' attention, the argument may need to be made on the basis that a dollar invested in occupational health and prevention of injury pays back much more in recovered costs than most investments.

In the new economy, some occupational hazards may be novel; some may be redistributed; and some may require specialized technology to control, which has been the historical experience in, say, the semiconductor industry. However, most of the major hazards are likely to be the same ones seen today in sectors such as construction. Serious risks will increasingly be concentrated in certain industries and groups of workers, among them disadvantaged and special populations. The practical management problem for occupational health and safety in the future, as in the past, will be to deal effectively with hazards that are fragmented and often irrelevant to the economy, and to deal with problems that are too often buried in aggregate statistics and nearly invisible from the outside—problems for which there is therefore little political will to do anything. But after an era of incentives for underreporting, apparently declining occupational injury rates, and competing priorities for management attention, will there be the will to do anything?

The Way Forward

What is the way forward? If society is to attain and, more importantly, sustain effective efforts in occupational health and safety, supporting a new priority for OEM, there need to be certain changes:

1. Consistency. OHS programs need long-term stability to thrive.
2. A stronger OHS infrastructure. Occupational health and safety needs a broader base in industry, government, labor, and academia.
3. Independent voices. New ideas usually come from small groups working intensively outside of day-to-day responsibilities. There needs to be respect for the role of university programs, union-sponsored institutes and centers, and worker-led organizations (such as the Committees for Occupational Safety and Health, social scientists, technical consultants, trade associations, and professional organizations), because these are society's think tanks for new ideas. The first rule of brainstorming for new concepts is to be wide open to new ideas and to evaluate them later. That is how practical, effective, and innovative ideas emerge.
4. Mainstream commitment. Special award programs and such are very good and have an attention-getting effect for a few years after their initiation. What really counts, however, is the integration of occupational health and safety into production and management: criteria for promotion, performance reviews, operating procedures, bidding on contracts, contractor performance, collective bargaining, fiscal projections, and operating

permits. The rest becomes window dressing after the first few years.

5. Disregard the distinction between safety and health. The professionals in each professional sector should be talking to one another all the time, regardless of their background and training.

6. Change the paradigm. Occupational health and safety is by rights a public health function, not a privilege or a negotiating position.

7. Return to the intellectual basics, but not to kindergarten. The blueprint for effective OHS regulations has already been written. Society does not need to reinvent it. The fundamental features of the Occupational Health and Safety Act of 1970, for example, are not the cause of OSHA's disappointing performance. Reform may be needed in OSHA, but the basic legislative philosophy has not failed.

8. Open the system. Occupational health and safety thrives when experiences are shared among professionals and especially among employers, and when management listens to its own workers. Occupational health and safety always falters when employers and professionals maintain strict isolation, refuse to share information, and take a top-down approach to the management of safety, acting by directive to their workers instead of learning from their workers' experiences.

9. Openness to new ideas. Canada and the United States represent two quite different traditions in occupational and environmental health protection. The United States itself has fifty experiments in state regulation and state-level workers' compensation. Much can be learned by comparing them and by examining other national models, such as the United Kingdom's Health and Safety Executive, which to most observers has been conspicuously more successful than OSHA.

10. Continuous improvement. For occupational health and safety standards as well as for environmental standards, a national policy

of continuous improvement makes sense. Standards are now proposed and adopted as if they are permanent and as if re-evaluation is an exceptional event. Standards do not stand for all time: they are superseded as more information becomes available, technology advances, and the economic cycle permits. Just now, the introduction of green technology and infrastructure reconstruction constitute one of the few optimistic lights in an otherwise dismal economic agenda. This is an historic opportunity to make things better. Why not institutionalize continuous progress and stop fighting it?

11. An end to environmental standards battles. Battles over new standards are, for the most part, ultimately delaying tactics. How much less disruptive economically and politically might it be to accept small and frequent incremental changes as natural steps, advancing a little more at every technological advance and opportunity without fighting individual battles over the documentation and justification for large-increment jumps in standards?

12. A unitary view of occupational and environmental health and medicine. It has been a consistent theme of this book that occupational medicine and environmental medicine are sister disciplines that in this age are merging, though that process is not yet complete. The next step in bringing these fields together may be to start thinking of occupational medicine as a subset of environmental medicine, a medical field concerned primarily with the built environment of the workplace and of sustainability. Sustainability in this sense is not environmental or ecological sustainability—preserving resources for future generations—nor is it economic sustainability—supporting the same harvesting (or exploitation) year after year. There is also a form of cultural sustainability, based on a shared vision of stewardship that keeps culture and values intact. Part of this vision of sustainability is that health should not be compromised for gain and that a sustainable society protects the health of those who make its wealth and continuity possible.

RESOURCES

Guidotti TL. Environmental and occupational health: a "critical science." *Int Arch Occup Environ Health*. 2005;60(2):59–60.

Guidotti TL, Hancock T, Bell W. Physicians and environmental change: what is our role and why should anyone listen to *us*? *Perspect Biol Med*. 1998;41:591–604.

Ravetz J: Towards critical science. *New Sci*. 1971;51:681–683.

NOTEWORTHY READINGS

Canadian Medical Association. *Health, the Environment and Sustainable Development: The Role of the Medical Profession*. Ottawa: CMA; 1991.

Dickens C. *Hard Times*. Mineola NY, Dover, republished 2001. [Classic novel, first published in 1854 in London, and generally considered to be Dickens' most severe condemnation of the Industrial Revolution. It satirizes the mindset of the "Strict Father" as described by Lakoff and in the text.]

Guidotti TL. Preventive medicine, public health, and the environmental movement. *Am J Prev Med*. 1991;7 :124–125.

Heilbroner RL. *The Great Ascent: The Struggle for Economic Development in Our Time*. New York: Harper and Row; 1963. [Robert Heilbroner had already predicted, in the 1960s, that economic growth and production would be limited by social restrictions on external costs, such as environmental degradation and occupational health and safety issues.]

Lakoff G. *Moral Politics: How Liberals and Conservatives Think*. Chicago, University of Chicago Press, 2002, 2nd ed. [First edition, published in 1996, was subtitled "What Conservatives Know that Liberals Don't".]

McCally M, Cassel CK. Medical responsibility and global environmental change. *Ann Intern Med*. 1990;113:467–473.

Ravetz JR. *The Merger of Knowledge with Power: Essays in Critical Science*. London: Continuum International;1989.

Ronchi D. The quality of working life movement: part I, history. *Employee Relations*. 1981;3(1):2–6.

Task Force on the Implications for Human Health of Global Ecological Change. *Human and Ecosystem Health: Canadian Perspectives, Canadian Action*. Ottawa: Canadian Public Health Association; 1992.

Weber M. *The Protestant Ethic and the Spirit of Capitalism*. Mineola NY, Dover, republished 2003. [Classic treatise in sociology discussing the influence of values and faith on economic bahavior. First published in German in 1905.]

Wells DM. *Empty Promises: Quality of Working Life Programs and the Labor Movement*. New York: Monthly Review Press; 1987.

26 GLOBAL OCCUPATIONAL AND ENVIRONMENTAL HEALTH

Occupational and environmental medicine (OEM) physicians, like the employers and workers they serve, are engaged on one level or another with the global economy by virtue of being in business. The rise of modern globalization, and of interdependence through trade and finance, connects most enterprises of any scale, directly or indirectly, and affects most workers in developed and developing countries. Occupational and environmental health problems also play an important role, generally unappreciated, in economic development, both as a drag on the national economy as it grows, a drain when it falters, and as a factor that always tragically limits the participation in modern life of those whom it affects when there is disability.

The word "global" is increasingly used to describe a broader range of issues and relationships, within and among countries, including those that affect minorities and vulnerable groups (such as indigenous peoples). In an increasingly integrated world, the word "international" is insufficient to describe common threats, risks, and responses, and it is also an insufficient word to describe the levels of cooperation and communication between peoples. "International" also implies, if only grammatically, bipartite or multipartite relationships between and among nations or countries, rather than the whole of health around the world, whereas "global health" as used today also applies to issues within countries and to vulnerable populations such as internally migrating populations, whether refugees or economic immigrants. Health issues are rarely unique to a particular country or society, but neither are they identical among different countries. With the exception of access to health care, health issues are rarely demarcated by a national border. The study of commonalities and differences in health and its determinants from one national community to the next, and how to change disparities in health, defines global health.

A small number of OEM physicians work mainly or exclusively for multinational companies or for international organizations in the global arena. Many have responsibilities for operations outside North America and for workers, including executives, who travel. Most provide services to the local workers of domestic employers, which are profoundly affected by globalization and international trade. Fewer physicians—but a significant number of them—work on environmental health issues around the world, usually through research. Whatever their level of involvement, an understanding and appreciation of global occupational and environmental health helps the OEM physician to see the big picture.

Global occupational and environmental health is the world perspective on determinants and problems of health relevant to OEM and other occupational and environmental health professions.

Global occupational and environmental health has many dimensions, among them:

- The role of occupational health in economic development worldwide
- The role of environmental health in economic development worldwide
- Management of occupational health in foreign subsidiaries and operations
- Health issues at international borders, associated with movement of people

- Travel medicine, as it applies to workers and management
- International agencies and organizations

ECONOMIC DEVELOPMENT

OEM physicians are concentrated in developed countries, of course, and are in short supply in developing countries. The OEM physician in North America is likely to be concerned primarily with occupational, rather than environmental, health in developing countries because demand for services is driven by the need to serve and address issues relating to foreign operations of the employer. It helps to understand the development process in a general way in order to visualize how occupational health services fit into development and play a role in economic development. The same overview helps in understanding the role of environmental health, which is less frequently a responsibility of the OEM physician with responsibilities in developing countries.

Attitudes toward occupational and environmental health are embedded in the social frameworks and public health systems of their societies and countries, as discussed in Chapter 25. Every country's approach to occupational and environmental health reflects its history, economic development, and culture—particularly attitudes toward risk—and is affected to some degree by its diversity. However, some generalizations can be made. One is that very few societies make occupational health a priority in their affairs (one exception is Finland). Its role in economic development is almost completely overlooked. Attitudes toward the environment are much better defined, however. As a society grows richer, it tends to become more risk-averse and insists on more protection. As a consequence, development tends to bring along with it, at least in later stages, an intolerance of personal risk and an insistence on public protection, whether from crime, pollution, or economic insecurity. Environmental protection also becomes a priority, because of a desire to prevent environmental health problems and a growing appreciation for environmental quality, both for its own sake and as an economic advantage. Within a given level of development, however, there seems to be almost no correlation between what priority a society places on environmental quality and the priority given to occupational health and safety, perhaps because occupational health is out of sight.

The Basics

Before undertaking any discussion of economic development, it is critical to think of the human faces behind it. Economic development too often reflects statistics and generalizations. The reality is that economic development is all about real people struggling to survive under difficult circumstances and how, how often, and how long the lives of some are made easier and the lives of others are made worse; because in any economy, there are winners and losers, and development is largely a matter of creating conditions to make more winners than losers.

Figure 26.1 shows a glimpse of the reality. The family in the photograph is working on the outskirts of Lusaka, the capital of Zambia. They are using a piece of scrap steel to break rocks into gravel. This is how they earn their living, every day, in the hot sun. They keep their children with them because there is no other way to look after them. They sell the gravel they make every day to a man who then sells it in bulk to a construction supplies dealer, who had a ready market when this photograph was taken because Lusaka at the time was experiencing a mild surge in building. If something goes wrong, and a rock chip flies into someone's eye, there is no health insurance or money for medical care. If the able-bodied adults who are strong enough to break the rocks are injured or become ill (in this country with a high rate of HIV/AIDS), who will earn the income for the family or look after the children? There is no safety net. This family is at an extreme end of poverty, trapped in an economic vise, and barely hanging on. Their survival as a family, if family members become sick or injured, is an open question. And yet this family is relatively fortunate because at least it has something to sell, a customer to buy the product, and income to share. Zambia once had a thriving economy based on copper, with a per capita income approaching European countries. After a series of reversals, including nationalization of the industry and collapse of commodity prices, the national economy crashed, thrusting Zambia into dire poverty. Commodity prices only recently recovered, due to demand from China. Were it not for this, there would be no housing construction and no demand for gravel. Both are ultimately dependent on economic trends on the other side of the world. Economic development is about people. Economic theory is an essential guide to how to create wealth that can be shared, and economic data are essential to test the reality. However, all too often the human face of economic development is lost in a fog of theory and statistics. At its core, economic development is about creating wealth for a purpose: so that all people can live their lives in a manner that frees them to pursue their own goals and aspirations, play the roles that they can play in their families and in society, and reach their own potential as human beings.

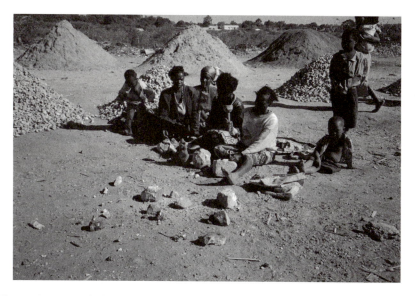

Figure 26.1. Family by the side of a road on the outskirts of Lusaka, Zambia. They are breaking rocks into gravel to sell for building material.

All countries are developing, in the sense that their economies are constantly changing into something else. The economy and level of technological and social development (a process often called "modernization" or "urbanization" in development shorthand) do not stand still. The United States, for example, moved in one century from an agriculture-dominated country of rural residents and small towns, through a robust manufacturing-dominated economy, to a service industry–dominated urban society, still with a large manufacturing sector, now caught, due to the world economic crisis, midway in transition to something resembling a greener economy dominated by information and innovation. Canada has experienced something similar, but together with Australia, it remains an anomaly among highly developed countries because extractive industries remain critical to the economy. In other words, economic development is not simply a process of countries ascending a stepwise ladder, getting richer in the process, until they are industrialized. It is a constant process of evolving that can go backward (as in the case of Zambia) as well as forward, and it does not stop with industrialization. Development also comes with an environmental cost that is rarely counted and evaluated.

Globalization is an economic regime that involves worldwide trade and a high degree of specialization by countries or regions in economic activities in which they have a natural advantage, such as natural resources (as in Australia), land (as in Brazil), or abundant intellectual talent (as in India). Countries that are highly dependent for their advantage on natural resources such as copper (Congo, Zambia) or crops such as coffee (Ethiopia, Guatemala, Ivory Coast) face great economic uncertainty when commodity prices fluctuate, which they always do over time. Another problem with resource-based relative advantage is that it creates a strong incentive for over-exploitation of resources, such as forest products in Indonesia and Thailand and overfishing in the world's oceans. The relative economic advantage of a country is not permanent. In the Arabian Gulf, Bahrain and Dubai (which is only one of the United Arab Emirates, but the one forced to develop more commercially) are running out of oil and so have diversified their economies. A relative advantage occurs when countries pass through a phase of high manufacturing capacity and low wages, making them exceptionally competitive for manufactured goods for export and for outsourcing production, as is the case in China in recent years and Vietnam today.

Outsourcing production creates jobs and raises wages in the countries doing the manufacturing, but the manufacturing step is very sensitive to costs and is not where the big returns lie in the value chain. Therefore, once wages rise to a certain level, the same countries try to outsource to other countries, as is seen historically with the movement of outsourced low-margin business in Asia from Japan to Taiwan or from Hong Kong to coastal China and now to interior (and poorer) China, Vietnam, and Cambodia. Unfortunately, as business moves from one country to the next, occupational hazards tend to follow the outsourcing in the form of unsafe work practices, unenforced occupational health standards, obsolete equipment, and untrained and unaware managers and workers.

Until 2009 it was relatively easy to categorize the winners and losers in the world economic system. The score was kept in terms of "gross domestic product" (GDP, the value of goods and services produced by the country), which is universally acknowledged to be deficient as a single metric for productive wealth and is used for that purpose anyway. GDP has many drawbacks, not least that it does not take into count, in some form of debit, the environmental and health costs of production, and it treats nonproductive and counterproductive costs—such as health care for preventable illness, tobacco consumption, and occupational disorders—as if they were productive economic activities. GDP is sometimes qualified by measures such as income distribution (the ratio of income of the highest earners to that of the lowest earners), which reflects social characteristics that relate to social cohesiveness and stability. The most important of these is the Human Development Index, which incorporates scales for per capita GDP, longevity, and standard of living (income taking into account "purchasing power parity," which is an adjustment for the cost of living).

The onset of the world recession has completely upset this neat way of thinking. Because of the initiating factors of the recession, economic instability began and was greatest at first in the most developed and richest economies. Countries that have been relatively isolated from global markets have tended to do better, at least in the early phases of the crisis. It is probably not an exaggeration to say that textbooks of economic development are now generally obsolete and will need to be rewritten. Although it is not clear that the current economic crisis represents the decline and fall of capitalism, as many radical critics believe, it is clear that the triumph of capitalism was declared prematurely. Two decades after the collapse of Marxist-Leninist socialism (the Soviet-style Communistic variety), capitalism itself is now in crisis. To be fair, the form of capitalism that is now in trouble was a largely unregulated, market-driven variety with many abuses, and it may be argued that it was a corrupt form that only needed reform. Whatever the verdict of history, what will come next in many countries is likely to be more regulated and *dirigiste* (state directed, as in the French system) than the old laissez-faire variety. If the economic future does involve more government oversight and regulation, environmental and occupational health may get more attention.

Terminology is important in global development work. Specific jargon is used by each international organization or country, such as the United Nations, the U.S. State Department, the U.S. Agency for International Development, and each of the numerous other governmental and nongovernmental organizations involved in global health. Some concepts and terms are common to each, however, and their strict meanings are not always familiar to Americans, who tend to use the words "nation," "country," and "state" more or less synonymously. A "nation" is properly a group of people with shared history, culture, and language, sometimes called a "people." However, not all such groupings are nations. Nations largely define themselves, such that even closely related peoples with a shared history or the same or almost identical languages, such as Czechs and Slovaks or, tragically, Hutu and Tutsi in Rwanda, may consider themselves to be separate nations. Within nations there may be tribes, a term that implies a self-recognized unit with a traditional, cohesive structure based on kinship ties and usually organized by clans. A "country" is a political entity that has defined borders. In most countries, the apparatus of governance has two parts: the "state" and the "government." The state is the corporate entity that represents and rules the people; the government is the specific apparatus of power that does the governing and can be changed without changing the state. There is a sharp distinction between governmental organizations (usually called ministries or departments), nongovernmental organizations (universally called "NGOs"; environmental NGOs are commonly called "ENGOs," although some of them think the term is pejorative), and UN or other "international" organizations or agencies. Very few NGOs are concerned with occupational health.

The terminology that describes developmental levels is constantly shifting. Countries that have developed an industrial or modern and urbanized infrastructure (in the sense of urban amenities and culture, not necessarily big cities) can be called industrialized, developed, advanced (the term is now out of favor), or more developed (the latter abbreviated MDs), terms that generally correspond to the level of income (as measured by gross domestic product, or GDP, per capita) of member countries of the Organization of Economic Cooperation and Development (OECD, twenty-seven member states), which includes western Europe, Japan, the United States, and Canada. Those that have achieved this level of infrastructure and income recently, such as Malaysia and Thailand, are called "newly developed countries." Which countries merit this label changes with each generation (newly developed countries of the previous generation included the "Asian tiger economies" of Hong Kong, Singapore, South Korea, and Taiwan).

Developing countries are those with infrastructure inadequate to need, a smaller level of economic activity, lower income, and often, but not always, fewer strong social institutions that are national in scope. The term "less developed countries" (abbreviated LDCs) is now out of fashion. There are no hard-and-fast criteria for the category, and the category is very heterogeneous: the World Trade Organization (WTO) allows countries to declare themselves "developing" as they see fit. Some developing countries have done well in terms of income and social services, such as Costa Rica and Botswana, and others have not, such as Bolivia. A few developing countries, such as Cuba, have experienced the special history of state socialism and Soviet-style Communism, whereas others, such as Georgia, Armenia, and Azerbaijan, have emerged from that history; China took a different path altogether. "Least developed countries" are those low-income countries that are recognized by the WTO as the poorest and most struggling, including Bangladesh, much of sub-Saharan Africa, Haiti, Nepal, and many isolated island countries. The recent world economic recession, however, has turned economic predictions for many of these countries upside down, because economic growth in some "less" developed countries, such as Togo, has been proportionately much greater than in stronger economies.

Every developing country has its own story. Economic profiles say little about how most countries arrived at their situation. Emerging economies are those undergoing a transformation, either breaking through to a middle-income level through a conventional development path or coming back after setbacks, such as those recovering from a history of Communism and the aftermath of the collapse of a Soviet-style system. The BRIC countries (Brazil, Russia, India, and China) are four large economies that play an increasingly important role in the world economy, but as a group they have nothing else in common. It is quite possible for countries to experience catastrophic reductions in income and economic development, as has been experienced in recent years, at different levels, by Argentina, Zambia, and, most recently and tragically, Zimbabwe. Some developing countries, such as Nigeria, Venezuela, and Kazakhstan, have oil resources; in development theory there is much talk of the "oil curse," because the commodity tends to distort national economies by preventing diversification and introducing opportunities for corruption, such that many of these countries fail to achieve their potential. Some countries inherited an infrastructure from colonization that proved useful in the postcolonial period (such as Ghana and India), and others were devastated by colonialism (such as Congo). These examples demonstrate that although there are similarities in the economics of developing countries, there are also many exceptions and special cases. China, the largest country of all, is also the greatest exception of all, having experienced in its long history almost every setback conceivable, including colonialism, yet having developed rapidly by following unique policies.

"Middle-income countries" are developing countries that are well along the path to development and have achieved much more than subsistence levels of income for their people, but that are below OECD income levels, such as Mexico and Iran. The World Bank and, for most purposes, the World Health Organization prefer to label countries by income level: low income (such as Pakistan, Myanmar, Laos, Mali), lower middle income (Indonesia, Colombia, Philippines, Moldova, Honduras, Ukraine), upper middle income (Belarus, Turkey, South Africa, Libya, Chile), and high income (New Zealand, Slovenia, Macao, Bahrain). However, this can be misleading. Most of the world's poor at present (2009) live in lower-middle-income countries. Some higher-middle- and upper-income countries are very small and depend on somewhat artificial economic foundations, such as tourism and financial services. The essential magazine for following world economic trends is the *Economist,* a British newsmagazine universally read in development circles, which simply calls countries "rich" or "poor" and otherwise avoids making too many generalizations.

Economic development proceeds along a political as well as an economic path. This must be understood by anyone working in global occupational and environmental health. National priorities may be very different in some countries: health is not necessarily the highest priority. Ministries of finance are always the most powerful government departments in their countries, and issues of occupational and environmental health, although not environmental protection, tend to be invisible to them. It is not unusual for the ministry of health to be low in status compared to other government departments or for the minister of health to be given the job for political reasons and to have no particular interest in health matters. Ministers of health rarely see environmental health and especially occupational health as falling within their mandate, although they may accept them as part of a comprehensive public-health program. Environmental health is often seen as a matter for the ministry of environment (particularly in countries with strong ENGO movements) and occupational health as a matter for the ministry of labor. Both of these ministries, in turn, tend to consider health to be outside their core mandates and almost always lack the required infrastructure in public health to do much anyway, with the possible exception of clean water and vector control.

It is important to distinguish between "population health risk" and "personal health risk," because the former is what is measured at the country level and the latter is what is experienced, especially by workers, and what drives occupational health issues at the local level. The difference is something like the difference between public health and medicine. Population health status reflects the health of the population on average or for the community as a whole, as reflected by the frequency of public health problems and the level of health according to various indicators related to personal risk and behavior, and how these health indicators are distributed. Personal health outcomes are individual illnesses or injuries that result from the interplay between the causes of the injury or illness and the risk factors present in the individual. For example, heart disease is more likely in people who smoke and who have a family history of smoking. Population health factors such as cholesterol in the diet are important for the population as a whole, but may or not be important for the individual. When such a person has a heart attack, it is a personal illness with specific implications for that one person; it may not have any particular implications for the risk of other people, especially if that person ate a different diet or had different life habits. Therefore, population health is not just the aggregate of personal health characteristics in the population, but a description of how the population behaves as an intact, organized community with different levels and subgroups. Measures of population health status represent the risk of poor health for the majority of people and the current state of poor health for a minority of sick people, who, at any one time, need access to health care. The total illness burden on society as translated to the level of population health is affected by how the society defines illness and chooses to accept or to act to prevent a burden of illness that results in disability. (This is one reason that the standard measure of the burden of disease in international comparisons has become the calculation of "disability-adjusted life years" [DALYs].)

The Development Cycle

Contemporary models of development have re-evaluated the fundamental relationships between economic expansion and social progress. The influential work of Amartya Sen has raised awareness on the true value of economic development, which is that it allows the individual to engage in social roles and personal aspirations and is therefore a community and a personal good. This line of reasoning places great emphasis on human rights and social development as an integral part of economic development. However, the predominant view among economists is still that economic growth is an end in itself.

Economists often speak of the "economic development cycle." This is the idea that economies progress stepwise through a predictable sequence of events that begins with a fundamental reliance on agriculture and a population living primarily in rural communities. This is called an "agrarian" economy. As productivity increases, more surplus crops can be sold and traded, but the basis of the society remains agrarian until it either reaches a point where it can support a process of industrialization, or industrialization is introduced. In the nineteenth century, industrialization (to a limited degree, so as to preserve most of the market for exports from the colonial power) was introduced by colonial powers. In the twentieth century, it was often financed by foreign aid and bank loans. In the twenty-first century, more industrial growth is the result of private debt, foreign direct investment, and domestic investment.

Industrialization yields products and services in anticipation of an excess of revenue over cost, which can then be invested back into the economy as capital for further development. Manufacturing also lowers the cost of finished goods and makes them more widely available at lower costs, eventually coming within reach of the average person, who becomes a consumer. However, economic development does not stop there. It is now known that the economic cycle progresses into an economic model based on services and information. At each step along the way, there are dislocations, disruptions, and instabilities, as well as advances in creating wealth. "Globalization" refers to trade and specialization of manufacturing and economic activity based on comparative advantage, such as access to resources, special talent, or low wages. The globalization of the manufacturing economy has also resulted in the export of numerous hazards in industry to countries poorly equipped to control them, among them asbestos. It has also resulted in the unsustainable exploitation of resources to meet a global demand, as in deforestation in Southeast Asia and overfishing in the world's oceans.

The history of how rich countries developed is an imperfect guide to what developing countries are experiencing. Developing countries develop differently than they did a few decades ago; for example, they skip steps in infrastructure development that are no longer relevant. Railroads are no longer considered critical to economic development; highways have taken their place. Technology—the cell phone even more than the Internet—has made a huge difference in the economics of developing countries. Because of the cell phone, citizens of developing countries are able to communicate easily, can learn about market prices for their commodities before they bring them in for sale, and can work through much larger social networks. Economists and decision makers know much more today and have access to much more information. It is not necessary to repeat mistakes of the past.

On a national level, finance ministers and development economists tend to believe that industrialization requires investment in production first and that once wealth is created, it can be invested in social goods such as improved health, worker protection, and protecting the environment. The fallacy is that by this theory, social goods, including health and work security, are amenities—nice but not essential. From the worker's point of view, however, a disabling injury usually means slipping back into poverty and social marginalization. Another way of looking at the problem is that basic occupational health services bring the workers and their families into full participation in the development process by protecting their lives, health, and income. The reasoning is the same as that underlying the theory of work capacity (see Chapter 18). In fact, the enhancement of health on a population level means the creation of opportunity and capacity, and provides the individual worker and his or her family with security, the potential for growth in income, and the capacity to do more in the community that merely subsist.

The key insight in new theories of development is that health and a decent income give a person the capacity and autonomy to function in society. This links the idea of economic development with human rights, which can be seen as a cluster of values that define the life and freedom of action of a citizen of the society. Of particular importance is the freedom and autonomy enjoyed by women. Social change becomes much more rapid and crosses generations more readily when women are empowered to engage in civic roles, to educate their children with different values, to obtain an education, to participate as partners in family decisions, to work in jobs out of the house or that are not necessarily traditional for women, to make reproductive choices, and to manage money. Gender equality shows a strong correlation with economic development.

The balance between population and available resources is another critical dimension in economic development. In the 1970s, there was much concern about overpopulation and the risk that increasing numbers of people in the world would outstrip the resources available. The imbalance between population and resources may seriously aggravate social and economic problems at a particular moment in time, but the trend over time has not been as dire as predicted. As it happened, the relationship turned out to be much more complicated, with population growth slowing and resource availability being profoundly affected by technology. That present trends, even though not as extreme as predicted, cannot continue indefinitely is clear, but the history of population issues over past decades shows that the issues are not a simple question of an arithmetic progression involving the availability of food and an exponentially increasing number of mouths, as famously described by Thomas Malthus. For one thing, increasing affluence and longevity tends to reduce population growth markedly by reducing fertility (in a demographic, not a biological, sense), providing at least a partial self-correction. In terms of fairness, access to the resources needed for an acceptable life is an issue of human rights.

The contribution of technology as a root cause of pollution and resource depletion was the other major theme of the environmental movement in the 1970s and, like population growth, has had to be revisited because the effects are much more complicated than projected at that time. Technology allows much greater efficiency and opportunity, which offset or mitigate its negative effects from the introduction of, for example, new products or processes that present risks. (See Chapter 25 for a discussion of "critical science" and the critique of technological progress.)

Urbanization (sometimes called "modernization," although this term has fallen out of favor) is the process of bringing together infrastructure, a critical density of people, political organization, a wage-based economy, and vastly greater social networks. It also incorporates the application of and access to technology in the lives of individuals and in society, during the initial years of agriculture and manufacturing. Urbanization as a social process is, obviously, concentrated in cities, but lines of communication, transportation, and migration also reach back to and affect rural life. There may be rapid incorporation of urban habits, lifestyles, tastes, and ideas into the life of villages and rural communities, often starting with fashion and music. Rural poverty is worse when the village is remote from towns, commodity prices are unstable (as they usually are), and infrastructure is poor (which it usually is). Rural areas also tend, as a rule, to be conservative and traditional. Urbanization brings in new ideas and new ways of thinking.

Globalization and Trade

The relationship between globalization and trade has been identified by many public health activists and some economists as a broad issue of concern, both as a public health issue and as part of a larger critique of globalization. The principal issues are:

- Trade agreements and the legislation to support them may subordinate national legislation on health and environmental standards.
- Trade agreements often do not acknowledge environmental protection, environmental health risks, workers' rights, or occupational health; or they manage them through weaker side agreements, as in the case of NAFTA.
- Financial policies imposed on countries in financial distress (historically by the International Monetary Fund, IMF) may reduce the ability of the population to purchase food and health care or to provide care for young children. (The IMF has reviewed and changed its policies.)
- National health systems or services that involve subsidies of government financing may be ruled an unfair trade advantage. (The issue was raised in the negotiations of NAFTA with regard to Canada's health care system.)
- Products imported from countries with lax inspection standards may present a risk to the public. (Imported toys that are contaminated or painted with lead have been a particular problem in North America.)
- Pressures to reduce costs and maintain high margins may result in exploitation of workers, unsafe working conditions, and adulteration of products (such as the addition of melamine to milk in China in order to fraudulently increase the apparent protein content).

- Patent protection and enforcement of intellectual property rights may limit availability of drugs and medical care in poor countries.

- The failure of the Doha round of trade talks, which involved reducing barriers to export of agricultural commodities from poor countries to rich countries, has locked many countries out of free trade and into poverty. (Doha, a city in Qatar, is where the agreement was negotiated.)

- Globalization has put intense pressure on many poor countries that deplete their resources in order to supply demand, especially if there is global competition. Deforestation is a common example.

The evidence for some of these charges, such as the perverse effects of the Doha round and deforestation, is strong. The role of globalization in some other issues is less clear.

Occupational Health

Occupational health protection is considered to be a "consumptive cost" by employers, a cost that is incurred by the employer for little or no gain, instead of as an investment that yields future benefit. The benefit is often difficult to quantify because it is expressed in terms of disability and health problems that have been avoided, not as a tangible return on investment. Employers often take the view that because their role in the economy is to create wealth, not to distribute benefits, it is not their job to protect the health of workers. This point of view ignores the ethical and social benefit of worker protection, but it finds some justification in the prevailing view in development economics that rising wages and economic development, on their own, do more than health interventions to improve health conditions.

On the other hand, the cost of health care for injured workers is low in developing countries, and workers are usually easily replaced. There is little economic incentive to invest in health protection, safety, or health services for injured workers. Although the costs of providing health care and measures for occupational health protection are minimal on an international scale of value, they are still seen to be an extra cost of production, particularly if an employer is in a competitive international market.

The primary health care system, where it functions, must accept the burden for occupational injuries and illness for most of the developing economy. There is usually no organized insurance or workers' compensation system, although employers may voluntarily pay some compensation to families of injured workers. Most enterprises in all economies, especially developing economies, are small and cannot support their own health care systems.

Most developing countries have sparsely developed occupational health and safety services. Such services are most likely to be available in the private sector because they are usually not given a high priority in the health care system. The World Health Organization (WHO) and the International Labour Organization (ILO) have therefore called for a commitment to "basic occupational health services" (BOHS), to be provided within the primary health care system through the training of health care providers (mostly physicians and nurses) and the addition of occupational health and safety personnel to primary care clinics and hospitals: a primary care level of occupational health, emphasizing primary prevention and hazard control, but integrated into the primary health care system. There is no question that BOHS is critically important to providing essential occupational health care to all workers, but whether it can be folded into a primary health care system, with its own priorities and limited resources, is still an open question. Prototype BOHS programs have succeeded, but most examples evaluated to date have been in China, which is not representative of other developing countries.

Lost income, in the form of wages that cannot be earned because the worker is disabled, can be devastating to the worker and his or her family, but in developing countries income levels are low to begin with. Because one worker easily replaces another, this disability-related loss is not perceived as an economic liability to the total economy. Over time, however, disability-related loss begins to become a drag on the economy. The problem becomes more acute and governments pay more attention as income levels rise and the losses become more apparent. Most national social security systems (such as Mexico's "Seguridad social") started at this stage, with coverage for the employed population in middle-income occupations and their dependents, at a time when the country had achieved at least lower-middle-income status.

As the economy develops, the cost of health care quickly rises. The burden of occupational injuries and illnesses increases health care costs and reduces productivity. When disability pension schemes, where they exist, are added, the cost becomes conspicuously higher because injured workers are younger than the disabled in the general population, whose disabilities are more often associated with aging, and therefore each injured worker is more costly to treat and support over his or her remaining lifetime if he or she cannot work.

Child Labor

Child labor is a huge humanitarian concern with great costs to society and the children themselves. However, child labor is difficult to eradicate because many families in some developing countries depend on the income. In most agrarian societies, children traditionally work in the fields and are an economic asset on farms. Seen through agrarian and village values and traditions, working outside the home does not seem abnormal, particularly where schooling is not valued highly. Children become economic liabilities when the economic level increases and attitudes change; then they are expected to stay in school. These changes in society do not happen uniformly or smoothly.

Historically, child labor was a mainstay in the new factories and mines of the Industrial Revolution and required a major social movement and landmark legislation to first control it (mostly by reducing work hours) and then effectively bring it to an end, which happened in the nineteenth century in Britain and in the 1920s in Canada as well as in several progressive states (especially Illinois and Massachusetts) in the United States. Child labor was controlled and then mostly ended in the United States as a whole in the mid-twentieth century, largely due to the work of a federal agency called the Children's Bureau. It took longer to end child labor in the United States because several early laws against it were declared unconstitutional on the grounds that the federal government was not deemed at the time to have authority over working conditions, only interstate commerce. Even today, child labor, without appropriate limits and controls, continues to be a problem, particularly in agriculture. Fatality statistics for the United States continue to record work-related deaths in workers seventeen years of age and younger, indicating that some young workers are still working in risky occupations.

In developing countries especially, children are employed in the informal economy, where wages are not recorded, no taxes are paid, and no standards are enforced. This tends to conceal the problem from view and cover up abuse. Families often send the child away to live with an employer as a sort of apprentice or indentured servant. A special problem occurs with socially disrupted or migrant populations and separated children or orphans. In countries with a high prevalence of HIV/AIDS, children who are orphaned are often left to support themselves. For girls, especially, this usually means domestic work, but sometimes prostitution is the only apparent option for earning enough money.

The costs are huge to society and even greater to the children themselves. Children who work instead of going to school for a full day lose education and miss opportunities. They are also more susceptible than adults to occupational health risks. The ILO estimated in 1997 that as many as a quarter of a billion children were working in jobs that presented some hazard or risk. Young bodies are more susceptible to hazards, and children injured at a young age may be disabled for life. Children, even if physically capable of the work expected of them, are impulsive and do not understand the nature of hazards or the need to work safely; they do not have the knowledge to protect themselves or the authority to insist that an employer protect them. The family, which may be far away, cannot effectively protect the child.

Child labor also leads to abusive situations because of the power relationship between adults and children, particularly if the children are employed outside the family, and because of the control over the child and his or her family exerted by money. Sometimes the family will turn a child over to an unrelated adult for money— virtually selling the child—expecting to receive an income from the child's work or, less commonly, in order to reduce the number of mouths to feed, with the expectation that the child will be taken care of. Girls are especially vulnerable to abuse because of gender discrimination in many traditional societies and because of the greater potential for sexual abuse and forced prostitution. At an extreme, the abuse can lead to child prostitution, crime, and virtual slavery. Children have even been kidnapped and forced into military service as child soldiers, with accompanying drug use, atrocities, and violence intended to keep them belligerent toward outsiders but pliant to authority.

The United Nations Children's Fund (UNICEF) monitors and documents trends in child labor and analyzes root causes in order to support efforts at prevention. It also administers the UN Convention on the Rights of the Child. ILO and UNICEF are particularly concerned that efforts to end child labor do not cause even more harm to children. UNICEF has compiled case studies where this has happened. Most involve dismissal and abandonment of the children when employers begin to feel pressure. The ILO sponsors the International Programme for the Elimination of Child Labor. One of the mainstays of the program is Convention 138, on the Minimum Age of Admission to Employment and Work (1973). Another is Convention 182, on the Worst Forms of Child Labour (1999), through which ILO seeks to eliminate the worst abuses first and then progressively raise awareness and change attitudes on child labor as a whole over time. In 2000 the United Nations adopted the "Palermo Protocol" (Protocol to Prevent, Suppress, and Punish Trafficking in Persons, Especially Women and Children); other conventions and protocols that deal with sexual abuse and illegal migration in general also apply to children.

Environmental Health

Environmental degradation is a predictable consequence of the development process in the absence of controls or a mature and inclusive civic culture. Environmental degradation is not exclusively the result of development, of course, and serious environmental health risks, particularly those involving water, are always present before economic development begins and can appear at any level of development. Clean water is critical for health, and control of contamination by human wastes is the most critical problem of all. Air pollution, in general, is more closely tied to the urbanization process and reflects the level of development of infrastructure, including the number of cars and trucks on the road and how energy is produced.

The most obvious impact of environmental degradation is illustrated by the severe air and water pollution encountered in many of the world's new megacities. Environmental degradation can also be seen as a cluster of issues that reflect potential adverse effects on health (which are usually difficult to prove); reduction of biodiversity and habitat (trading short-term economic gain for long-term destruction of potentially renewable resources); depletion of nonrenewable resources; limitations on future land use; risks to agricultural productivity and food supply; and diminished appeal for tourism, trade, and quality of life. Environmental degradation restricts future economic options, which is generally what gets the attention of ministries of finance.

At one time, the predominant attitude was that protecting the environment was something that only rich countries could afford to do, so developing economies tried to get rich first before making an effort to protect the environment. The global increase in awareness of the environment for its own sake—because of media attention, the risk of ecological catastrophe, and the desire to exploit commercial opportunities—has changed that, and now most governments at least nominally support environmental protection, although they do not all follow through with support for that protection. Most societies are less interested in environmental health than in environmental quality. This is because in the political and social agenda of most countries today, environmental quality issues are increasingly seen as critical to the development of a sustainable economic base (and often tourism), but environmental health is seen as old-fashioned, particularly with respect to clean water, and tends to be seen as a by-product of an earlier generation of progress, particularly with respect to air pollution. These attitudes are not particularly rational, but they are deep, and they influence political priorities and decision makers. During the severe recession that is ongoing as this is being written (2009), more attention has been given to the prospects of economic recovery through rebuilding infrastructure and public investment to support a sustainable, "green" economy. This is new, at least on the present scale.

Environmental health, however, does not usually benefit from the attention paid to environmental quality as a whole. Relationships between human health and ecosystem conservation, biodiversity, and wildlife protection exist, but they are indirect. The constituencies and incentives to protect the rain forest and to protect human health from water in urban slums contaminated with feces are usually very different, and the former is generally much more appealing to politicians and business interests. (It should be noted that in recent years there has been a paradigm shift in the private sector, and more business interests are shifting to at least acknowledge the benefits of environmental protection, often seeing it as the basis for new industries such as ecotourism. It is also hard to sustain a tourist industry when there are periodic outbreaks of diarrhea.)

Issues of environmental health in developing countries are dominated, reasonably, by the need for a secure and clean water supply. Beyond that, the agenda is diverse and driven in large part by the concerns of the community as they understand the environment, not necessarily any objective standard. ENGOs play a disproportionate role in setting the environmental agendas of many emerging or developing countries. For example, during the reconstruction of Eastern Europe following the collapse of the Soviet Union, much attention was paid to environmental issues that might have seemed marginal as health risks by North American standards, but that had been heavily publicized by ENGOs. One such issue involved opposition to a high-temperature incinerator for toxic wastes in a situation where no other disposal option was available, creating a bigger risk of dumping and uncontrolled release.

FOREIGN OPERATIONS

OEM physicians who serve as medical directors in their organizations may have responsibilities for managing occupational and environmental health in foreign operations. For those companies based in the United States, Canada, the European Union, or another developed country, the corporate infrastructure for occupational and environmental health is normally already in place and functioning, and the challenge is to apply the same standards as in the home country while being responsive to the local situation. However, as business changes, it is increasingly common for large corporations to be truly multinational and for companies based in emerging and developing countries (such as Brazil and India) to own American subsidiaries and even parent companies. Then the challenge becomes to harmonize upward to the highest standard whenever possible over time.

Few multinational corporations have a simple corporate medical department anymore. More often, these departments include some responsibility for environmental health as well as other responsibilities: often product liability, sometimes safety (which is more often centralized), and occasionally security. The manager, often but not always an OEM physician, must, with a limited staff, simultaneously oversee and monitor the provision of medical services at the local level, manage corporate liability and compliance with policy, troubleshoot problems, anticipate and prepare for emergencies, and work closely with management to ensure that occupational and environmental concerns are reflected in corporate decisions, some of which (such as new plant design) are not primarily about health. In addition to all this, there must be time to cultivate working relationships with other senior managers and to learn the culture and policies of the organization.

Managing foreign operations presents a number of challenges:

- Policy development
- Compliance with standards and best practices within the parent company
- Compliance with local standards and best practices, especially by audits
- Organizing an occupational health service that conforms to the corporate organization and is still responsive to local needs
- Identifying service providers at the local level
- Managing health issues for visitors
- Managing endemic disease in high-risk locations

Although mission and vision statements are important in every large organization, they are particularly important in defining occupational and environmental health policy in far-flung multinational corporations. Essential in all such policies is a commitment to comply with all applicable regulatory requirements, but there must also be a clear commitment on the part of the employer to occupational health and safety and environmental health protection as values. Without a clear statement of intent and unambiguous policies that support enforcement, local operations invariably go their own way, and compliance becomes inconsistent. This places the organization at extreme risk, for several reasons. The employer without tight control over local operations may inadvertently violate local regulatory laws, may have difficulty with quality assurance and exports, may lose control over occupational health protection and workforce health, and may face serious reputational damage, especially if the company is seen as applying different standards away from home. Strong and well-monitored policies that honor a commitment to occupational and environmental protection are therefore fundamental to managing foreign operations.

A convenient approach to ensuring consistency of standards is to adopt well-recognized global standards, such as those of the International Organization for Standardization (ISO—the acronym is a pun on the prefix *iso-,* meaning "same" in Greek); the British Standards Institute's OHSAS 18000 (which has applied for ISO recognition, but this has not yet been granted); the voluntary ILO Guidelines on Occupational Health Management Systems (ILO opposes ISO adoption of OHSAS 18000); or DEKRA Certification (particularly popular in German-speaking countries), depending on the function. The largest multinational employers often have internal occupational health and safety standards that are applied throughout the organization, rather than relying on local regulations. These are normally chosen to be lower than the lowest regulatory standards. In the past, they often conformed to standards recommended by the American Conference of Governmental Industrial Hygienists (ACGIH), but increasingly the harmonized standards of the European Union are being adopted.

The single most important tool for ensuring consistency in compliance with standards, corporate policy, and best practices is the audit. Audits should be undertaken at reasonable intervals, such as every few years, and should, ideally, examine outcomes (reportable injuries and illnesses, fatalities, near misses); reporting relationships; performance indicators; facilities and resources; budget; personnel; qualifications of professional staff; quality of case management; measures for quality assurance; training; adherence to procedures; disaster preparedness; availability of technical assistance for mitigating hazards; and actual performance in key functions: occupational health and safety hazards in place, environmental emissions and effluent, safety hazards, fire and hazardous materials management, engineering controls, management of personal protection, and housekeeping. In practice, the audit has to conform to the scope of the management unit or department, but it can uncover many gaps, and this information can be used to propose needed changes to management.

The occupational health and safety management structure must conform to the general pattern of organization of the company, or it will be out of step with general management. A company may have regional or national medical directors or a centralized corporate medical department that tries to do it all by managing hired local physicians. Which structure is preferable depends on how the corporation is organized and where it is operating. This may change over time, sometimes abruptly. For example, for most of its history Shell Oil was among the most decentralized of large companies, but in recent years it suddenly set out to restructure itself to a more traditional organization. Management of occupational and environmental health must follow.

Finding trained occupational health and safety professionals and environmental managers can be difficult in developing countries. One approach is to bring in expatriates to do the work, but this is often unsustainable over the long term. Expatriates should be partnered whenever possible to local talent so that the expertise can be transferred. Such an arrangement ultimately expands the talent pool in the country, raises awareness, and may even create new career opportunities in health and, particularly, safety. There is a strong temptation to "raid" academic programs for faculty talent, but this may have the unfortunate effect of destroying the program. A better option is to provide material support for whatever academic programs exist and to hire the students they produce.

Inevitably, a business visitor—such as a customer, government official, or corporate official from a partnering company—to the home country or to a hosted meeting held in a third country will fall ill or seek medical care. In general, there is no problem with the company providing emergency care, but it is always advisable to carry insurance to cover such situations. It may be very difficult for the company to stop providing care to a valued contact after the initial emergency is over, but the terms of the insurance policy set limits, making this easier. Some visitors will request medical care for themselves or their families as a quid pro quo of doing business. The OEM physician must be very careful about complying with such requests.

The Foreign Corrupt Practices Act of 1977 carries tough criminal sanctions against any employee or agent of an American company who provides or offers "anything of value" to a foreign official to influence decisions or to direct business. Similar legislation has been adopted by other OECD countries, including Canada. Bribery of foreign corporate officials is also against the law in the United States and Canada. Elective medical services are very high in value and clearly fall under these laws.

Foreign operations are sometimes located in zones of endemic disease that threaten employees, the local community, and business travelers to foreign operations. The most common serious situation of this nature occurs with operations in locations where malaria is endemic or where HIV/AIDS infection is prevalent. Where the local infrastructure is lacking, the employer may have to be proactive in establishing health services for the local population. Malaria illustrates this problem well and is a severe problem in several tropical regions where, for example, oil and gas are produced. It can best be controlled by the application of a series of partial measures for primary prevention (vector control, insecticide-treated mosquito netting, and long-sleeved shirts and long pants, as well as DEET and chemoprophylaxis for visitors), none of which are complete defenses but which together greatly reduce the risk. Some cases will occur, so access to effective diagnosis and treatment is required (diagnostic testing, first- and second-line chemotherapy) to prevent disability (particularly from falciparum malaria). If the local health care system cannot support malaria management programs, the employer may have to. Oil companies are in a position to do this, but many other industries are not. Likewise, HIV/AIDS and related problems such as infection with tuberculosis represent a major challenge in southern Africa—a challenge that has been met by a concerted and sustained campaign of prevention, medical treatment, and aggressive case management by the South African mining company Anglo American. Anglo American has emerged, of necessity, as a global leader in workforce health and disease management.

Ultimately, however, the only sure way of monitoring foreign operations is to visit. The OEM physician who assumes responsibility for widely distributed foreign operations should normally plan on spending 30 to 50 percent of his or her time traveling in order to do so.

BORDER HEALTH AND MIGRATING POPULATIONS

Issues of border health and immigration are as critical within North America as anywhere in the world, and they are of particular interest in global environmental and occupational health. This is unusual in global health as a whole, which has traditionally not concerned itself with health issues in the United States and Canada (with the possible exception of aboriginal health issues) and has generally considered Mexico to be too developed, on a relative scale, to be of real interest.

Global health as a field has an informal specialization in migrant populations that is mostly concerned with refugees—who by definition are outside their country of nationality—and internally displaced persons. This often involves camps and involuntary population movement across international borders, and the driving issues are usually political or related to warfare or civil unrest. In general, border issues have not been of much interest otherwise in mainstream global health, with the exception of the U.S.-Mexico border. That particular border has attracted serious scholarship in global health, and in many other fields, because of its unique characteristics and because for so many years it was the most stark example to be found of countries at different levels of development in intimate contact. In part for this reason, this border area has experienced a plethora of health-related studies, demonstration projects, and commissions, mostly devoted to infectious disease, health promotion, and access to health care.

Global environmental and occupational health has a very different perspective, which places more emphasis on economic refugees and the problems of coordinating environmental and occupational health where two very different systems come together.

Border Health

Occupational and environmental health along international borders presents many special issues. Because of the similarity in legal tradition, level of development, and economic organization, managing health issues along the U.S.-Canada border is mostly a matter of respecting the differences in authority and legislation (as covered in Chapter 24). The United States and Mexico are rather more different and at very different levels of economic development. Therefore, as a practical matter, the principal border health issues in North America requiring active management are those along the U.S.-Mexico border.

It should be noted that throughout this book, "North America" is used to refer to the United States and Canada, without reference to Mexico. Obviously, Mexico is part of North America geographically, but culturally it is part of Latin America, and the Spanish word *norteamericano* refers to American (some Mexicans prefer *estadounidense,* in recognition of the fact that they also share the continent and consider themselves *americano*) and, usually, to Canadians also.

The U.S.-Mexico border extends for 2,000 miles between San Ysidro, California, and Tijuana, Baja California, in the west and Brownsville, Texas, and Matamoros, Tamaulipas, in the east. It is the second-most-transited border in the world, after the U.S.-Canada border. There are four American states to the north of the border (California, Arizona, New Mexico, and Texas) and six Mexican states to the south (Baja California, Sonora, Chihuahua, Coahuila, Nuevo León, and Tamaulipas). The border area (often called *la frontera*) by convention (agreed to in the 1983 "La Paz" Agreement between the two countries) extends 100 kilometers, or roughly 63 miles, on either side of the international border itself. It is an area of intense cultural mixing, where English and Spanish are used interchangeably and daily life blends American and Mexican customs. Much of the area is sparsely populated, but there are several large, interfacing cities on opposite sides of the border, particularly San Diego and Tijuana, the two cities of Nogales (Arizona and Sonora), El Paso (Texas) and Ciudad Juárez (Chihuahua), Laredo (Texas) and Nuevo Laredo (Nuevo León), and the larger cities of the Rio Grande River Valley (Texas and Tamaulipas). There are also numerous indigenous communities on both sides, most of them very small.

The border is also an area of unusual contradictions, where rich cities (including some urban areas on the Mexican side, which has a higher per capita income than the rest of Mexico) abut impoverished communities, including poor towns and Indian reservations in the United States and *colonias* (informal shantytowns) in Mexico. It is also an area beset by interrelated social problems, including high crime rates, drug use and smuggling, illegal immigration, trafficking in people, and high unemployment. Most of these problems affect both sides of the border and have proven rather intractable over the years. At the same time, economic development has been led, especially on the Mexican side, by the North American Free Trade Agreement (NAFTA, 1994) and by considerable cross-border local trade. Americans seek Mexican specialties, cheaper prices on high-value products (including pharmaceuticals), and low-cost services. Mexicans patronize stores in the United States for lower prices and a greater variety of merchandise.

As in most arid regions, the principal environmental health problem along the border is water supply and quality. Much of the U.S.-Mexico border is defined by the Rio Grande ("Rio Bravo" on the Mexican side), which has a very low flow and is inadequate to supply the growing population. There is a constant risk of fecal contamination due to sewer line breaks and spillover during flooding in many border communities. Substandard housing is a serious problem on both sides of the border. Air pollution levels have tended to abate over the years, especially with the closing of a smeltery near El Paso that had been the cause of local lead contamination for many years. Heavy pesticide use in agriculture, especially in the Imperial Valley (California), Mexicali Valley (Baja California), and Rio Grande Valley (Texas), has made the area a "hot spot" for pesticide toxicity and has raised issues of chronic toxicity. Toxic waste from local industry has created a serious local disposal problem, with several incidents of dumping, illegal discharge into water, and illegal transport into Mexico.

Some Mexican consumer products and folk medicines have been found to contain toxic levels of metals (especially *greta,* which contains lead). In the early 1990s, a cluster of cases of neural tube defects in children born in Matamoros raised concerns over pollution levels in water and possible exposure to toxic substances, such as solvents, during pregnancy. The issue was never resolved.

In 1965 the government of Mexico introduced a program to stabilize employment, promote economic development, and reduce economic migration to the United States in the border area. The plan facilitated the establishment of assembly plants and small factories, called *maquiladoras,* in duty-free zones such that American companies could bring unfinished products and components over the border, have them assembled by Mexican workers who were paid lower wages, and then have the assembled products returned to the American side of the border, again duty free on the U.S. side, for incorporation into the finished product and distribution. From the beginning, it was highly successful and attracted many companies. Over the four decades following, the *maquiladora* system came to employ over 1.2 million workers (one-third of Mexico's manufacturing workforce) and made northern Mexico more prosperous. It also created a trained and reliable workforce that provided a platform for economic development. However, the revenue generated by the *maquiladoras* was highly cyclical and depended almost completely on the U.S. economy. Employment tended to swing wildly between boom and bust, most spectacularly in 2001, when *maquiladora* employment dropped by almost a quarter within the year. Even so, the economy remains stronger and wages are higher in the border area than in most of Mexico.

The current outlook for *maquiladoras* is uncertain because wage levels on the border have risen out of competitive range for low-margin assembly and low-cost production work, with such work now being outsourced to China. On the other hand, productivity (per worker) has continued to rise and the workforce, after forty years, is now experienced, well trained, and adaptable, while still demographically young. The *maquiladora* sector is still competing successfully in more high-value products, such as surgical instruments, and where proximity to the U.S. market is important—either because transportation costs are high relative to the value of the product, as is the case with durable goods such as appliances, or because product styles change rapidly, such as denim pants. Production requiring protection of intellectual property is also undertaken in the *maquiladoras,* because Mexican legal protection is stronger than in other countries with more competitive wages.

Despite the economic success of the *maquiladora* model, it has been very controversial. Many critics accuse it of exploiting Mexican workers, which is not surprising given that wage disparities are so obvious when so close in geographic proximity. Although occupational health protection is strong in Mexican legislation, enforcement is often lacking, creating a vacuum for compliance that companies could exploit in the *maquiladora.* Documentation of elevated rates of occupational injury and illness is hard to find for the region, and there are many anecdotal and unconfirmed reports. It seems clear that occupational health protection has not been as stringent in Mexico, but how this may have affected morbidity and disability rates is not documented.

Many government-sponsored binational and multilateral organizations are active on the border, most in a coordinating rather than an executive or operational role because of the fragmentation of authority. Because of the priority placed on the region, the Pan American Health Organization maintains an office in El Paso, Texas, to deal with U.S.-Mexico border issues. The U.S.-Mexico Border Health Commission, established by agreement in 2000, is a bilateral council of government officials with the objective of addressing shared health issues. The Border Legislative Conference is a forum for state legislators in both countries with the goal of sharing solutions and coordinating legislation. There is also a U.S.-Mexico Border Governors Health Table, established in 1980, and a U.S.-Mexico Border Counties Coalition, established in 1998. These official bodies have a similar agenda: emergency preparedness (terrorism being the priority on the U.S. side, natural disasters on the Mexican side, especially where there is a flood risk), control of communicable diseases, and strengthening infrastructure; environmental health has not been as much of a focus, and there has been essentially no activity in occupational health. Despite this impressive structure of coordinating bodies, effective coordination has been elusive.

The U.S.-Mexico Border Health Association, established in 1943, is the professional organization devoted to issues of border health. It is headquartered in El Paso.

Immigration

Immigration into the United States comes from all nations, but Mexico is the single largest source of immigrants, as it has been historically. The distribution of new immigrants to the United States, including those from Mexico, is now widespread rather than concentrated just north of the border area. Canada is similar in the diversity and wide distribution of its immigrants, but the distribution by country of origin is different (Canada draws primarily from China and India). In both countries many of the immigrants are highly skilled and well paid, but most are not.

Immigrant health issues have been a recurring theme in public and occupational health. In the late nineteenth and early twentieth century, there was much concern over the introduction of disease into the United States by recent immigrants, most of whom had poorer health status than native-born Americans and acculturated immigrants. Some of this concern was valid (although tuberculosis rates, of particular concern, were already high in the United States), though much of it was a cover for anti-immigrant politics.

Much of the U.S. economy has become dependent on lower-wage immigrant labor, including more hazardous industries such as poultry and meat packing (which has a very high rate of musculoskeletal injuries), construction, and agriculture (where risks include pesticide exposure as well as traumatic injury). Although the perception of poverty may be different relative to an immigrant's experience in the country of origin, in U.S. terms many of these workers are poor in a country with relatively high costs of living and therefore experience barriers such as poor transportation and inadequate health care. Immigrant workers in low-wage positions may be highly vulnerable because of language barriers, illiteracy (they may not be able to read easily in their own language), low levels of education, discrimination, dependence on their employers, the rural location of many jobs and communities, and lack of political representation. They often lack the protection of workers' compensation and unemployment insurance because of their work in agriculture and in domestic work, where workers are not usually covered. Occupational health and safety training may be rudimentary or lacking entirely, and when given, it may be ineffective if not colloquially translated and provided in an accessible and culturally sensitive manner.

Agricultural workers in particular may be migrants with no settled home and may reside with their children in camps with poor sanitation and close proximity to sprayed fields and other hazards. The Migrant Clinicians Network (MCN) was established in 1984 to address the health needs of migrant (moving from place to place) and seasonal (traveling to a place to pick a particular crop) farmworkers and their families in the United States. MCN is national in scope and manages a variety of funded programs to help member physicians provide prevention and health care services.

All of these problems are much worse if the immigrant does not have legal status. Illegal, or "undocumented," immigrants lack basic protection under the law and are easily exploited because they can be turned in and forcibly repatriated at any time. A particularly egregious incident occurred in 2005, when Immigration and Customs Enforcement (ICE) tricked undocumented immigrants in North Carolina into assembling for what was billed to be a mandatory occupational health and safety training meeting sponsored by OSHA—a meeting that was then raided. Prior to the incident, OSHA had been making a considerable effort to reach out to immigrant workers, undocumented or documented, in order to raise awareness and elicit cooperation and compliance with occupational health and safety protection. There was concern that the ICE action would not only negate this effort, but would also discourage even legal immigrants, who fear harassment and job discrimination. A more detailed discussion of the plight of undocumented aliens is beyond the scope of this text, because the core problems are social rather than environmental or occupational.

TRAVEL MEDICINE

Because of globalized trade, the need for travel to foreign operations by executive and technical staff, and the occasional case of an introduced disease in a returning tourist or business traveler, travel medicine has entered the mainstream of OEM. This section is only a very broad overview, because a detailed exposition of travel medicine would be vast and well beyond the scope of this book. Also, it is generally a mistake to rely on a book for information on travel medicine, unless it is updated very frequently. This section should therefore be considered a discussion of travel medicine as it pertains to OEM physicians; it is not an introduction to travel medicine.

Any OEM physician with responsibilities that include travel medicine must regularly consult the relevant authoritative sources for current information, without exception:

- Centers for Disease Control and Prevention: www.cdc.gov/travel
- Public Health Agency of Canada: www.phac-aspc.gc.ca/tmp-pmv/index/html
- World Health Organization: www.who.int/en, which allows access to the Weekly Epidemiological Record and other documents
- ProMed-Mail (sponsored by the International Society of Infectious Diseases): www.promedmail.org

These sources provide current information on trends around the world and recommendations on appropriate immunizations.

Some generalizations can be made that narrow the scope of concern for routine and predictable travel. For example, yellow fever, although an important cause of disease, is not a common threat for business travelers, who rarely travel into endemic areas and are likely to be aware of it if they do. Likewise, high-altitude sickness, though very serious for the mountaineer, is unlikely to be a concern of the business traveler.

The role of the OEM physician is primarily in managing prevention, not diagnosis and treatment, which are best left to the infectious disease specialists. However, in managing prevention, the OEM physician does not have to do it alone: every substantial city in North America now has a travel clinic to which business travelers can be referred, and even when such a clinic is not at hand, guidance on prevention is freely available from sources such as those listed above.

The majority of business travel by North Americans is to Europe and elsewhere within North America. Most frequent business travelers are healthier and fitter than the average tourist, simply because of self-selection. Automobile injures are the single most-common serious threat to health while traveling. Unsafe sexual behavior remains a leading cause of acquired infection among travelers, despite the well-known and ubiquitous threat of HIV/AIDS. Waterborne disease and poor sanitation are major problems not only in developing countries, but also in less-developed regions of many middle- and high-income countries as well as remote areas of all countries.

Higher-risk areas for business travel tend to be clustered as follows:

- Regions where malaria is endemic—chiefly the tropics—present a major risk to business travelers and to local residents, including employees.
- Hepatitis A is the most common vaccine-preventable illness among travelers; immunization should be routine for business travelers.
- Hepatitis B remains a serious and potentially life-threatening risk in much of the world and is easily prevented by immunization, which should be routine for business travelers.
- Influenza is a very common disease transmitted to travelers, who may not be protected by influenza vaccine designed for the Northern Hemisphere if they travel in the Southern Hemisphere, where strains are often different in a given year.
- Meningococcal disease is uncommon, especially outside equatorial Africa, but it is a significant risk for religious pilgrims

making the hajj to Mecca, in Saudi Arabia, whatever their socioeconomic class. Business travelers are unlikely to be at risk, but hajji (pilgrims) should be protected.

As noted earlier in this chapter, malaria is a major problem in global health and therefore travel medicine, and it is a practical problem in many industries with operations in endemic areas. Malaria is a risk in urban as well as rural areas. High frequencies of chloroquine resistance are now found widely throughout the tropics and southern Africa, including northern South America, central Africa, southern Asia, and Southeast Asia. Chloroquine sensitivity is confined largely to Central America, the west coast of Mexico, central and southern South America, the Middle East, western North Africa, and scattered locations in China.

Prevention is a major challenge for business travelers in all malaria-endemic areas. The OEM physician should follow authoritative guidelines for prophylaxis, but certain facts are noteworthy. The first line of protection against malaria is for the traveler to practice primary prevention against mosquito bites by reliably using DEET on clothing, sleeping inside permethrin-impregnated mosquito netting, wearing long-sleeved shirts and long pants, and spraying small spaces with DEET before occupying them; adherence to these measures is poor. Not taking malarial prophylaxis should not be considered an option for the business traveler: the risk is too high, especially where falciparum malaria is involved. On the other hand, the state of the art of chloroquine-resistant malarial prophylaxis is not ideal, and all viable choices involve trade-offs in terms of the risk of side effects and sufficient inconvenience to discourage adherence, which is generally poor. Mefloquine, an earlier drug of choice for prophylaxis, has become highly controversial after reports of serious behavioral side effects, and may be considered to present an unacceptable risk of liability. Resistance to doxycycline has not been reported. It is highly effective in the prevention of falciparum malaria, and it is usually readily tolerated by travelers, although it is photosensitizing; it may be considered to be underutilized. Most prophylactic drugs need to be continued for four weeks after departure from the high-risk area, which often leads to adherence failure, but atovaquone-proguanil and primaquine require only a single week after departure, making them attractive options for short trips to high-risk areas. Standby emergency treatment (SBET) of suspected malaria is a relatively new strategy, which requires the traveler to be alert to early symptoms and to take an antimalarial drug at therapeutic doses at the first sign of fever. Recommendations vary, but the SBET strategy is designed for travelers who do not wish to take chemoprophylaxis (arguably a bad idea), who will be in endemic but low-risk areas, or who will be more than twenty-four hours away from medical care; it is not necessarily recommended.

Travelers' diarrhea without blood is an almost ubiquitous risk, even occurring at times in North America and western Europe, but it is rarely threatening to the healthy business traveler if he or she can remain hydrated. Bloody diarrhea is another problem altogether. Prevention of each involves avoiding potential fecal-oral contamination, which can be achieved by eating only well-cooked foods and consuming either heated or commercially bottled beverages. Iced beverages and salads present particular risks.

Emergency medical evacuation by air is a logistical nightmare. Commercial airlines vary in their policies otherwise, but they will never transport unstable patients. Air ambulance services and U.S. military aircraft (which charge by the hour) are extremely expensive. Emergency air evacuation only makes sense when the risks of remaining in the country are greater than the risk of making the trip, the patient is sufficiently stable to survive the trip, the treatment facilities at the destination are both superior and necessary for survival, and the disease is not readily communicable. A particular wrinkle in such services is that insurance policies and service contracts may be written either for "repatriation," which means transport to the patient's home country, or for transport to the closest facility providing adequate care, which may be the nearest adequate hospital, from where the recovering traveler must then find a way back home. There are commercial medical evacuation and advisory services, such as International SOS, that manage such situations and other difficult situations under contract.

Routine travel by air carries a risk of deep-vein thrombosis. This problem is greater in economy class and on budget airlines, where it is more difficult to stretch out and to move one's legs. Travelers should flex their feet at the ankle periodically and move around to prevent venous stasis. Anti-thrombosis support hose pulled smoothly around the calf (never bunched to form a constrictive band, which has a tourniquet effect) reduces venous pooling, risk of thrombosis, and dependent swelling and discomfort.

Finally, jet lag—sometimes but not often called "circadian dyschronism"—is a familiar phenomenon for international travelers crossing longitudinal meridians and time zones, and there are many explanations for it. Discordance with circadian rhythm patterns (as discussed in Chapter 13) is probably the most important mechanism, but mild hypoxia, dehydration, sleep deprivation, and irregular mealtimes undoubtedly play a role. There are many folk remedies, and some progress has been made toward pharmaceutical treatment, particularly with melatonin (which seems to be effective in about half of users, as judged by a Cochrane review). The most reliable and nondisruptive measures to minimize jet lag, admittedly only partial in their effectiveness, include the following:

- Set watches to the destination time on takeoff and begin to think in terms of the time zone to be entered.
- Avoid all caffeinated and alcoholic beverages from several hours before departure to several hours after arrival.
- Eat in moderation when hungry and sleep when tired on the plane and in transit, but begin to eat meals on local time on arrival.
- Expose oneself to intense light during daylight hours on arrival, whether by going outdoors or using a commercial phototherapy device.

- Use sedatives or hypnotics for sleep sparingly if at all and only on arrival, never before or during a flight.

- Manage jet lag, whenever possible, with short naps or by scheduling time to adjust before any activity requiring mental acuity or high performance.

- When traveling westward, try to stay awake until bedtime at the destination. When traveling eastward, which is usually harder, do the best one can.

INTERNATIONAL AND GLOBAL ORGANIZATIONS

The United Nations was established in 1945 in the aftermath of World War II in an effort to secure peace permanently, to protect human rights, and to make a better world. Regarding the latter, it has been remarkably successful, and although often criticized for being imperfect in regard to the first two goals, its humanitarian interventions, moral influence, and contribution to world stability have created conditions that allow progress in the human condition. The Universal Declaration of Human Rights (1948), together with revolutionary France's Declaration of the Rights of Man (1789) and the statements defining freedom in the Anglo-American tradition from the Magna Carta to the Bill of Rights (and including, most recently, the Canadian Charter of Rights and Freedoms, 1982), stand as milestones in the history of human rights and cornerstones of human rights law. Not surprisingly, within the United Nations, issues of environmental health and occupational health are perceived as human rights issues and are understood in terms of equity, ethics, and access, not unlike the emerging view of environmental justice in the United States, but with the addition that material security and protection are seen as basic human rights and not just a matter of fairness. The United Nations operates through the "UN system," a network of specialized bodies and subsidiary agencies, or "organs," which have complicated reporting and governance structures. The principal organizations for environmental health are the World

Health Organization (WHO), the United Nations Environment Programme (UNEP), and the United Nations Development Programme (UNDP, which usually takes the lead in coordinating UN activities in developing countries). Other agencies may have some role as well: the World Bank Group (which has played a critical role in environmental issues worldwide); the United Nations Children's Fund (UNICEF has been involved in children's environmental health, including water issues); the Food and Agricultural Organization (FAO); the International Atomic Energy Agency (IAEA); UN Habitat (which focuses on housing); the World Trade Organization (globalization); and others have all had important roles in environmental and occupational health. Where their writs overlap, as in occupational health, UN agencies typically coordinate: WHO and the International Labour Organization (ILO) are the lead agencies in occupational health.

WHO is the United Nations agency for health issues and should already be familiar to any OEM physician. WHO is the single authoritative source for national and global health data. WHO (www.who.int) is essential for monitoring disease outbreaks worldwide, international travel recommendations, global environmental health, global environmental change as it affects health (UNEP is the lead for environmental issues in general), and global occupational health. WHO is managed by a director-general who, together with an executive board, is responsible to the World Health Assembly: a directing committee that meets every year with representation from all UN member states. Although many activities are centralized at the headquarters in Geneva, WHO has six regional offices and conducts much of its work, especially training, at the regional level. The WHO Regional Office for Europe is especially large and widespread (encompassing forty-two countries across Europe and Asia, because it includes Russia and the Asian states of the former Soviet Union) and is a leader within WHO in taking initiative and producing materials. There are many environmental initiatives. Occupational health is guided by a decade-long Global Plan of Action on Workers' Health; work in occupational health is closely coordinated with the

ILO. Much of the environmental and occupational health work sponsored by WHO is undertaken by a network of Collaborating Centers, which are centers of excellence located mostly at academic institutions; these centers conduct research, provide training, and produce literature and other tools to support WHO initiatives. These Collaborating Centers do not receive regular funding from WHO (although some expenses may be reimbursed), but the status is coveted as recognition of their contribution on a global scale.

The Pan American Health Organization (PAHO) serves the Western Hemisphere, having been founded in 1902 as the Pan American Sanitary Conference (later "Bureau"), with an initial emphasis on control of yellow fever. (As the construction of the Panama Canal illustrated, yellow fever was recognized as profoundly an occupational hazard.) The creation of WHO in 1946, a year after the United Nations itself, centralized world health initiatives as WHO absorbed preexisting international agencies. PAHO retained its autonomy, however, and in 1949 entered into an agreement by which it would serve as WHO's regional office for the Americas, but would retain its preexisting structure, which is similar to WHO, and identity. PAHO also has programs in environmental health and occupational health.

The European Union (EU) currently (as of 2009) contains thirty-two member states and is mentioned many times in this book. Because of the size of the single, common European market and its purchasing power, EU standards have become the new de facto regulatory standards for world trade. Countries outside the EU, particularly Canada, have largely adopted EU standards in order to ensure access to the European market for their exports, knowing that those standards generally exceed those in other countries—including the counterpart American standards, which are increasingly dated—and are consistent with "greening" the economy over time. Prior to this, the EU had positioned itself as the world leader in standards setting in environmental and occupational health by harmonizing internal standards among its member states, a contentious but often very boring—and much mocked— process but one that has left it with a comprehensive body of regulatory documentation, reporting requirements, and legal precedents for other countries to draw on, as they once drew on ACGIH for comparable documentation. The result is that world standards are being harmonized upward (in a positive sense). The EU has its own network of organizations in the field, including the European Environmental Agency and the EU-OSHA (the European Agency for Health and Safety at Work), among others.

Elsewhere, as in the Association of Southeast Asian Nations, environmental health and certainly occupational health are treated as national issues.

There are so many nongovernmental organizations (NGOs) dedicated to environmental health that it is impractical to list them. It is much more useful for the OEM physician to choose the area of interest and then to search for the relevant organization on the Internet.

There is only one global organization for occupational health, but it is very active. The International Commission on Occupational Health (ICOH) was founded in 1906 as the Permanent Commission on Occupational Health, in order to create a sustainable organization to carry on the work of a major international conference held that year on occupational injuries and illnesses. ICOH hosts thirty-six scientific committees, through which it does most of its work disseminating scientific research, providing training, and providing assistance, especially in developing countries. ICOH itself convenes the World (previously "International") Congress on Occupational Health every three years, and many of the scientific committees hold important conferences on occupational health topics, some of them annually on off years from the congress. At the national level, ICOH has a network of national secretaries and is establishing organizations for some regions, such as the Asian region. ICOH's Code of Ethics (discussed in detail in Chapter 25) is the global standard of practice and is acknowledged as such in the laws of some countries. The practical working language of ICOH is English, although it has also been bilingual in French, but key documents are available in many languages. ICOH is recognized as an NGO by the United Nations and has a close working relationship with WHO, ILO, and other global organizations with interests in the field, particularly the International

Social Security Association and the International Occupational Hygiene Association. ICOH is headquartered in Rome and can be reached at icoh@ispesl.it or www.icohweb.net. Membership is open to all professionals in occupational safety and health, and the application process requires the endorsement of three current members.

RESOURCES

Amick BC III, Levine S, Tarlov AR, Walsh DC, eds. *Society and Health.* New York: Oxford University Press; 1995.

Bim A-E, Pillay Y, Holz TH. *Textbook of International Health: Global Health in a Dynamic World.* London: Oxford University Press; 2009. [This is the standard text in global health and is most useful to the OEM physician as general background.]

Humphries J. Child labor: lessons from the historical experience of today's industrial economies. *World Bank Econ Rev.* 2003;17(3):175–196.

Keystone JS, Kozarsky PE, Freedman DO, Northdurft HD, Connor BA. *Travel Medicine.* 2nd ed. St Louis, MO: Mosby Elsevier; 2008.

[Current statistics and guidance on the current policy of governments, UN agencies, and most major organizations in the field change rapidly and can be obtained only on the Internet. This is particularly true during the current economic recession. The OEM physician is encouraged to access authoritative Web sites for any factual information.]

NOTEWORTHY READINGS

Buttel FH, McMichael P, eds. *New Directions in the Sociology of Global Development: Research in Rural Sociology and Development.* Vol 11. New York: Elsevier; 2005.

Caplan AL, McCartney JJ, Sisti, DA, eds. *Health, Illness, and Disease: Concepts in Medicine.* Washington, DC: Georgetown University Press; 2004.

Feachem RG, Kjellström T, Murray CJL, Over M, Phillips MA. *Health of Adults in the Developing World.* New York: World Bank / Oxford University Press; 1992.

Guidotti TL. Development, health and the environment: one model. *OSH & Development* (Swedish Association for Occupational and Environmental Health and Development). May 2002;4:43-54.

Guidotti TL. Occupational health and economic development. In: *Basic Occupational Health.* New York: Oxford University Press; 2010 (projected).

Guidotti TL, Goldsmith DF. Occupational medicine in a developing society: a case study of Venezuela. *J Occup Med.* 1980; 22 (1):30–34.

Keating DP, Hertzman C, eds. *Developmental Health and the Wealth of Nations: Social, Biological, and Educational Dynamics.* New York: Guilford; 1999.

Lane RE. *The Loss of Happiness in Market Economies.* New Haven, CT: Yale University Press; 2000.

Marmot M, Wilkinson RG. *Social Determinants of Health.* Oxford: Oxford University Press; 1999.

Roberts MJ, Tybout JR, eds. *Industrial Evolution in Developing Countries: Micro Patterns of Turnover, Productivity, and Market Structure.* New York: World Bank / Oxford University Press; 1996.

Rodriguez-García R, Goldman A. *The Health-Development Link.* Washington, DC: Pan American Health Organization; 1994.

Rotberg RI, ed. *Health and Disease in Human History.* Cambridge: MIT Press; 2000.

Xue SZ, Liang YX. *Occupational Health in Industrialization and Modernization.* Shanghai: Shanghai Medical University Press; 1988. [This is an outstanding, now scarce, reference on China's early experience with modernization. Shanghai Medical University is now Fudan University.]

CONCLUSION

TO THE NEXT GENERATION OF OEM PHYSICIANS

The new physician in occupational and environmental medicine (OEM) has an opportunity to shape the future of field and through the field to shape occupational health and environmental health and integrity for the next generation. This conclusion is therefore written as a charge for the new OEM physician and the next generation. It is an opinionated, personal message from an author who is in sight of the end of his career to physicians who are just starting down this rewarding but unusual path. Unlike the rest of the book, it uses the first person plural, partly to cast what is said in the author's "authoritative" voice, but also to emphasize that many leaders in OEM share these views, at least individually, publicly or privately.

Occupational and environmental medicine (OEM) is unique in medicine because the field looks outward to society and technology for change and not inward to the next new drug or biomedical breakthrough. OEM is practiced in the world, not in the hospital, so it is a paradigm of the ambulatory, client- (if not necessarily patient-) centered style of medicine that the profession now strives for. OEM, or at least the occupational pole of it, has gone as far or farther than any other medical specialty in defining evidence-based guidelines. The environmental pole presents an opportunity to apply medical knowledge in new ways in and out of the clinic.

With all this potential, OEM can be a model for the medicine of the future. We are focused on the individual in the office or clinic, but we can deal with population health and the big picture. Our field keeps people out of the hospital and gives them the opportunity for better lives. We apply the knowledge of medicine outside medical practice, in different and innovative ways. Our training model emphasizes experience in the community and with people as they live, not as they are come to us in the hospital, feeling at their worst, often helpless and separated from their real lives. Seen this way, OEM is a model for the medicine of the future—proactive, individualized, and evidence-based—rather than a relic of the past.

Fundamentally, OEM may have its ups and downs, but it will always be needed because there will always be a role for the physician in managing aspects of health and work and the environment will always have an influence on health. OEM matters to people because we all live in the environment and we all either work or depend on someone who does.

A Paean to Occupational Medicine

Imagine that the scope of medicine suddenly doubled, creating new practice possibilities, ways of applying medical knowledge outside of the clinic, and an abundance of challenging cases. Imagine every day in clinic being different. Imagine the impact on medical practice of a demographic shift that suddenly brought large numbers of young adults back into primary care and that supported older citizens and encouraged them to be vigorous and productive. Imagine the problems of geriatrics given a new dimension in which life experience is considered an asset and retirement is optional, not forced by disability. Imagine new means of prevention opening up to public health and preventive medicine as well as new opportunities for the physician to practice prevention. Imagine public health and medicine joined together in a partnership where prevention and treatment go hand in hand. Imagine the vision of Kerr White, who advocated a union of medicine and public health, come to life.

Occupational medicine does all this for medicine and as much again for public health. As a specialty in practice, it is typically visible to primary care practitioners only in fleeting glimpses, yet it affects most patients from young adulthood and adolescence to well beyond retirement age. As an academic specialty of medicine it overlaps much of general medicine yet incorporates its own unique content and principles, creating an opportunity to apply old knowledge in new ways. It is the field of medicine most directly in touch with changes in technology and the economy, and together with preventive medicine and family practice it is arguably the field most in touch with society generally. It is certainly the least inwardly looking and "ivory tower" because it is practiced entirely in the "real world." It is essentially defined by its social dimensions and draws its knowledge base from the study of populations and communities, yet it is highly technical and may be heavily clinical in some practice settings. It is a type of medical practice that is distinct in its challenges but includes elements that most physicians practice every day without realizing it. It is a medical specialty in form and content but with so few specialists in practice that other physicians for years to come will handle more cases than the specialists themselves. Intellectually, it is a bounty, with new issues and challenges that make every day unlike the one before.

Specialties are distinguished by the unique nature of their subject matter or practice. Most specialists are defined by organ system, such as cardiology or orthopedics; some by anatomy, such as otolaryngology; some by age group, such as pediatrics; and some by technique or mechanics of practice, such as anesthesiology. A few are defined by etiology or type of pathology, such as infectious disease and oncology. Others are defined by the need for a particular type of health care, such as family practice. Occupational medicine has been predominantly a specialty of the latter type but also has similarities to the etiology-based specialties in its emphasis on toxic and physical exposures.

As societies mature and become richer, they grow more averse to risk. The question is whether members of society who avoid a risk to themselves have a right or a privilege to impose it on others. Fundamentally, occupational medicine is about how we value our lives, how we treat those who create wealth and support us, and the risks we wish to take with our lives.

A Paean to Environmental Medicine

The overarching mission of environmental medicine is to create a world fit to live and to raise children in, one in which all people are free to reach their biological and personal potential. The OEM physician helps to achieve this by identifying, understanding, and then correcting preventable external threats, hazards, and risk factors to health.

OEM is primarily defined by the study of tangible, material influences on the body that come from the outside world and the body's responses to these influences. The term "influences" is used here rather than "exposures" because it is a more general term and sidesteps the implication that the only relevant influences are chemical exposures or forms of energy. Some influences are personal and interactional, such as psychogenic stress, but they are just as relevant. However, a large class of influences does not fit this model. These are the effects of ecosystem disruption that may, for example, result in favorable conditions for disease transmission or lead to secondary effects mediated by the economy or social disruption. The influence of cultural change affects health through lifestyle and attitudes toward health-related behaviors. The influence of social equity and civil society makes it safe to create and to be more open with others. The influence of environmental quality and positive determinants of health gives people a reason to sustain rather than exploit communities, confident that their needs will be met and that the communities can become or remain good places to live.

One of the great unrealized opportunities in environmental health is to address the challenges of the built environment. We fuss on the edges with building-related problems and ignore the many subtle ways that urbanization and land use affect our health and lock us into energy, transportation, and residential patterns that perpetuate health risks. Cities are artificial ecosystems, built by people but preserving remnants of natural ecosystems as part of their structure. Sustainability is just as important for these urban ecosystems as for natural ecosystems. A sustainable urban ecosystem, conceptually, has a lesser impact on the environment (footprint) as a whole than does a conventional city; it is a more pleasant and creative place to live, so that residents are motivated to preserve its features rather than overbuild; and it is an efficient structure that concentrates human impact and spares the negative consequences on less dense parts of its region. Above all, it is healthy and attractive, and its citizens sustain it because they want to and because of deeply held values, not because they are fearful. If the people who live in a place are not healthy and their aspirations are not fulfilled, why would they want to continue to live there or try to sustain it? This approach to enhancing the urban environment and making it compatible with, rather than antagonistic to, environmental protection is consistent with the principles of sustainable development and with environmental medicine. It is a fundamental issue in further progress and an unresolved problem in urban and regional planning. It connects the environment with help at a deeper level. This is an old idea, by the way. It was the view of the great public health advocate Max Joseph von Pettenkofer in the nineteenth century.

The environment or global ecosystem (which some more mystical environmentalists personify as Gaia, for those who need to attach a name or a face to big ideas) has value in itself apart from its utility to human beings. However, most people are concrete, not abstract. They are concerned most with how the environment affects them and their family and close others. Protecting the environment begins with protecting people so that people will see their interest in protecting the environment.

If people are harmed by what they encounter in the world of daily life or work, we all lose. If people are affected adversely, even a little, by environmental exposures, then we fail to reach our full potential as a community, as a society, or as individuals. If we do not invest in our environment, our lives will be the poorer. The question, therefore, is how much we value our lives. If we do not place a value on our lives, we will not invest in the environment.

As societies mature and become richer, we know that they grow more averse to risk. Members of society may choose to avoid risks for themselves by choosing where they live and insulating themselves with the protection they can afford, but the question is whether we would be better off lowering the level of risk for all of us. Fundamentally, environmental medicine, and all of environmental health, is about how we value our lives, how responsible we choose to be, and how we wish to live.

OEM AND ITS DISCONTENTS

OEM at its best also represents a side of medicine that is the opposite of treating disease: the preservation of wellness. For all the time that medical students spend studying sick people, they are rarely asked to consider the objective of maintaining health. There is little place for the healthy in medicine, it would appear. The public and the health care system do not demand its inclusion in the medical curriculum.

For physicians who care about providing care to keep people healthy, rather than only treating them for illness, OEM is one way, and a very good way, to do this. However getting started in the field and ultimately reaching this potential is not so easy.

Getting Started

As explained in Chapters 1 and 12, few physicians practice mainstream environmental medicine exclusively. The field merges into occupational medicine, and it is in the latter pole of the combined field that the OEM physician usually supports the practice. Thus, for all but a few practitioners, plus those who work in government and the few doing academic research on environmental topics alone, the key to a successful career is to become very good at occupational medicine and to leverage one's interests in environmental medicine.

Certain steps should be taken by every physician seeking to enter OEM practice:

1. Become informed about the field.
2. Define objectives.
3. Review the profile of local industry.
4. Become knowledgeable regarding local occupational health problems.
5. Plan the proposed service.
6. Identify staff, facilities, and resources.

Ideally, these steps should be taken in the order given. However, the sequence actually taken is usually the reverse. Hospitals, clinics, and groups tend to use whatever equipment and whichever staff are available to start a service (usually poorly planned), and they end up learning through their mistakes what the community does *not* want. The aspiring OEM physician often has to learn to make do, innovate, persuade, and inveigle to create a service he or she can be proud of.

It is often wise in the beginning to target a specific industry, employer, or common occupation, such as firefighters or police or health care workers, and to become known as the local expert. Department of Transportation commercial driver certification (see Chapter 18) has been the mainstay of satisfying careers. This is a surer path than becoming the expert on a particular hazard or clinical condition, which can be very limiting.

A good way to start in occupational medicine is to assume responsibility for the employee health service of a medium-size hospital. However, the alert OEM physician will quickly recognize that this can be very limiting. Hospitals tend to be very conservative employers. However, they are good training grounds. Directing a hospital employee health service is a good way to observe both the good and the bad in occupational medicine practice. It also provides a "captive" patient base on which to build for later expansion of services. The major disadvantage of getting started in hospital employee health is that "familiarity breeds contempt." The occupational physician for a hospital is often a lone voice.

For an occupational health service is to be responsive to local employers, the OEM physician must understand the hazards in local industries, the major employers in the area, the organization and ownership of local industries and their suppliers, and the special features of the work force. The economic base of the community holds many surprises. The presence of one or two major factories with obvious or unusual hazards (perhaps confined to a few workers) may blind one to the reality that most workers in those factories are exposed to more conventional hazards, such as noise. In many industries, such as the oil and gas and the chemical industries, the number of workers is very small compared to the volume of production. Many workers in any local economy are employed in automotive repair and servicing, fast food operations, agriculture, tourism (including hotels and motels), and even healthcare, usually outnumbering those in the "dominant" industry of the community. Each of these local industries generates sufficient injuries and illnesses, workers' compensation issues, and fitness-for-duty problems to require medical services on a frequent basis. Because of their small scale, these industries also need help and have trouble getting what they need from consultants at a price they can afford.

New Thinking

There are so many areas in which advances can be made in OEM. This is truly a field in which an individual physician can make a difference for an entire community, can discover a "new" disease (often entirely new, if associated with a new process or chemical), can introduce new ideas, and can successfully challenge authority (although perhaps not in the world of workers' compensation—but that is another story).

The field of OEM needs to reexamine and rethink issues of professional training, the relationship between OEM physicians and departments of human resources, the balance between prevention and case management, teamwork and competition among occupational health professions, cross-training in professional competence, and especially the balance between occupational and environmental medicine. The author of these volumes served as president of the American College of Occupational and Environmental Medicine (ACOEM), which has made a start on these issues. But the natural tendency of the OEM physician, guarding a small specialty, is to patch things up at the top rather than try to fix the foundation, which is what is needed.

Little effort has been made in the United States to study the experience of other countries with similar problems that have pursued different paths. France, Canada, Germany, Sweden, and Finland, in particular, have adopted different models for occupational health and hygiene services and have experienced their own transitions and troubles (especially Sweden). Some of their systems, such as physician training, work better than the American version and should be studied as adaptable models. Others may not work as well, such as the French preoccupation with periodic health surveillance, but we stand to learn from the experience of others. Certainly there is much in the performance of Britain's Health and Safety Executive that could be of value to OSHA.

Welcoming the New OEM Physician

The field remains wide open to motivated physicians who wish to enter the practice in a credible manner and deliver service of high quality. Most occupational health care will continue to be provided by primary care physicians in the community rather than by formally trained specialists. There are now and will for many years be many opportunities for these physicians to develop their skills in occupational health care conscientiously and to incorporate occupational medicine into their practices as an integral and challenging part of primary health care.

However, organized occupational medicine (except for ACOEM) has not always been welcoming to these physicians. Some specialists in occupational medicine (to use the formal name of the specialty) see them as a threat. However, they are keeping OEM alive. Physicians who enter the field in mid-career bring life experience, medical and surgical skills, and knowledge of the community that helps the field succeed and stay relevant. In many places that do not have specialists, these physicians represent the standard of practice and uphold it perfectly well; most of them are already specialists in other fields. These physicians also expand the ranks of providers to meet the demand that specialists never can and to be a presence in places where there are no qualified specialists and probably never will be. Without them, demand would dry up for lack of supply, with employers turning to anyone with an MD and neglecting credentials and special expertise entirely.

There will always be a small number of young physicians who wish to train for highly specialized and academic careers. They will continue to be attracted by the intellectual richness and challenge of the field. Because the field has such a low profile in medical school and in the community, however, there will never be many of them. It is highly unlikely that the few physicians who have an interest in this field will be diverted from specialty training simply because they do not need it to practice occupational medicine. Their motivation and the achievement of their goals require the challenge and the prestige of a recognized specialty. They are the future leaders and they know it.

What visibility the field of occupational and environmental medicine does enjoy in medical school and to the public is largely due to those same physicians practicing in the field who entered in mid-career. Rather than treat this as a problem of intrusion on the specialty from the outside, diffusion into the field in mid-career should be considered an opportunity to expand the ranks of active, engaged, and experienced practitioners. The majority of practitioners who enter occupational medicine do so without taking residencies, for very good and practical reasons. It is currently nearly impossible for most physicians who enter the field in mid-career to earn a credential that would attest to their competence. This is a formula for losing all control over quality assurance and continuing the marginal-ization of the practice of occupational medicine.

Toward a Renewed Specialty

Key to addressing this problem is establishing appropriate creden-tials. At present, physicians who enter the field in mid-career do not have an opportunity to demonstrate that their preparation is sound and to prove their practice skills in the field. Until recently, the dis-cussion in this area has been about whether to allow or restore some lateral pathway to board certification, a move that would be blocked as a bad precedent by the American Board of Medical Specialties anyway. But why should specialists who train in a residency hold the same credential as physicians who enter in mid-career, and who are usually interested more in practice than in a specialty-based career? Maybe the pathways need to diverge.

There needs to be fresh air brought to this stale debate. There is considerable merit in a two-tier system, in which a separately titled, meaningful, rigorous, examination-based credential is made available for those physicians who enter the field laterally. The new credential would recognize added competence, not specialty certification, at approximately the current level expected by the current American Board of Preventive Medicine (ABPM).

Another key to addressing this problem of credentials that match competence is training. Regardless of whether a two-tier system is considered, the specialty should upgrade the existing residency in occupational medicine into a fellowship, one that matches the tech-nical complexity and breadth of content of the field, by requiring candidates for the specialist credential to have three years of medical training, for a total of five years in training. This higher level of train-ing would also be certified at a higher level, again by the ABPM but perhaps with a new designation of "occupational and environmental medicine." What would be the practical and funding impact of this radical change? Almost nothing. Since virtually all OEM specialists already complete at least three years of medical training before they enter an occupational medicine residency, nothing would actually change, except that perception would match reality. So why not?

The two tiers already combine in one system for occupational medicine. This is, in fact, the system in place right now in both Canada and the United Kingdom, and it works well in both. (Both countries have their issues, but this is not one of them.)

We need new thinking in OEM to break through the impasse in training and credentialing. We have lived too long with a system that has been not only an imperfect compromise, but a dysfunctional straitjacket that has distorted, stunted, and deformed the specialty of OEM.

EPIPHANIES

Sound decisions on health protection can be made only when the science if right. But even if the science is right, it does not by any means guarantee that the policy decision will be right. If the science is wrong, however, the policy decision is always wrong, and if it happens to be right for the wrong reason, nobody who understands will believe it. That is why OEM, which is profoundly social in its consciousness and history, must be based on science. Research is the taproot of OEM and the source of its strength. However, that is not what OEM is really about, no more than a tree is just about its roots and photosynthesis. Science without a social consciousness leads to a neglect of values, which lie at the core of medicine in the form of the relief of suffering, the provision of comfort, and the injunction to do no harm.

OEM is really about values. It has to do with how we choose to live and work. It is about how we treat the planet and whether we care about people we have not met yet who share it with us. It is about those who provide us with the goods and services we need and whether we need to know their names to be concerned with their health and well-being. It is about what we think is fair and right. It is about respect for the worker, about respect for the fellow citizens of the planet, and ultimately about respect for ourselves.

THE ESSENTIAL LIBRARY FOR THE OCCUPATIONAL AND ENVIRONMENTAL PHYSICIAN

Occupational and environmental medicine (OEM) physicians are advised to refer first to these sources for reference and guidance, and to the "Resources" list at the end of each chapter.

All physicians engaged in the practice of OEM are advised to subscribe to the Occupational and Environmental Medicine List (Occ-Env-Med-L), which is an indispensable means of communication for health professionals in the field. Occ-Env-Med-L reaches approximately 4,000 recipients in seventy-five countries. Content includes announcements, important new developments, discussions of professional topics, and requests for information. The list is hosted by the University of North Carolina and has been moderated since 1993 by Dr. Gary Greenberg. It can be accessed at http://occhealthnews.net/occ-env-.htm. The archives of the List are particularly useful for locating current commentary on a particular topic.

Other invaluable sources include the following:
American College of Occupational and Environmental Medicine (ACOEM). *Occupational Medicine Practice Guidelines*. Chicago: American College of Occupational and Environmental Medicine. Produced as a series with sequential revision. See www.acoem.org.

The Essential Library for the Occupational and Environmental Physician

ACOEM Health and Productivity Toolkit. Chicago: American College of Occupational and Environmental Medicine. Produced as an online resource available by subscription. See www.acoem.org.

AMA Guides to the Evaluation of Disease and Injury Causation. Chicago: American Medical Association; 2008.

AMA Guides to the Evaluation of Permanent Impairment. Chicago: American Medical Association. Updated every few years. Use either the most current edition or the edition mandated by state law (in Texas, for example, the fourth).

Greenberg MI, Hamilton R, Phillips S, McCluskey GJ. *Occupational, Industrial, and Environmental Toxicology.* 2nd ed. St Louis: Mosby; 2003.

Hathaway GJ, Proctor NH. *Proctor and Hughes' Chemical Hazards of the Workplace.* 5th ed. New York: Van Nostrand; 2004.

ILO Encyclopaedia of Occupational Health. Geneva: International Labor Organization. 5th edition in preparation.

International Commission on Occupational Health. ICOH Code of Ethics for Occupational Health Professionals. Rome. www.icohweb.org.

Last JM. *A Dictionary of Epidemiology.* New York: Oxford University Press; 2007.

Lauwerys RR, Hoet P. *Industrial Chemical Exposure: Guidelines for Biological Monitoring.* Boca Raton, FL: Lewis; 2001.

Lippman M, Cohen BS, Schlesinger RB. *Environmental Health Science: Recognition, Evaluation and Control of Chemical and Physical Health Hazards.* New York: Oxford University Press; 2003.

Rom WN. *Environmental and Occupational Medicine.* 4th ed. Philadelphia: Lippincott Williams & Wilkins: 2007.

Rosenstock L, Cullen MR, Brodkin CA, Redlich CA. *Textbook of Clinical Occupational and Environmental Medicine.* Philadelphia: Elsevier; 2005.

INDEX

Note: Page numbers followed by "t" indicate that the reference is to a table on the indicated page.

Index

ABOUT THE AUTHOR

TEE L. GUIDOTTI, MD, MPH is currently an international consultant in occupational and environmental health and medicine. He is the former Professor and Chair of the Department of Environmental and Occupational Health in the School of Public Health and Health Services, The George Washington University Medical Center, Washington D.C., and Director of the Division of Occupational Medicine and Toxicology in the Department of Medicine, School of Medicine and Health Sciences. Prior to taking that position in 1999, he was for fourteen years Professor of Occupational and Environmental Medicine and Director of the Occupational Health Program in the Department of Public Health Sciences at the University of Alberta in Edmonton, Canada. He completed medical school at the University of California at San Diego, trained at the Johns Hopkins Hospital, and obtained his degree in public health at the Johns Hopkins School of Hygiene and Public Health. He holds board certification in the United States in internal medicine, pulmonary medicine, and occupational and environmental medicine and a fellowship in occupational medicine in Canada and the United Kingdom. He also holds professional credentials in toxicology (DABT) and environmental science (QEP). His research interests include occupational and environmental lung diseases and inhalation toxicology. His career has been unusually balanced in occupational and environmental medicine. He is best known in occupational medicine for his expertise on the occupational health problems of firefighters and oil and gas workers. His environmental interests include air quality, risk science, ecosystem and human health, and child health and the environment. He has published over 250 papers and book chapters and produced six books. He has written extensively on the evaluation of scientific evidence in litigation, adjudication, and policy. Dr. Guidotti has served as President of the American College of Occupational and Environmental Medicine and holds many fellowships and awards. He is Editor-in-Chief of the *Archives of Environmental and Occupational Health.* He is the recipient of many awards and honors.